# Dyslexia
# A Psychosocial Perspective

# Dyslexia
# A Psychosocial
# Perspective

*Edited by*

MORAG HUNTER-CARSCH

University of Leicester

**W**

WHURR PUBLISHERS
LONDON AND PHILADELPHIA

© 2001 Whurr Publishers

First published 2001 by
Whurr Publishers Ltd
19b Compton Terrace, London N1 2UN, England
325 Chestnut Street, Philadelphia PA19106, USA

**British Library Cataloguing in Publication Data**

A catalogue record for this book is available from the British Library.

ISBN 1 86156 194 6

Printed and bound in the UK by Athenaeum Press Limited, Gateshead, Tyne & Wear.

# Contents

## Chapter 14                                                         245

The role of counselling in supporting adults with dyslexia
  *Charmaine McKissock*

## Chapter 15                                                         254

Specialist teacher-training in the UK: issues, considerations
and future directions
  *Gavin Reid*

# DEDICATION

TO HENRY

# Acknowledgements

The Editor's thanks are due to:

- All the contributing writers and, in particular, Margaret Herrington who also assisted with editing selected chapters and in the discussion of an earlier draft of the manuscript.
- The team of organizers and helpers for the 'Sharing Good Practice' series of inspirational conferences at Leicester University School of Education, Ted Hartshorn, Aubrey Nicholls, Fiona and Chris Hossack and their fellow members of the Leicestershire Dyslexia Association, Maureen Hardy and her supporters in the UK Reading Association for their collaborative work on behalf of promoting the understanding of literacy difficulties, dyslexia, and specific learning difficulties.
- The delegates at the 'Sharing Good Practice' conferences who have shared their thoughts and experience and all the teachers, parents and students who have similarly contributed in the course of working together.
- Professor Ken Fogelman, Dean of Education, Leicester University; Tom Whiteside, Director of the School of Education; and Wasyl Cajkler, Head of Continuing Professional Development, for their support and encouragement.
- Professors Jean and Geoff Underwood, for their interest and kind introduction to Professor Pekka Niemi and the researchers at Turku University, Finland.
- Professor Pekka Niemi and colleagues at the Centre for Learning Research, Turku University, and Professor Katri Sarmavuori, Turku University.
- Dr Greg Robinson, Newcastle University, Australia, for discussion of research into visual difficulties.
- Dr Henry Carsch for his translation of the Beqiraj–Carsch model which formed the basis for the extended theoretical model in the chapter on

meta-cognition and for his sustaining encouragement through the production of this volume.

- All who assisted with aspects of the production of the manuscript: Linda Basey, Chac in Lam, Sue Mailley, Judith Schofield; and very special thanks to Carole Fitzpatrick for her assistance with the final production.
- Whurr Publishers and their adviser, Professor Margaret Snowling.

# Contributors

**Alan Crombie**
Independent ICT Consultant, Bridge of Weir, Scotland

**Margaret Crombie**
Network Support Manager, East Renfrewshire Local Education Authority, Scotland

**Gilly Czerwonka**
Co-ordinating Teacher (Specific Learning Difficulties), Blackburn with Darwen Local Education Authority, Lancashire, England

**Anne Henderson**
Education Consultant, Tutor in Mathematics and Dyslexia at University of Wales, Bangor, Wales

**Margaret Herrington**
Director of the Study Support Centre, University of Nottingham, School of Continuing Education, Nottingham, England

**Morag Hunter-Carsch**
Lecturer in Education at Leicester University School of Education, Leicester, England

**Sue Mailley**
Education Consultant, Stamford, England

**Charmaine McKissock**
Consultant, writer, trainer and assessor specialising in adult dyslexia

**Tim Miles**
Professor Emeritus of Psychology, University of Wales, Bangor, Wales

**Lindsay Peer**
Education Director of the British Dyslexia Association, Reading,
England

**Hanna-Sofia Poussu-Olli**
Senior Lecturer in The Institute of Education, Turku University, Turku,
Finland

**Peter Pumfrey**
Professor Emeritus, former Dean of the School of Education, The
University of Manchester and currently Visiting Professor at University
College, Worcester, England

**Gavin Reid**
Senior Lecturer, Department of Equity Studies and Special Education,
University of Edinburgh, Scotland

**Jean Robertson**
Lecturer, Manchester Metropolitan University, Manchester, England

# Preface

At the time of going to press, awareness of the new working definition of dyslexia by the British Psychological Society's working party on dyslexia, literacy and psychological assessment is just beginning to be felt (BPS/DECP 1999). The impact of the definition itself, and perhaps more crucially, the shift of focus away from the broader field of specific learning difficulties (SpLDs) as defined by Pumfrey and Reason (1991, 1996) and in the 1994 DfEE Code of Practice, to one example of a SpLD, dyslexia, has yet to be felt.

The OFSTED (1999) report on SpLDs in mainstream schools has been published, and the government is in the process of revising the *Code of Practice on the Identification and Assessment of Pupils with Special Educational Needs* (DfEE 1994). It seems likely that the definition of SpLDs and the relationship of certain categories of 'special need' may be affected not only by the BPS new working definition of dyslexia but also by a range of developments and research in education and related fields (for example, the literacy strategy (DfEE 1998a), the curriculum for citizenship and the human rights framework, ICT and new literacies, including emotional literacy (Sharp in press) and perhaps also by shifts in public opinion as a result of successful media campaigns (such as the dyslexia television season, summer 1999).

This is a book for teachers at all levels. It addresses vital questions in the field of SpLDs such as dyslexia. Among them are the following:

- Are we moving away from understanding the relationship of dyslexia to the wider field of SpLDs?
- Does the new definition promote a more accurate understanding of dyslexia and of the range of literacy difficulties?
- What are the implications of the research findings, the definitions and their revisions for teachers and learning support staff for educational psychologists and all multidisciplinary specialists?

- How will it affect parents, and most crucially, the identification, assessment and teaching of children who may or may not be considered to be 'dyslexic'?
- In what ways will attitudes and expectations about teaching (a) dyslexic and (b) 'non'- dyslexic children be affected?

In order to address these questions there is an urgent need for teachers to create an opportunity to pause in their hectic chase to deliver the curriculum and raise standards in order to look and 'see the wood *as well as* the trees' and to listen in order to 'hear themselves think'. Most of all, there is a need for conversations which lead to deeper understanding of teachers' own teaching and its relationship to the diversity of experiences which are called 'learning'. In the words of Harold Shapiro, President of Princeton University, USA:

> ... the special role played by conversations in one's education ... includes ... very particular kinds of exchanges, either between individuals or between individuals and cultural artifacts such as books, new ideas, works of art and musical masterpieces. The unique context that defines these types of conversations is that the individual or individuals involved expect, through their reflective and thoughtful engagement with the work and ideas of others, to expand their imaginations, enlarge their awareness, deepen their understanding and hone their ability to perceive new possibilities of all kinds.
> (Shapiro 1998)

Shapiro was addressing the Princeton University community. Yet, for teachers and learners everywhere, at all stages, including the stage of continuing professional development education, it is the quality of the engagement in conversation and the experience of the imagery and imagination at work which can contribute indirectly as well as directly to understanding matters which affect personal, interpersonal and wider human communication and well-being. It is this quality experience which constitutes the stuff of 'getting to grips with dyslexia', learning and teaching.

This book invites readers to engage with this kind of experience, through conversation with the contributors. It seeks to provide a kind of practical support which derives from sharing perspectives presented by a range of experienced practitioners and researchers and, in so doing, not only reviewing their perspectives critically but also possibly discovering confirmations of personal professional perspectives in the light of sharpened vision from experiencing a different stance.

It aims to address the problem of clarifying some of the questions and, by juxtaposition of a range of perspectives, to offer a possibility of expanding understanding of our experience of SpLDs, including dyslexia, through the perspectives of skilled workers in the field. Although there is much in the book that illustrates and illuminates good classroom practice, its main concern is the thinking about practice, the kind of thinking that informs teaching so that it results in a deepening of quality of the learning experience for the learner.

An orientation towards the questions addressed in the first part of the book, on 'central issues', is introduced in the first chapter, in terms of the 'wood *and* the trees' imagery. The questions of which perspective, and where a teacher's focus should be at any moment in the interactive learning process, especially with dyslexic learners, leads to the central discussion with Tim Miles, a distinguished pioneer in the field, about the core matter of the research findings relating to causal factors and the physical basis for SpLDs such as dyslexia (Chapter 2). The context of the conversation, still involving the 'landscape' of recent research into the physical basis for dyslexia, then sharpens focus on the presence or absence of visual difficulties. This discussion (Chapter 3), is with Sue Mailley, a teacher—researcher with a keen interest in observation and an emphasis on fundamentals such as whether children in primary class-rooms are actually able to see comfortably.

Moving from the focus on vision and visual difficulties, the discussion about another fundamental question, 'What characterizes effective special teaching of learners with SpLDs such as dyslexia?', invites readers to take a shared journey in order to reconnect the pioneers' principles and practices of structured multisensory teaching with what is understood in the current scene, to be 'structured multisensory teaching':

> The training of SENCOs should include guidance on the nature and implica-
> tions of specific learning difficulties and the structured multisensory
> programmes that are of benefit to pupils with such difficulties.
> (OFSTED 1999, para 24)

The conversation with Morag Hunter-Carsch (Chapter 4), brings together experience of teaching children, adolescents and teachers from both sides of the Atlantic, and involves some pauses on this route for thought about the relationship between structuring thinking and struc-turing feelings. These matters are discussed more fully in Chapter 5 in which she seeks to go 'beyond meta-cognition' to explore the re-integra-tion of meta-affectivity as a component of meta-comprehension. The issues are then viewed from a social interactive perspective (Chapter 6) with Margaret Herrington, a specialist teacher of adults. The two authors explore a range of questions, sharing their conversation in the course of their own professional quest.

In the journey and conversation through the second part of the book, the leader and guide is Peter Pumfrey who, with Tim Miles, has a penetrating perspective in the field. In Chapter 7, his vision probes deeply into the recesses of memory. Conversation with him sets the scene for questioning 'What basics to back?' and inspires readers with confidence to scale the heights of integrating wider perspectives and increase their skill in sharpening focus on detail.

The shared discussion of 'the roots and branches' of 'the trees and the wood' then turns to conversation with Hanna Poussu-Olli, a university lecturer and researcher. In Chapter 8, she looks closely at what is involved in adult dyslexia and, remarkably, finds that although some dyslexic learners can seem to have overcome their literacy difficulties, evidence of phonological processing delays can still be traced by use of sophisticated technology for diagnostic assessment.

In Chapter 9, Morag Hunter-Carsch reflects on her conversations with parents and with adult literacy education advisers, illuminating ways in which, through partnerships between parents and teachers, parents' questions may be answered and their children's literacy difficulties and SpLDs eased. Chapter 10 continues the theme of communication; Lindsay Peer, a teacher, researcher and Education Director for the British Dyslexia Association, shares her deep concern for dyslexic learners who are multilingual and opens up the conversation to invite all with an interest in dyslexia and multilingualism to share their experience and contribute to collaborative research.

The following two chapters (11 and 12) invite readers to consider a different form of communication, by 'thinking mathematically' with Ann Henderson, a teacher and teacher–trainer, and to converse with Alan and Margaret Crombie about the potential of information and communication technology (ICT) to assist dyslexic learners. Bringing together Alan's expertise in information technology, and Margaret, a specialist teacher and administrator, aims to share with readers their confidence and enthusiasm about the world our youngsters may face, and to look positively towards their potential access to expert and individualized learning support.

In a similarly confident mood, the conversation is joined by two teachers with a shared interest working in different professional contexts. Jean Robertson, a lecturer and researcher, and Gilly Czerwonka, a specialist (SpLD) teacher, independently became interested in the Balance Theory propounded by Dirk Bakker. In Chapter 13, they discuss the findings of their research informed by Bakker's theory and their adaptations of neuropsychological approaches for teaching in the classroom in ways which employ ICT.

We then return to a major theme of the book — the *affective* as well as *cognitive* concerns in the context of providing appropriate learning support for dyslexic adults and children. Charmaine McKissock shares her experience as a counsellor and illustrates in her own way the importance of listening to learners. This 'branch' (and all other 'branches') are revealed as needing to be connected firmly to the 'roots' and fed through the central issues in the notional trees and woods analogy of the book. They are finally brought together in the messages from Gavin Reid, an eminent teacher–trainer, who shares his catalytic and illuminating perspectives on specialist teacher training and its future directions.

**Morag Hunter-Carsch**
**Leicester**
**December 2000**

# Part I
# Central issues

# Chapter 1
# Seeing the wood *and* the trees: specific learning difficulties and dyslexia

MORAG HUNTER-CARSCH

---

Questions addressed in this chapter include:

- How might a psychosocial perspective contribute to understanding of specific learning difficulties, dyslexia and other literacy and learning difficulties?
- What are the priorities for teachers in relation to teaching students with specific learning difficulties and those with literacy difficulties?
- What role does motivation play in overcoming reluctance to read and write for dyslexic students and for those with more general literacy difficulties?

---

## Introduction

This chapter develops the theme of the importance of **conversation** and introduces other themes which also permeate the book. These include awareness of the wider issues relating to **communication**, individual differences in mental imagery, and the importance of **relating cognitive and affective dimensions of learning**. Collectively, these themes draw attention to the relevance of the **psychosocial perspective**.

This chapter is organized into three parts. The first discusses matters of communication in terms of perspectives which writers, researchers, teachers and students bring to learning interactions and which determine the individual's stance. The second considers priorities for teachers with regard to the relative emphasis they place on teaching literacy or on teaching about the learning *process* as distinct from its *content*. Recognition is made of the tensions between class teaching and the provision of individualized learning support across the curriculum. The third part addresses the problem of the relationship between expectations and motivation, with particular reference to success with literacy learning. It offers a model for the understanding and motivating of reluctant readers and writers. The model is discussed in terms of its relevance for learners with specific learning difficulties (SpLDs) and for others with more general literacy difficulties.

# Specific learning difficulties and dyslexia: a psychosocial perspective

### Themes, imagery, perspectives and stance

In the chapter title, reference to the 'wood *and* the trees', broadly involves representation of the concept of SpLDs, as 'the wood' (an umbrella term for many kinds of difficulties, such as dyslexia, dyscalculia, developmental motor disorder, dyspraxia, speech, language and communication disorders) with dyslexia as one of the 'trees'. The intended inference in adapting a familiar phrase is, simply, that attention is being drawn to the relationship between the two parts.

In this connection it is useful to be aware that the diversity of direction of current research provides a substantial challenge just to keep abreast of developments, for both the specialist SpLD teacher as well as the class teacher. However, matters of terminology and definitions are dealt with elsewhere in this book (see chapters 2, 4 and 7) and reference is made in several places to the British Psychological Society working party report which provides a helpful overview of definitions and research (BPS, 1999). In Chapter 2, Miles draws attention to neurological findings (magnetic resonance imaging (MRI), positron emission tomography (PET) scans and computer assessment) and provides a commentary on the current interest in 'the phonological basis of dyslexia'. For example Frith, in Hulme and Snowling (1997) notes that the major presenting symptom of dyslexia involves unusual and severe difficulties in learning to read and spell, that is an emphasis on literacy difficulties). Later on, in Chapter 8, Poussu-Olli reports on discovering phonological problems underlying adult dyslexia even after successful basic literacy learning.

The complexity of the field is also illustrated by the trend to have specialist teachers for each of the following diagnostic categories which are regarded variously as subsets of SpLDs (dyspraxia, speech, language and communication problems) or as independent areas. Furthermore, there is a tendency for behavioural difficulties, which may be considered by some to include attention deficit hyperactivity disorder (ADHD) to be separately classified from SpLDs.

Although it might be suggested that, collectively, these trends (like new 'woods' with different kinds of 'trees' which have outgrowing 'branches') extend knowledge about many facets of SpLDs, it becomes more difficult for the practising teacher to recognize where the diversity of specialisms come together in the process of planning for teaching and learning through teaching. The original path to – and through – the 'woods' has become so overgrown in the density of the 'forest' that it is hardly even a matter of 'seeing the wood for the trees' – there are many 'woods' growing within this 'forest'. For the teacher, the challenge is to connect the paths and make their own maps, possibly having to combine sections of maps from various sources (see chapters 4 and 7 for reconnecting with earlier routes (and roots), in a conservation mode, and chapters 10 and 15 for perspectives on new directions).

The use of the 'tree *and* wood' imagery also provides an example which can be explored in terms of individual differences in mental imagery. At one level, the question is how the reader 'sees' the wood and the trees (i.e. what mental imagery is prompted by the phrase). At another level, it prompts consideration of what is involved in the relationship of SpLDs to dyslexia. Why therefore stress the 'and' in the title? Should the 'wood and the trees' be seen both at once, and if so, where is the focus and what is the picture? When they are discussed, do these terms evoke associated feelings which illuminate experiences felt by the people to whom they refer (people with SpLDs … dyslexic people)?

It is *how* the words are experienced, as distinct from the assumed instant 'communication' of their intended meaning that becomes the focus of this chapter. This aims to heighten awareness of symbols and referents, and the possibility of loss of clarity as the popularity of certain words and changing fashions in use of prefered terminology may bring about losses as well as gains in shared understanding. The question is 'How have the terms "specific learning difficulty" and "dyslexia" been affected by cultural contexts as well as the passage of time? Do they mean the same thing, and evoke the same associations, today as they did almost a century ago'? Perhaps more vitally 'How are these terms experienced in the minds of their users, whether they are themselves "dyslexic" or not? In this wider sense, this book is about language and thought and the attribution of meaning and values as well as about learning and learning difficulties.

The act of picturing 'woods' and 'trees' is intended to evoke a sense of the experience of being able to focus selectively on the foreground and to alter/adjust mental focus, at will, in order to look at the background. Thus either a cluster of 'trees' or any one of the 'trees' or parts of 'trees' can be given attention. Similarly, by moving and adjusting focus, the 'wood *and* the trees' can be viewed sequentially or simultaneously. In the analogy, parts of the tree e.g. branches or protruding roots might represent the characteristics or clusters of symptoms from which the nature, construction and strength of the 'tree' and the 'wood' might be gauged. The 'pictures' conjured up mentally may not be 'visual' for some readers. It is only by exploring our shared mental imagery that we can begin to approach some appreciation of individual differences in comprehension and the potential for confusion and misunderstanding which surrounds the mediation of thought through language.

A different and parallel analogy to that of trees and wood (which relies on the sense of vision) might be constructed so that it relies, for example, on the sense of hearing. The use of this mode (the creation of auditory imagery) might lead to greater appreciation of the musicality of speakers' and writers' expressions and their capacity for creating imagery through sound by their use of voice, linguistic patterns and the precision of their choice of vocabulary.

The theme of exploration of imagery might, at this point, be pursued beyond visual and auditory imagery to consider motor-kinesthetic representations. It is perhaps less easy to represent through words 'picturing' movements, the dynamics of shifting mental imagery and the recognition of what it is that prompts a movement in a particular direction and what impedes progress along the path of communication whether through speech or writing, listening or reading. The kinds of questions which are prompted include: why is it so much easier for a reader to 'walk along' with some speakers or writers and not with others? Is 'pace' a factor? Are their 'steps' too long? Do they pause and then take too long to 'get started' and does that affect the listeners' rhythms? It may be that certain kinds of motor-kinesthetic imagery are less well understood by those with a preference for seemingly more readily accessible auditory or visual imagery. It may be that such dimensions of experiencing are seldom explored except, perhaps by poets, who may also be dancers.

With reference to this particular analogy, examples of teachers' 'pictures' include detailed visual images of (for example) oak trees, and emergent discussions on the characteristics, outlines and growth patterns of deciduous and coniferous trees. For some teachers, the images were less visual than verbal, drawing upon associations with biology texts, and for some they involved recollections of walks through particular woods, and keen motor memory, tactile imagery of leaves with sharp points, such as holly. For all, the distinctiveness of their individual conceptual material became evident in sharp contradistinction from the extent of the assumptions which we were each making about shared understandings (see Chapter 6 re levels of metacognition).

Understanding the range of individuals' ways of experiencing learning is at the heart of effective teaching for those described as '*having* SpLDs' or '*being* dyslexic' or 'dyscalculic' or any number of such descriptors. It becomes clear in the course of working with dyslexic learners that individual dyslexic students' learning experiences and diversity of experiencing learning are seldom shared sufficiently between students and teachers in mainstream classrooms in primary and secondary schools. Nevertheless, it is encouraging to learn that dyslexic students in tertiary education are being encouraged to explore such parameters within highly specialized one-to-one tutoring and/or counselling contexts (see for example Herrington 2001a; 2001b).

The following discussion aims to illustrate the perspectives of dyslexic adults and of learners with 'different' styles of learning. Although only a small sample is included here (three dyslexic adults and one adult with a 'non-visual' learning style), many others clearly reflect their views. The subsequent chapters provide diverse perspectives from which to explore both the 'woods' and the 'trees'. In the first part there are neurological-biochemical perspectives (Chapter 2); sensory-physical perspectives (Chapter 3); social-interactionist perspectives (Chapter 4); educational perspectives (Chapter 5) and psychosocial perspectives (Chapter 6). The second part of the book begins with historical, medical and psycho-educational perspectives (Chapter 7) concerning 'roots' and looking also to 'branches'. Further 'branches' then explore different modes of communication, thinking, learning support (including counselling), different research traditions and modes of training (chapters 8-15).

## Messages from three dyslexic adults: attitudes, self-esteem and success

ANNA: *'I'm very fortunate. I've had excellent help from my teachers and my parents and have learned to think about dyslexia in a very positive way.'*

On the basis of her work with dyslexic university students, Margaret Herrington, who provided the above example, suggests that Anna's comment is a typical response to earlier learning support. Herrington wished to draw the attention of secondary and primary school teachers to adult dyslexic students' views of the importance of early intervention and effective learning support in their personal histories.

If we are to understand, from an educational point of view, which factors contribute to the effectiveness of support experienced by dyslexic students, there are many questions to pursue. Might not dyslexic students be the most reliable source to approach in order to inform teachers (and parents) about ways of encouraging the development and sustainance of such characteristically positive atttitudes to their dyslexia? It may be helpful also to find out from teachers their relevant perspectives on planning, teaching and recording the nature and extent of learning support and the kinds of questions/research questions which arise. In following this line of investigation, it is easy for teachers to begin to formulate questions about learning support that students have experienced in school, e.g.:

- When did the students first receive learning support?
- Was it in primary school?
- Was it a 'normal' part of classroom interaction or 'special' provision?
- Were there continuities or changes in the support on transition to secondary school or to tertiary education?

And, clearly, questions also need to be asked about learning support beyond school or college and into the home and life in the community:

- What is it that guides and informs students' relevant expectations of others and of themselves as learners (and of others) with regard to their attitude to dyslexia?
- In what ways might the 'culture of learning' in different contexts affect the development of a positive attitude towards dyslexia?

Although questions about effectivenesss of schools are explored elsewhere (e.g. Duffield 1998), the focus has not been on learning support and dyslexia in and beyond school. There remains a need for investigation and longer-term studies to explore the relevant dynamics more fully.

The fact that these matters are complex should not permit their dismissal. Two brief illustrations may serve to point towards the range and relationship of factors which may play a part in developing and sustaining a positive attitude to dyslexia by those who experience 'the condition' as well as by those who do not. (The bold type is used for the speaker's own emphasis in the examples.)

> ANDREW: *'Could you just say to teachers, please, not, ever, to ask dyslexic students like me to read out in class. It is too much to bear, to be unable to do it properly. The shame is awful. It just made me want to run away and not come back to school.'*

This plea, made by a young man, Andrew, in his twenties, now working in the fashion industry, was made in the context of an interview about his school days and in response to questions about how he managed to cope with what he described as repeated failures to carry out required written work and to read at school and at home (study). These problems persisted in contrast to his verbal fluency, general knowledge and considerable personal charm. He explained further, in response to questions about his demonstrable persistence with his schoolwork, despite his difficulties:

*'You see, if it hadn't been for my mother, I wouldn't have stuck it out and eventually finished school with some exams passed, nor would I have become a voluntary reader – I really love reading now! Nor would I have picked myself up when I lost my first job because I was not quick enough at making notes and all the records that were needed beyond the beginning stage of being an assistant. I simply wouldn't have kept on thinking of other ways I could manage the tasks. It was my mother who helped me when I had such awful temper outbursts in primary school and explained to the teachers and helped the teachers to help me. I don't think it was just because she was a teacher that they respected what she said. She was able to explain what they could do and they felt they could do something.'*

Many dyslexic students require an advocate, even when they have superb skills to make their own case. Not all teachers are prepared to listen, and some teachers might dismiss any such approach by a student as 'making excuses and seeking special attention'.

MICHAEL, a successful university lecturer involved in training teachers commented on his own dyslexia:

*'It was "discovered" in primary school, largely as a result of my mother's efforts but I was put into a remedial class in secondary school and had a tough time coming to terms with the fact that I just had to concentrate on finding ways of getting around problems, emphasizing what I was good at and drawing upon my strengths. The school didn't seem to know what to do. I was helped greatly by weekly visits which my parents organized, to an excellent counsellor who helped me to find out more about my strengths and to feel good about myself. I realized that it was no good wearing it like a badge on my sleeve, making an excuse out of it, or getting depressed about it. I simply had to get on with finding out about doing things the best way I could and getting around the bits I recognized that I did not do so efficiently. It helps to have a sense of humour too!'*

These messages are from people who are now developing their careers successfully. The attitudes of peers and teachers during schooling, and of 'significant others' at work, may be seen to be important but for all three adults, parental contribution to their success appears to have been vital to their success and was recognized and warmly acknowledged.

Personal experience through formal interviewing and informal conversations, supports the belief that these three responses are frequently replicated by 'successful' adults who are dyslexic. The overwhelming impression from dyslexic learners' reflections about their school experiences is one of deep appreciation of the individuals who 'noticed' and 'did not make it too noticeable to others'. Such teachers (and later work supervisors) made it possible to rescue self-esteem and to maintain a sense of hope. It was their attitude which was felt to be invaluable and to counterbalance the memories of frustration, anger and sense of injustice.

Recalling the feelings of having to go into classrooms in secondary schools where teachers 'did not understand' independently prompted memories of wishing to truant. Others report their accounts of actual truanting, as a result of their frustrations at school. Such recollections raise the vital question of what is it that makes the difference between leaving the school premises during the compulsory hours and managing to stay in school despite the difficulties?

### A 'non-visualizer' employing a different learning style

A further example relating to individual differences in imagery within learning experience is offered as a bridge between the above section containing the words of dyslexic learners and the subsequent discussion about implications for teachers of individual differences in learning, SpLDs and dyslexia. It concerns 'non-visualizers', whose different learning styles may not be identified without careful observation and extended conversations with their teachers.

Some time ago Sue Palmer, then a primary school teacher, attended a guest lecture by Helen McLullich at Leicester University. In the course of the lecture, Sue found that she was unable to visualize in the manner that Helen and many other teachers who were present almost 'took for granted'. Helen, a skilled teacher with specialist knowledge about teaching young children, music and multi-sensory teaching approaches, has both keen auditory and visual memory. In the course of written correspondence after the lecture, Sue explored with Helen the fact that, although she could not 'see in her head', she had become an 'ace-speller'. Sue attributed her spelling skill and her keen interest in words to the fact that she 'had been taught by her brilliant, intuitive mother' and was enabled to compensate for her 'non-visualizer' learning style through a keen sense of meanings of words:

> *'If it hadn't been for my mother I might well have been unable to read and write – but I can't summon up a picture of her, no matter how hard I try!'*

The above extract is from reported correspondence between Sue Palmer and Helen McLullich (Hunter-Carsch 1989). Sue, who is now a specialist consultant in literacy, a writer and a mother, continues to share her interest and understanding about dyslexia both as a professional and in the light of her personal experience, as she has a dyslexic daughter.

Although the three cases (Andrew, Michael and Sue (who was not considered to be a dyslexic learner but did learn differently)) cannot be taken to be representative of all positive and successful 'achievers', the importance of their mothers' support is noteworthy (see Chapter 9).

Teachers and the research community owe a debt of gratitude to parents and families who continue to share their understanding in a range of ways including voluntary work with professional associations, e.g. local branches of the British Dyslexia Association.

## Literacy difficulties, SpLDs and dyslexia

### Literacy and/or learning emphasis?

The challenge facing the class teacher, as a teacher of literacy whether in primary or secondary school, is that of managing to provide appropriate learning support for students at all levels of literacy. Since access to a mainly academic curriculum depends on successful development of reading and writing skills to 'automatic level', anyone with literacy difficulties will require support with learning literacy. For those with SpLDs such as dyslexia the emphasis becomes one of directing support towards literacy learning rather than towards the perceptual, cognitive processing and organizational problems which may underlie literacy difficulties, and for some of these pupils, the compounding behavioural difficulties which may derive from frustration when faced with their learning difficulties.

The fact that the new working definition of dyslexia (BPS/DCEP 1999) specifies its focus on literacy learning at the 'word level' is likely to increase this emphasis on literacy (rather than learning). This will be further endorsed by the 'non-exclusive' emphasis of the new working definition ('pupils with moderate learning difficulties or sensory impairments can also be described as dyslexic if they cannot read'; Greaney and Reason 1999). Thus, although teachers are expected to deal with literacy teaching, it is important for them to recognize also that there are different types and degrees of learning difficulties among pupils.

For teaching purposes teachers also have to recognize characteristics of individual differences amongst those who are described, (in the Code of Practice, DfEE 1994), as having 'mild learning difficulties', and to deal with the problems which the new working definition presents as it affects the still-operational 'exclusionary' (discrepancy-based) definition of SpLDs (DfEE 1994) until and unless the revision of the Code of Practice (anticipated in 2002) alters the current definitions and categories of 'special need'. As several other chapters in this volume address issues of definition (see chapters 2, 6 and most especially Chapter 7), here the intention is simply to draw attention to the need for teachers to adopt the stance of a researcher in attempting to formulate hypotheses about how best to assist individual learners. This will require teachers to 'go behind or beyond' their students' words in order to ensure that there is shared understanding of intended meaning and to discover students' optimal modes of learning, as well as to 'go behind and beyond' the literature's use of definitive terminology in the sense of becoming aware of the trajectory of meaning (the direction from which understanding comes, historically and in terms of academic discipline, orientation of study or experience, and the direction in which that 'gaze' is moving).

A broad approach is required for teaching (traditional) literacy across the curriculum (not only in the Literacy Hour in England and Wales and not only in primary school) in a manner that includes pupils with high literacy achievements as well as those with literacy difficulties (i.e. all those who came within the BPS (1999) working definition of dyslexia which might include some who might otherwise be described as pupils with SpLDs and may also have SpLDs beyond literacy). Although the national literacy strategy framework provides teachers with helpful information about developmental expectations and 'normal' patterns for teaching, especially within the Literacy Hour, more information is needed about strategies for promoting individualized teaching, especially of writing and spelling.

### Differentiation: where to begin?

*Handwriting speed, fluency, listening comprehension, written language*

Experience suggests that one of the most practical steps towards managing individual differences (differentiation) in the classroom with schoolchildren of any age, involves establishing awareness of children's characteristic differences in speed of completion of different kinds of work. This is especially useful with regard to handwriting speed. The point is not to suggest that speedy completion is a valued skill, as such, but that it is essential to be aware of variations in the range of time required by different children for routine tasks. This can be done by baseline screening of handwriting speed for the entire class (easily completed in less than half an hour by use of perceptual forms copying for young children up to seven years of age and the handwriting test for older pupils who have been introduced to the alphabet and copy writing; Hunter-Carsch 1993). The main diagnostic indicators readily observable at this level of screening are:

- Individuals who lag behind the others (slow copy-writers).
- Those whose writing lacks fluency and 'good form' (and who may have difficulty in employing 'automatically' a mental model of the shape or letter formation and who may have directional and/or kinesthetic memory difficulties).

At this very simple level of screening, the class' written work on any simple writing task such as the screening tests, can be allocated to three piles for speed of completion ('fastest', 'average' and 'slower') and also for form/legibility and fluency ('good', 'average' and 'strugglers'). Once rough 'norms' are compiled for the class, the teacher can scan the range of the students' work and make a closer examination of the 'bottom third' ('Slingerland's rule') for both categories ('speed of completion' and 'form/legibility and fluency'). The samples may then be ranked, informal identification can be made of students about whom further efforts need to be made by the teacher to monitortheir written work in class in order to sense whether their sample work was representative of their usual efforts. Diagnostic assessment should be undertaken to discern the severity of their difficulties. Where further advice is required, more experienced teachers, special educational needs co-ordinators (SENCOs) and possibly educational psychologists might be approached for advice (see also Alston and Taylor 1990; Markee 1993; Smith 1994; Chapman 1997 and the literature on dyspraxia).

Another often overlooked indicator of vital individual differences is listening comprehension (which correlates highly with 'general intelligence'). Teachers may have a good working knowledge of children's responsiveness and may be able to carry out an informal assessment by asking questions about a story read to the class during the Literacy Hour. Clearly, this assessment is best carried out on a one-to-one basis and teachers may require some assistance to administer e.g. the Narrative Retelling Test (Sage 1995). Meanwhile, there is increasing evidence to suggest that it is possible to discover more about the nature of any difficulties if screening procedures are carried out by classroom learning support assistants (LSAs) after a brief training course together with the teacher. At a very basic level, some students have difficulties knowing what exactly they should be attending to. Their seeming 'lack of concentration' may reflect uncertainty about instructions and a lack of confidence about attempting tasks lest they fail. The fact that an adult is giving attention and assisting in directing their attention may go some way towards carrying out a more detailed exploration of possible listening comprehension difficulties. When the focus is on exploring listening, and especially with students with literacy difficulties, it is best to avoid requiring written responses to any investigatory survey.

If Slingerland's 'rule of the bottom third' is followed and the lowest third of the class for listening comprehension is identified, the next level of exploratory diagnostic monitoring can proceed. When planning their teaching, teachers would then be aware of which students are likely to require more than spoken information (such as assistance from visual supporting cues and clues, additional information, slowing down and repetitions of instructions).

Teachers are often anxious about spelling and are encouraged to be so in the climate of concern to raise standards of literacy. However, spelling (in English) requires a solid underpinning of awareness of the operation of 'Phonics 44' (Morris 1984; 1993), which, for dyslexic students, may require multi-sensory teaching (e.g. Hornsby 1991; Augur and Briggs 1993; Johnson et al. 1999). In the absence of specialist teaching, however, dyslexic students may be helped by working in peer pairs (a stronger speller with a weaker speller) using Prompt Spelling (Watkins and Hunter-Carsch 1995).

It is striking to discover that if a written language approach is employed, both spelling and handwriting can improve, seemingly spontaneously, as long as the pressure on both skills is relieved. Within the parameters of a teaching approach such as systematic drafting and redrafting (Binns 1978, 1989), there is a clear recognition that in teaching written language ('creative writing') the focus must be firstly on the writer's intended meaning and the importance of reaching the intended audience. The emphasis is thus on clarifying the message, employing visual sketching, drawing, mind-mapping or noting of rough ideas from which a selection is made of the part to be developed; this is then 'redrafted' with frequent work in pairs and whole-class work on reading drafts aloud in order to listen and hear where there are areas that are not clear in meaning.

Brackets are placed around such areas (words or phrases) to signal that they are not clear and need to be redrafted. But, it is the confidence with which writers can continue unimpeded by 'surface-feature' problems of spelling and handwriting that normally brings about keen interest and enthusiasm to communicate in writing. Binns models the 'expert listener' and does not make corrections mainly on the page of students' written work. His discussions, hearing students and attending to what they want to say, whether they want to use brackets for spelling or for adding more descriptive wording, inevitably lead students to discover for themselves what kind of assistance they need. They become self-directed, find their 'voice' and work well with others to develop their ideas. Students have shown that they do this during examinations as well as in classwork and homework and that they can dramatically increase their sense of control and calm during examinations through recognition of the value of signalling through brackets that they are unsure of spellings.

This 'bracket' technique works well as a diagnostic approach for surveying students' awareness of their own spelling difficulties. Typically, dyslexic students tend to bracket as many words spelled correctly as misspelled. Teachers may observe whether there are patterns of difficulty among other students' bracketed words and so identify the extent of uncertainties about correct or incorrect spelling. These problems, however, are likely to diminish with access to word processors with spellcheckers and (eventually) speech-to-text systems (see Chapter 10; for further information about teaching spelling see Montgomery 1999; Ott 1997; Hughes and Hunter-Carsch 2001).

## Help with reading

In secondary schools, students should have ready access to all-important texts on audio-tapes not just printed texts. Short sections of taped material (e.g. five-minute tapes) are easier to manage than hour-long tapes. Parents are often willing to assist with the preparation of audio-tapes of books and worksheets and capable students with pleasant clear voices may also find reading aloud useful for their own revision. By using headsets or earplugs, there need be no interference from audiotaped materials during routine classroom work. Access to such material is important not only for dyslexic students but also for students with English as a second language, who may benefit from hearing models of intonation and stress patterns in spoken English, matching it to printed text and being able to repeat material as required. More sophisticated technology and computer programs for learning to read and write are likely to be available in the near future (see Chapter 10 and Haase 1999, 2000).

If teachers are to be effective in teaching literacy in secondary school they need to understand the normal developmental process as well as know what to do to support learning for those who are dyslexic. Yet in the literature most models of reading development relate to 'young literacy learners' (Clark 1994) (see also Adams 1990; Clay 1991; Owen and Pumfrey 1995; Funnell and Stuart 1995). One model which looks at teachers' conceptual maps of literacy in and beyond primary school and across subject areas has been generated by Reid et al. (1993). Their model employs four dimensions on two axes:

- High or low levels of mediation, control, structure or management exercised by the teacher.
- High or low levels of initiative, engagement, collaboration and active involvement enjoyed by the learner in the learning process (Figure 1.1).

These authors stress the point that their model is aimed to assist description, rather than for judgement. They make no assumptions about which quadrants are 'best'. They state:

'We would expect teachers to locate some of what they do at different times and for different purposes, in a range of quadrants.' (Reed et al. 1993, p.171)

Figure 1.1 may be useful in pinpointing some areas of difference in viewpoint, stance or emphasis. If, for example, a parent has in mind the picture of 'Abstracted Literacy' and the teacher centres on 'Immersed

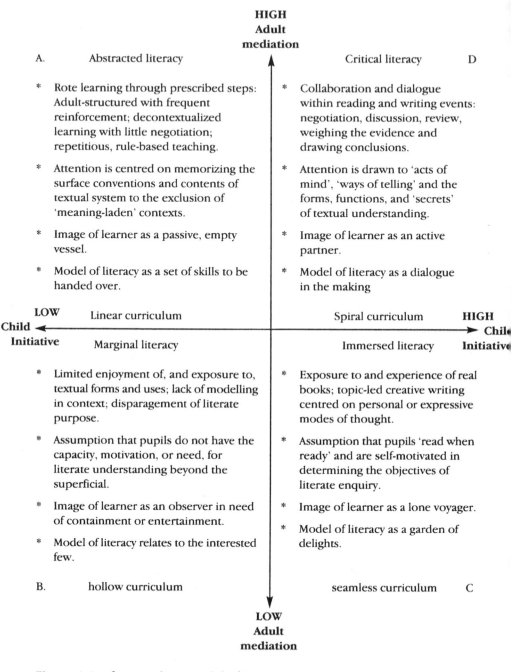

**HIGH**
**Adult**
**mediation**

A.              Abstracted literacy                                    Critical literacy         D

*   Rote learning through prescribed steps:        *   Collaboration and dialogue
    Adult-structured with frequent                     within reading and writing events:
    reinforcement; decontextualized                    negotiation, discussion, review,
    learning with little negotiation;                  weighing the evidence and
    repetitious, rule-based teaching.                  drawing conclusions.

*   Attention is centred on memorizing the         *   Attention is drawn to 'acts of
    surface conventions and contents of                mind', 'ways of telling' and the
    textual system to the exclusion of                 forms, functions, and 'secrets'
    'meaning-laden' contexts.                          of textual understanding.

*   Image of learner as a passive, empty           *   Image of learner as an active
    vessel.                                            partner.

*   Model of literacy as a set of skills to be     *   Model of literacy as a dialogue
    handed over.                                       in the making

**LOW**       Linear curriculum                        Spiral curriculum          **HIGH**
**Child** ◄─────────────────────────────────────────────────────────────► **Chil‹**
**Initiative**   Marginal literacy                       Immersed literacy       **Initiative**

*   Limited enjoyment of, and exposure to,         *   Exposure to and experience of real
    textual forms and uses; lack of modelling          books; topic-led creative writing
    in context; disparagement of literate              centred on personal or expressive
    purpose.                                            modes of thought.

*   Assumption that pupils do not have the         *   Assumption that pupils 'read when
    capacity, motivation, or need, for                 ready' and are self-motivated in
    literate understanding beyond the                  determining the objectives of
    superficial.                                       literate enquiry.

*   Image of learner as an observer in need        *   Image of learner as a lone voyager.
    of containment or entertainment.
                                                   *   Model of literacy as a garden of
*   Model of literacy relates to the interested        delights.
    few.

B.              hollow curriculum                        seamless curriculum        C

**LOW**
**Adult**
**mediation**

**Figure 1.1** A four-quadrant model of teaching through adult–child proximation through literacy learning. (Reed et al. 1993, p. 172, in Owen and Pumfrey 1995) (Reproduced with kind permission of The Falmer Press.)

Literacy', their dialogue will require careful navigation around their personal conceptual maps of literacy if the student's journey is to be their shared concern. Their mutual re-fuelling of the youngster in his or her personal quest may take skill in shared navigation from the parent–teacher team and a clear recognition of the role played by peer groups and colleagues.

### Changing attitudes of students with literacy difficulties

Findings of research evaluating summer literacy schools held in Leicester in 1998, with a population of lower literacy achievers (not including Statemented dyslexic students) revealed the tenacity of some students' views of themselves as 'other than achievers'. In this they share with some dyslexic learners, a low self-concept and limited self-esteem. To shift this impression may require more than the impact of skilled teachers and helpers at school. It may also require evidence of actual increments in learning and a response of recognition and respect from parents – understanding the meaning of students' progress even in what may be quite small steps. This recognition is hard to gain, especially during a phase in schooling when peer pressure tends to constitute a major influence and demonstrating being co-operative in the learning process at school does not always rank highly in some of the toughest school contexts. 'Being part of the crowd' and conforming to peer group pressure becomes vital during this sensitive stage of removal of the security of being 'top' of the primary school and entering the beginning of a phase of being 'bottom' of a vast new, and for some, overwhelming secondary school environment. This move entails a shift in scale not only in size of school buildings and potential for getting lost but in the mind-mapping of how to judge success as a person, not only as a reader and writer.

The question of identity is central for all (not just for dyslexic students). This does not solely concern 'attitude to reading', nor the capacity of the individual to discern what is socially aceptable to the peer group. It involves a deeper level of a sense of the relative prevalence or absence of hope, and with that, that of motivation. Whereas the motivational dimension may be readily apparent, it is difficult to measure its effect reliably solely in terms of a group survey or questionnaire responses, or even in terms of two short interviews. An attempt has been made, however, to explore relevant issues in a contextualized manner, in greater depth, by following up points of discussion and emergent views of a sample of 24 students' accounts of themselves during six summer literacy schools. Their views are related to those of a group total of 162 students who attended the 1998 summer literacy schools at Leicester.

*Research findings about prerequisites for literacy development at 11*

What becomes evident as essential for the success of summer literacy schools is the communication from staff to pupils of an increased sense of 'being in control' of their own literacy development and their own ability to make choices. This finding was made independently of studies associated with dyslexic learners but might be regarded as suggesting that in this respect dyslexic learners locate their relevant feelings at an even more extreme point in the relevant notional continuum (see chapters 4 re. the 'C' (control factor) and re. continua and Chapter 6).

For individual students there are related prerequisites for becoming confident voluntary readers and writers. These include discovery of their own 'voice', believing in themselves, and sensing what they want for themselves. The opening up of possibilities not previously entertained appears to depend on students' recognition and appreciation of their own imagination at work – and being able to organize their thoughts in a way which requires not only efficient and effective listening to others, but 'hearing themselves think'. But, the increased level of meta-cognitive awareness that is necessary to do this is closely linked to recognition of feelings (not only thinking). This 'meta-affectivity' (see Chapter 5) concerns self-recognition (awareness of 'This is how I feel') in relation to acceptance that it is alright to feel that way. This 'personal permission' to acknowledge feelings and to link them to thinking, is intimately bound up with the development of identity.

Since children choose to read 'in order to become' (i.e. to expand their sense of their own identity), the reading choices of youngsters who are initially lacking the self-confidence which generates the curiosity 'to seek to become' will often be limited to a cursory look at a book cover and flicking through the pages. The potential for engagement in dialogue with a book's contents is simply not there. The expectation that there might be an intellectual (and affective) response to self, by self, is absent. Before the choosing of books can become real (i.e. done deliberately with a sense of purpose) there is a need for engagement with 'reading life' (situations, events, stories) and 'reading self' (not books) at a more direct level and responding consciously to personal feelings and choices. This is vital for dyslexic learners who show reluctance to continue experience with printed texts when these are associated with physical discomfort (for example, Michael revealed in discussion that he experienced a pain in his head when faced with print).

One demonstrably effective way of promoting such engagement is through role-play, drama and a balance of opportunity to observe and join in with increasing recognition of the effect of choice in so-doing. There is a substantial difference between the child's efforts to join in, to be one of the group, and their choice to engage in the action itself – directly contributing to the dynamics of the dialogue. Becoming a participant rather than an observer is only one step. The choices include: to contribute either more or less, to adjust and respond, to appreciate leadership and accept and support a leader, to justify alternative viewpoints, to take on leadership or to share leadership. Without experiencing the responses of 'others who are valued and who care', the learner's explorations of these positions and their related responsibilities, the imagination of the learner-reader remains unharnessed for the task of self-directed learning in the course of developing a personal 'voice'. It is essentially a matter of self-determination which plays a role in facilitating or impeding learning to become literate to the automatic level (i.e. to the point at which the purposes of literacy can be grasped and it can be easefully employed).

For dyslexic learners, who include some who are very able speakers and actors, it is vital to provide recognition of areas of strength (for example, Susan Hampshire's success as an actress and her public sharing of the struggles she has had as a dyslexic learner), thus, to help learners to become confident readers in the quest of 'becoming' (i.e. achieving their identity as autonomous individuals not only as readers and writers (Riesman 1950)). Hence, teachers and literacy assistants may need to step back from the printed text and build up students' relevant shared experiences, the relationships which promote the application of imagination to the task of reading. It is through supported shared experience of literature and non-fiction through 'Talking with Books', that they may become self-directed (Hunter-Carsch 1984).

For many struggling readers, appreciation of what is involved in reading is limited – and that is where their seeming lack of effort may often conceal an absence of the essential awareness of what reading actually involves in terms of personal growth (*'enteliche'*). To generate an internal picture of how to get at intended meaning requires direction of learners' effort towards building whole pictures (perhaps not details or single facts initially). It is essentially a matter of 'getting the pieces together'. It is in this way that reading comprehension is closely related to listening comprehension.

This is not to suggest that decontextualized listening comprehension exercises will be successful in contributing directly to improving reading comprehension (they may even have the opposite effect), but to draw attention to the fact that many of the summer literacy schools' pupils moved from a position of not being 'centred' (focused) in their attempts to improve their reading to a point at which they could become 'centred' (really engaged with the content of the text – the 'ideas' and 'story'). This process of 'centering' is perhaps a part of what is broadly termed 'concentrating'. It concerns having the mind on the job. But it does not usually respond to attempts to command the minds to attend. These are children who are not so much 'truanting in mind' (Collins 1996) because they do not choose to truant, or to 'be elsewhere', they are simply **absent in mind** but not aware of the fact that their minds are not 'present' because they do not appreciate what the reading task requires in terms of 'engaging the mind'. They may not be aware that they need to engage with the larger ideas – the storyline created through the emerging pictures in words - not just the words themselves. **Their concentration on the mustering of the effort they have to put into the task of 'decoding' the text is so great that the reasons for trying to do so become lost.**

This is not simply a limit in word-level understanding of the process of decoding (or encoding), nor even a limitation of facility to grasp the sentence-level of understanding texts, but of **grappling with the whole text level and the rationale for so-doing** (Jackson 1985; Binns 1989; Sage 2001).

Why summer literacy schools worked so well for so many may not relate to teaching of component skills or vocabulary, nor to incentives, but to the fact that their **context made it acceptable to talk about tackling reading, writing and spelling (personal learning targets) without embarrassment** and with an optimal staff:pupil ratio so that plenty of help was available and it was seen to be appropriate to ask for assistance (an essential point indicating a special need for dyslexic learners, perhaps to an even greater level of intensity). The social acceptability of engaging with imagination while wrestling with following text in plenary sessions in the Literacy Hour, and having the chance to read along, but not being forced to read aloud alone, was all part of what was described by the pupils in interviews as 'good', valuable and useful to them. They enjoyed the 'permission' to engage with the relevant experiences (actually listening and recalling events in stories which had some intrinsic interest). This was strikingly evident in responses to the theatre company's performance of a play that brought together a number of themes with which many of the pupils could identify. They were **helped into the text**.

Once real questions were being asked, the road to independent self-directed reading was within view as an idea – a possibility, not because of any printed words but because of the stimulation of curiosity about ideas which were being experienced in a dynamic manner and requiring a personal response. The pupils were on the road to **recognizing the existence of questions about their role as determined by their identity**.

## Especially difficult for dyslexic girls

A further factor for discussion and further research is a trend mentioned earlier as observable among girls with lower literacy levels. Although there was no statistically significant gender difference in attitude to literacy, there appeared to be a tendency for girls to have a more negative attitude, perhaps more easily identifiable in interview data, which was reflected in a wish to adopt boys' forms of presentation, to prefer boys' games and to retain a stronger and more negative attitude to literacy. It is as if members of this subgroup, failing to see themselves as part of the 'normal' expectation for girls to be more readily literate and fond of literature, had turned elsewhere to find a sense of identity.

In summary, the evidence from this study supports the suggestions that:

- **Voluntary reading and writing is closely related to recognizing that reading (literacy) helps the reader/writer to 'become', perhaps to realize, or at least approximate his or her ideal.**
- **Attitude to literacy is thus bound up with 'sense of identity' and hopefulness which depends on 'being able to hear yourself thinking' which depends on 'being listened to' and recognizing that one has to make choices (and being able to engage in an internal dialogue).**

The comments of Andrew and Michael are echoed in these findings. Whatever the reasons for limited progress in literacy learning (whether related to situational, constitutional, traumatic or attitudinal factors) the relationship between motivation to read and write and the feelings evoked by attempts to read and write vitally affect learners' willingness to continue with the process of learning to become literate. For dyslexic students, where there may be a degree of physical discomfort associated with the act of reading, it becomes vital to find ways of overcoming physical discomfort (see Chapter 3).

## A model for motivating reluctant readers and writers

The psychosocial needs of different subgroups of students with literacy difficulties (whether described as 'students with reading difficulties' or 'dyslexic learners') may be more closely related (at the level of understanding motivation to read and write) than has been recognized previously. However, the teaching routes through which to support the effective development of the relevant subskills to the automatic level may differ. The teacher of reluctant readers (who may be reluctant for a range of reasons) requires to have a well-grounded, theoretically based, yet attractively and imaginatively differentiated teaching approach for different subgroups and for individuals. Further research is needed in this area, possibly exploring selected aspects of recent work on cognitive and learning styles (Riding and Rayner 1998; Reid 1997; 1998; also Chapter 5).

## Links between components

The three words 'motivate', 'reluctant' and 'readers' are analysed below in Table 1.1 in terms of their underlying meanings. The main ideas represented may be connected by 'reading downwards'. The links between each step of the larger argument can be 'read' through the links across the Table. The following descriptions trace the argument, first, by exploring the columns then by tracing the links across the Table (clusters of words sometimes taking more than one line in space).

Table 1.1 concentrates on the reading process rather than attempting to make reference in full to both writing and reading which would require substantially more space than is available in this book. It is recognized, however, that the reading process is mainly one of working with 'given' materials (text), whereas writing involves creation of text itself. Although the 'decoding' and 'encoding' processes cannot simply be regarded as reciprocal, they do have complementary aspects. In particular, the underlying motivational factors may be strongly related in the learner's developing attitude to literacy as a whole. Table 1.1 and this discussion thus refer primarily to reading but may be generally taken to provide guidelines which may be adapted for investigation of attitudes to writing.

**The left-hand column relates to the action required in order to achieve the aim (to motivate the reader).** It is essentially about what has to be done (the verb component) to motivate readers. It has in mind the position of the teacher or parent who wishes to encourage a learner-reader who is struggling and does not apear to be developing into a voluntary reader. The idea of 'motivation' is traced downwards under nine interrelated questions and responses. Following the line of argument traced (downwards) by the nine questions and responses (points) in the column, it becomes evident that teachers (or parents) who wish to understand how to motivate reluctant readers need to be aware of the connections between these points. The reasoning is as follows:

In order to grasp the reasons for the seeming reluctance to read (Point 1 'Why?'), the question must be posed (Point 2 'What do they read?') and the further and closely related question: if not books, what do they actually 'read', i.e. respond to with intent to understand? (Point 3 'Not only printed texts'). Facility in dealing with printed texts is dependent on prior experience and associated sense of the social aspects of reading (i.e. a social-interactive model of reading (Point 4).

Such a model, internalized through positive early experiences of interacting with texts and people, especially one well-loved and/or respected person, normally bonds the act of reading with purposes which include shared (social) enjoyment and anticipation of pleasure personally. The purpose of reading then comes to be self-directed to seek repetition of this

**Table 1.1** Motivating reluctant readers

| How motivated is the learner? | What is their 'stance'; attitude, feelings? | How close is the learner to doing what successful readers do? |
| --- | --- | --- |
| 1 Why do they seem to lack motivation to read? | *Why are they reluctant?* | Can they read? Can't? Won't? Don't? |
| 2 What do they 'read'? | *Who/what is it about?* | How do they do it? |
| 3 NOT ONLY PRINTED TEXTS | *IMAGES, IDENTITY* | BECOMING AND BEING |
| 4 Social-interactive model of reading | *Role model: learner/teacher* | Competent, automatic |
| 5 Purposes for reading texts | *Creating texts, de-centring, centring and deep centring* | Mastery of 'Phonics 44' |
| 6 RECOGNIZING | *LEARNING PREFERENCES* | LEARNING DIFFICULTIES (+SpLD e.g. dyslexia) |
| 7 Self-advocacy | *Self-confidence* | Literacy |
| 8 LOVE OF LANGUAGE | *LOVE OF LEARNING* | COMMUNICATION |
| 9 Meta-linguistics | *Meta-affectivity* | Meta-cognition |

experience (Point 5) for personally defined purposes (which diversify with widening experience of texts). The continuing developmental sequence involves the developing reader in becoming aware of what the process of independent reading actually requires of the reader (Point 6 'Recognition') and the gradually increased confidence to choose to ask for repeated experiences of 'reading' together (at the early stages simply, an aspect of 'being' together, company and shared experience). As the learner-reader develops a sense of power over choice about the reading experience and what brings about pleasure as well as 'answers' to questions, fulfilment of needs and resolution of conflicts, the appreciation of this process can come to generate an increased appreciation of how language works (Point 8), especially in terms of how poetic language relates to evocation of feelings and how precision in choice of words assists thinking and achieves (for example) economies in communicating exactly what is intended. Such niceties of communication require their own vocabulary to describe and work with the linguistic notions which convey meaning, i.e. 'meta-linguistic awareness' (Point 9).

The nine points in the right-hand column are related to questions and responses which trace connected aspects of the wider argument about how to promote voluntary reading. This column connects ideas concerned with the reader's state or situation rather than the purpose of the intervention which is the concern of the left-hand column. Reading downwards, to connect the lines of points in the right-hand column, the argument would run as follows.

**This column is concerned with what successful readers do**. The first question in relation to a seemingly unsuccessful reader is to check the facts about whether they see themselves as able to read, not able or not wanting to read, for whatever reasons (Line 1). A quick observation of attempts to read may provide opportunities for 'miscue analysis' or lead to shared discussion about what actually happens when they try to read (Line 2). It can soon become evident whether they have any sense of purpose in undertaking reading, for example, do they want to experience the story content or to relive a shared experience (remembering the story as read to them by someone, or told them, or as seen on a film, video or television)? That is, is their sense of what it is to be a reader, one which takes into account the fact that reading can help readers to become more knowledgeable (Line 3). Mastery of the act of reading involves not only automatic decoding skills but being able to connect beyond the word level to make sense of threads of arguments and connected ideas in larger chunks of text (lines 4 and 5).

For some readers this can present difficulties, for example in relation to limited experience of the content being presented in printed text, limited speed of connecting ideas requiring additional learning support, possibly additional sensory input and reinforcement and substantially extended practice (Line 6) or differently presented and practised learning strategies activated in collaboration with appropriate resources, such as plastic letters, Edith Norrie lettercase, speech mirrors, audiotapes, slowed down speech-to-text, ICT systems involving slowing or lengthening the phonemes (Haase 1999) for SpLD, e.g. dyslexic learners. For learner-readers (and writer/spellers) to be able to employ these complex skills in an integrated manner, awareness of how 'literacy' (Line 7) relates to 'communication' (Line 8) is required.

To do this requires meta-cognitive awareness (thinking about thinking) which itself requires a vocabulary to deal with the component parts of the process. This is not a simple matter of 'recall' but involves understanding exactly how the recall of perhaps seemingly unrelated 'facts' or notions (phonenes, graphemes) can be related to meaning units (morphemes) and this sense can be made of the system employed for going beyond decoding or encoding 'speech written down' to the mastery of the rules and conventions of written language and the range of text types (genres) employed for a range of purposes.

**The centre column deals with attitudes and feelings involved in making the necessary links to becoming a voluntary reader and writer.** Essentially, these concern the learner's awareness of how they fit into the social picture, what is expected, how this should feel, where to look for help and models and how to summon up the necessary courage to explore the process from different points of view (inside it, outside it, and what it does to the person and to others). In short, this column draws attention to the central role of feelings in the whole learning process. Awareness of feelings may not only be helpful but may be essential to free emotional 'blocks' or overcome hurdles in mastering the learning process.

The following paragraphs present these ideas in a different but related manner, by reading across Table 1.1. Some of the ideas may be repeated, but are linked in a way which may make the connections between components more readily accessible for diagnostic purposes. The identification of 'problem areas' in the learner's approach to reading is easier if there is an attitude of flexibility on the part of the diagnostician and provider of learning support (whether class teacher, specialist teacher, parent or peer), if they are aware of the links between ideas and have a sense of the fact that most learners' attitudes to reading/literacy learning and their prior experiences are intimately connected and 'overdetermine' their responses. It is seldom simply a matter of providing one link or line of information or practice.

Each 'line' is linked in the following manner:

| Line 1: | Why do they seem to lack motivation to read? | *Why are they reluctant?* | Can they read? Can't? Won't? Don't? |

Questions which are implicit in the title words are drawn out. If we do not recognize the different strands of meaning, the connections between the three ideas remain a mystery.

Line 2:    What do they 'read'?    *Who/what is it about?*    How do they do it?

This level of logical follow-up questioning sets the scene for finding out about the realities of readers' experiences and, by taking a wider view of reading to include reading of pictures, television, videos, faces, music and movement, provides access to a way of finding out where their basic curiosities about life lie or how damaged these have become. The aim at this level is to locate a starting point of shared interest in learning.

Line 3:    NOT ONLY              *IMAGES,*            BECOMING
           PRINTED TEXTS         *IDENTITY*           AND BEING

These words are capitalized as they relate to the central thesis of this model (the dynamics which connect the individual's views with attaining their sense of successful membership of the social group). The ideas behind the words direct attention to the possible focus of the underlying will to learn (it is something to do with looking at life not only as an outsider but wanting to be part of it and having pictures in mind and hopes about what might be good to be able to do or to become – models who are admired and loved – and aspirations). Sometimes this 'will to learn' needs to be re-connected with the underlying motivational strands which may not be readily available at conscious level in some circumstances.

Line 4:    Social-interactive    *Role model*         Competent/
           model of reading      *learner/teacher*     automatic

This line provides labels which may be helpful for exploring the connections between components in the minds of teachers as well as learners (what do teachers think reading is and does for readers?; what kind of model is the teacher providing – does it fire the student's imaginations and help them to connect with other desirable models?; how clearly can the learner conceptualize what is involved in becoming competent to the level of 'automatic rapid word reading' and processing (comprehending) the text?).

Line 5:    Purposes for          *Creating texts,*    Mastery of
           reading texts         *de-centring, centring*  'Phonics 44'
                                 *and deep centring*

Motivating any reader to pick up a text involves having a sufficiently appreciated purpose for potential readers to wish to engage with it. If the purposes for reading are insufficiently clearly articulated or not acceptable to readers, there may be problems to be resolved at this level. Problems can sometimes be resolved by moving away from pre-printed texts to creating readers' own texts as writers. Relating the two strands of literacy (reading and writing) can often be usefully and effectively accomplished by working as an artist (Binns 1989), painting or drawing texts which may be static or moving, or dictating narrative or instructions so that the words can be transcribed (easy with speech-to-text systems). Adapting a stance as an observer or storyteller (often requiring de-centring) to that of an experiencer of something which requires deeper engagement with feelings in order to explore it (often requiring deep-centring) points also to a need to be 'on task' (simply 'there in mind', that is 'centred'). Mastery of the code for encoding as a writer requires a degree of phonological awareness (or compensatory sensory awarenesses) to recognize the component sounds (phonemes)in the English language and knowledge, and skills to be able to match these with the letters (graphemes) and letter strings. This process is commonly called 'Phonics 44' (Morris 1990).

| Line 6: | RECOGNIZING | *LEARNING* | LEARNING |
|---------|-------------|-------------|----------|
|         |             | *PREFERENCES* | DIFFICULTIES |
|         |             |             | (+ SpLD, e.g. |
|         |             |             | dyslexia) |

These words seek to remind us that it is necessary to bring the relevant awarenesses to the conscious level. This may involve simply sharing the fact in a non-punitive manner, that it is understood that the 'reluctant reader' is 'reluctant', that there are very likely good reasons for this and that with relevant insights (into self) the learner's learning preferences may emerge, revealing avenues for making learning easier. This level involves a sense of tolerance and acceptance of individual differences and interest in exploring together the nature of learning. This is particularly important in situations in which reluctance to read (or do any literacy-related work) relates to experience of inappropriate teaching methods and unrealistic imposed learning requirements (such as mastery of a set number of spellings on a daily or weekly basis). These experiences may often be shared by students with SpLDs such as dyslexia. They also affect any student with literacy learning difficulty in the sense that it is often necessary to show (demonstrate) and even explain to the student the acceptance of them as individuals, as they are – they will have a need to feel in control of the situation in a learning interaction in which they feel very much 'out of control'. They will need the skills which are labelled in the following line.

| Line 7: | Self- advocacy | *Self-confidence* | Literacy |
|---------|----------------|-------------------|----------|

Learning how to ask for help and to state needs where relevant is very challenging for some youngsters. It is virtually taboo in certain social situations in our school and classroom culture from the point of view of the adolescent learner (whatever the strength of teachers' interests and attempts to make it otherwise). Peer group views are an essential component in making it permissable/acceptable to work together in pairs, groups or to employ self-help approaches. One-to-one tutoring by a peer or an older student may be acceptable. Acceptance of assistance from an ancillary or a teacher involves prior creation of a culture in which this is acceptable. Working towards this can be demanding for all concerned. The extent of parents' and teachers' shared understanding of 'the dangers in these waters' varies. Self-advocacy and self-confidence (based on recognition of needs and preferences), however, may be essential prerequisites for independent continuing development of the requisite levels of literacy for 'launching into voluntary reading'.

Line 8:     LOVE OF LANGUAGE     *LOVE OF LEARNING*     COMMUNICATION

These words, again capitalized as centrally connected strands of the thesis, relate to factors which are required to keep the system going once the new start has been made. If a genuine love of language may be fostered through, for example, finding the right poet or writer to express the learner's feelings or promoting the learner's own texts as sources of celebration of communication, it is more likely to encourage a more general will to learn and to go on learning. This wider love of learning may be communicated through any of the language modes, speech, writing or reading, and involves connecting with 'real-life' concerns (as in the summer literacy schools in Leicester). The communication of the Speak-Easy Theatre Company with students who recognized reflection of some of their experiences in the life of 'Citizen Kim' provides an example of the way in which the circuit needs to be connected in order for the message to go right through the system. Separate lessons on communication, learning about a selected topic or the manner of expresson exemplified by a particular piece of writing do not make the necessary connections. It is the integration of the experiences of all three which promotes the relevant will to repeat the experience.

Line 9:     Meta-linguistics          *Meta-affectivity*          Meta-cognition

The final line underlines and connects the range of ideas through the three main strands. It provide terms for describing facets of the strands. The three terms concern: first, language for negotiating our concepts of what is involved (meta-linguistic awareness); second, awareness of the feelings which are experienced, in this case in association with literacy tasks (frustration or delight (meta-affectivity)); third, recognition of the *thinking about thinking* which is needed to manage to develop and deal with concepts, ideas and the further dynamics of what goes on in the mind of learners, readers, writers or teachers which it may be necessary or helpful to share in the course of learning interactions and which render the process understandable in itself (meta-cognition).

The above account of 'reading' Table 1.1 provides a basis for consideration of the potential of the model for guiding observations, discussions and one-to-one interviews with students so that its diagnostic dimensions may be applied. The teacher/diagnostician may mentally run through the questions prompted by each set of lines (moving across the Table) and, considering the lines as 'levels', attempt to locate a starter level at which there is clarity about what students experience and think, and to establish those areas about which there may be some uncertainty as to how learner-readers feel and what might constitute evidence to back up decisions that a student was not entirely confident and independent at the relevant level.

The way forward for both teachers and students through conversations and 'talking with books' may involve consolidation of the base level before moving to the next level. With students as adventurers in charge of moving forward in this shared quest, the role of teachers becomes one of listening keenly, facilitating discussion and following the learner's inclinations in order to work with texts chosen by them (and scaffolded by the teacher). This is not the same as the work of the individual teachers in selecting and matching the level of text difficulty to the learner-reader's current capabilities (as would likely be the procedure in the Reading Recovery Approach as employed in primary schools). This involves shared exploring of potentially very challenging texts or 'too easy texts' in the light of the learner's selection.

The context for talking about books is just that – a way of establishing a discourse. The issues of how challenging is the text, the teaching and learning of subskills, including the combining of analytic and synthetic phonics in the course of exploring words, are all matters for deepening the engagement with the literacy experience. This approach does not rely on a single prescribed route for teaching (although there are helpful guidelines from the wealth of materials on teaching the 'new' phonics (Adams 1990; Bielby 1994). Its strength rests in the flexibility which it affords teacher-learner pairs (or groups). There is also a substantial (and overlapping) body of resources relating to the teaching of dyslexic students (e.g. Hornsby 1982; Augur and Briggs 1993; Lannen et al. 1997; Ott 1997; Reid 1998). The framework for the emotional (psychosocial) development must be such that the questions and issues which are noted on the chart, guide teachers' enquiries (which are likely to be most effective when the following learner-reader's direction of discussion rather than taking over and developing or endorsing dependence on teachers or even 'learner helplessness').

As learner-readers acquire confidence in their teachers, it is likely that the pace of learning will escalate substantially. For learner-readers to experience taking the lead in asking 'how to' deal with hurdles, is vital. This is in direct distinction to the apprenticeship reading approach and to the direct teaching approach as used with young learner-readers. It requires the older learner-reader to become progressively more aware of what the reading process involves, to explore the technical aspects of constructing meaning from the whole text, sentence structure and word-level work. It complements the approach outlined in the guidelines for the Literacy Hour and can usefully draw upon resource materials from the in-service pack designed as part of the 1998 National Literacy Strategy publications (DfEE 1998a).

Implicit in this approach is recognition of the logical sequential basis for the generation: first, of a sense of trust between learner-readers and teachers; second, sufficient will-power to see the learning task through to its conclusion; and third, a sense of purposefulnes and hope that the success in so-doing can carry learner-readers on to mastery of further learning and beyond matters of self-concern to care for others. In the words of Erikson (1968):

> 'Psycho-social strength, we conclude, depends on a total process which regulates individual life cycles, the sequence of generations, and the structure of society simultaneously: for all three have evolved together.' (p. 141)

## Conclusion

To return to the questions posed at the beginning of this chapter.

### How might a psychosocial perspective contribute to understanding of specific learning difficulties, dyslexia and other literacy and learning difficulties?

The answer involves recognition that dyslexia may be regarded as a 'social construct' in response to which individuals, whether formally diagnosed as 'dyslexic' or who consider themselves to be 'non-dyslexic', can generate personal attitudinal responses to the 'condition'. Whether they regard dyslexia as a matter of 'difference' or as a 'disability' may be influenced by, and influence, others in their families, schools and communities. Responses of researchers to research findings are also contextualized culturally. Through awareness of the psychosocial perspective, attitudinal factors may be examined and their effects considered as a part of the educational process and of processes which have an impact on individuals' educational success.

**What are the priorities for teachers in relation to teaching students with specific learning difficulties and those with literacy difficulties?**

This question has been considered broadly from the perspective of changing expectations about literacy requirements, literacies and multi-literacies in a multi-lingual global context. Teaching approaches based on systematic research and classroom experience have been illustrated along with material from case studies. It is suggested that teachers' priorities at primary and secondary level should include not only basic 'traditional literacy' but also ensuring that students have a will to read and write and the self-confidence to wish to relate to and communicate with a chosen audience. The importance of oracy and communication skills which underpin literacy skills is indicated.

**What role does motivation play in overcoming reluctance to read and write for dyslexic students and for those with more general literacy difficulties?**

The answer to this question has been attempted by sharing a diagnostic sequence of questions designed to ascertain at what levels there appear to be more or less intense difficulties in raising students' and teachers' expectations of themselves towards realistic levels for achievement and success in integrating a sufficient number of positive experiences and retrievable memory traces in pursuit of these achievements, to become able to build a sense of identity as readers and writers. The teacher's facilitatory rather than direct instructional role has been illustrated along with recognition that for some dyslexic learners there will also be a need for a direct teaching component but that may require to be grounded within the wider context of the positive self-perception as a reader and writer.

# Chapter 2
# Reflections and research

TIM MILES

Questions addressed in this chapter include:

- How do recent research findings explain the nature of dyslexia?
- How do different kinds of research illuminate the problem?
- What is the evidence for a phonological deficit?
- What is the evidence from brain research?
- Is there a theory which makes sense of the different manifestations of dyslexia?

## Introduction

This chapter reviews some of the recent research into dyslexia. It is divided into four sections, entitled respectively, *Informal observations, Evidence for a phonological deficit, Evidence from brain research, and Concluding remarks.* Emphasis is placed on the need to understand the many stresses that dyslexic children and adults undergo and on the fact that some of them can be very talented. It is now established beyond doubt that dyslexia has a physical basis.

## Informal observations

I should like to begin by sharing with you some of my general impressions of dyslexia, based largely on informal observations. My aim is to give you something of the 'flavour' of what dyslexic children and adults are like at different ages.

It is possible to pick out those 'at risk' as early as three years old (Augur 1990), although how soon dyslexia is thought of as a problem is hard to say.

It must be supposed that, when reading lessons start an intelligent dyslexic child soon notices that their classmates are able to 'please teacher' by responding appropriately to the baffling marks found on paper or on the blackboard, whereas they have no idea what response is needed. That these marks represent speech sounds is something that dyslexic children can be taught, but one cannot count on them picking this up automatically.

Even when – by age 9 or later – some proficiency at reading has been acquired, it is still difficult for many dyslexics to read for pleasure. Many of them are capable of appreciating good literature – when it is read to them; but the effort involved in having to decipher text for themselves, particularly after a tiring day at school, is likely to be too great to be tolerable. Spelling is yet more of a problem, and even with systematic structured teaching and the use of compensatory strategies and specially taught mnemonics most dyslexics remain poor spellers. Among older children there is also the problem of essay writing: it is possible to be brim-full of exciting and original ideas and yet not be able to set them out in an orderly fashion on paper; and because of weak presentation examination candidates sometimes experience the frustration of receiving a lower mark than their overall knowledge of the subject seems to merit.

The problems do not stop here. The basics of mathematics sometimes present difficulty: understanding the symbols used may give rise to problems, while the memorizing of number facts (for example that $8 \times 7 = 56$) is usually far from easy, even though – once the initial problems are overcome – dyslexics can be highly successful mathematicians. Musical notation may present problems, not because the child is insensitive to music as such, but because to read music (as opposed to the playing of it 'by ear') a large number of symbols, representing tempo, rhythm, duration etc., have to be named and their functions understood (see also Miles and Westcombe, in press).

In addition there are the inevitable social problems – forgotten messages, mistaking the time of an appointment or taking 'the first turn left' instead of the 'first turn right'. Teachers who are unaware of the distinctive needs of dyslexics can sometimes compound the problem by accusing them of laziness, carelessness, cussedness and the like – with the result that they feel even more discouraged and frustrated.

The themes of this book include awareness of what is involved in learning and what constitutes 'effective learning'. I would argue that if learning is to be effective for dyslexic adults in particular, one should be specially aware of the frustrations and humiliations which many of them will have experienced earlier in life. I am not, of course, saying that it is necessary to be perpetually harping on about them, only that it is very easy for a tutor to unwittingly re-open old wounds, as recorded, for example, by Gilroy and Miles (1996, pp 48-9). Two further books seem important in this connection: *The Scars of Dyslexia* (Edwards 1994) and *Dyslexia and Stress* (Miles and Varma, 1995). In both cases emphasis is laid on the personal feelings of dyslexics rather than on their literacy problems as such; and I have met dyslexics who have told me that they have been more damaged by the unsympathetic treatment that they have received than by the literacy problems themselves (see also chapters 1 and 14).

It is sometimes said that in adulthood the signs of dyslexia are not so obvious – that they are masked by the fact that it is possible to learn all kinds of compensatory strategies. It is true that if one looked simply for poor reading one would miss many people who were obviously dyslexic in other ways but who had taught themselves to read adequately. This however, merely underlines the absurdity of equating dyslexia with 'poor reading' – a mistake which, sadly, is still prevalent among some researchers (Henry et al., 2000, pp. 40–42). Despite the variety between individuals and despite the many compensatory skills which dyslexics can acquire, it remains true that even in adulthood the basic pattern in dyslexia does not change (Miles, T.R. 1993, Chapter 31)).

I shall pass now to some findings about dyslexia which have come to light as a result of systematic research and are now considered. This will comprise a brief review of the evidence for a deficiency at the phonological level, followed by an account of some recent neurological evidence and some concluding remarks.

## The evidence for a phonological deficit

For our purposes 'phonology' may be defined as the science of speech sounds in so far as they convey meaning. There is wide agreement among researchers that in some way or other the conversion of stimuli in the environment into speech sounds takes longer for dyslexics and is relatively difficult for them to acquire.

Some of the more important points are as follows:

- When they are tested on immediate recall of auditorily presented digits dyslexics tend to have a shorter memory span than suitably matched controls. This is in line with the familiar observation that when dyslexics are given a series of instructions they tend (more than non-dyslexics) to 'lose track' and forget some of the things which they were told. An interesting recent development has been the claim that in the case of younger children recall of nonsense words is an even more effective measure than recall of digits (Gathercole and Baddeley 1996).

- If the digits are presented visually the amount which dyslexics can reproduce again tends to be less than that for controls. For example, in one of their early studies, Ellis and Miles (1977) presented their subjects with strings of five, six and seven digits and found that dyslexics aged about twelve and a half recalled fewer digits than younger non-dyslexics aged about eight who were matched for spelling age. Not only does this finding confirm the idea that dyslexia involves some kind of anomaly and is not simply the consequence of late development; it also lends support to the idea that the problems for the dyslexic are not 'visual' or 'auditory' as such but arise from a weakness at verbal labelling (Vellutino 1979; Liberman 1985; Miles, E. 1991).
- There is also evidence that dyslexics tend to be less sensitive than non-dyslexics in recognizing that words rhyme and in dividing words up into their component  phonemes. (For relevant sources the reader is referred in particular to Catts 1989; Rack 1994.)

However, it should not be assumed that a difficulty at the phonological level accounts for all the manifestations of dyslexia. An exciting recent development has been evidence adduced by Nicolson et al. (1995) and Nicolson and Fawcett (1999) that some minor dysfunction of the cerebellum may be involved. This hypothesis has been confirmed by brain scan techniques (Nicolson et al. 1999) and also makes sense of an earlier claim by two of these authors (Nicolson and Fawcett 1990) that dyslexics have a distinctive difficulty in acquiring 'automaticity', that is, in making their responses so ingrained that they become automatic. This is an interesting notion which requires further research.

## The evidence from brain research

One of the most exciting discoveries of the 1980s was that when post mortem examinations were carried out on the brains of those known to have been dyslexic in their lifetime specific abnormalities were found (Galaburda et al. 1987). In the 1990s it has been possible to examine living brains by the techniques known collectively as 'neuroimaging'. The main techniques are positron emission tomography (PET), suitable for use only with adults, and magnetic resonance imaging (MRI), suitable for all ages. Those interested in further details may wish to consult Reid, Lyon and Rumsey (1996).

To return to the post mortem research, Galaburda and colleagues (1987) made a special study of the *planum temporale*, which is part of the surface of the temporal lobe on each side of the brain. During the course of their investigations they discovered *ectopias* (intrusions of cells from one layer to another) and *dysplasias* (disorganizations of cells within a cell layer). Even more strikingly, they found that in eight cases out of eight the plana on the two sides of the brain were symmetrical, even though in unselected cases such symmetry had been found to occur only about 20-25% of the time.

In the concluding section of their paper Galaburda et al. (1987) wrote as follows:

'Indirect evidence suggests that asymmetry of the planum results from the greater pruning down of one of the sides during late fetal life and infancy, a process that implicates asymmetry of developmental neuronal loss. Symmetry, on the other hand, reflects failure of asymmetrical cell loss to occur. The exuberant growth of the otherwise smaller side in the symmetrical cases might produce complex qualitative alterations in the functional properties of the system.' (p. 867)

This could mean that the exceptional talents shown by some dyslexics in certain areas, such as art, architecture and engineering, are no accident but are the consequence of a different balance of skills in the brain. At the risk of oversimplifying one might say that in the majority of cases language skills are mediated by the left hemisphere, whereas 'holistic thinking' (recognition of patterns etc.) is mediated by the right hemisphere. It has therefore been suggested that so-called 'lateral' thinking (including creative thinking) comes easily to dyslexics, whereas 'linear' thinking – for example, arranging symbols in a correct linear order – presents them with difficulty. In a very challenging book, West (1997) has suggested that the special talents observed in some dyslexics are the consequence of this distinctive brain organization. He then argues that, since computer technology can now take care of the 'clerical' skills (copying text, adding up figures and the like) which were important in previous generations, dyslexics are no longer at the same disadvantage; on the contrary, they have a distinct *advantage* in jobs which require creative thinking and viewing situations as a whole.

A further exciting development occurred when comparisons were made between dyslexics and non-dyslexics in respect of the *magnocellular* and *parvocellular* divisions of the visual system. These two terms can be explained as follows:

'In primates fast low-contrast visual information is carried by the magnocellular division ... and slow, high-contrast information ... by the parvocellular division.' (Livingstone et al. 1991)

When Galaburda re-examined some of the brains on which he had earlier carried out post mortem analysis he found that the parvocellular layers were not unusual but that there was considerable disorganization in the magnocellular layers, with the cell bodies being of a much smaller size than would have been expected. It was then not long before the suggestion was made that there could be a similar subdivision within the auditory system (Galaburda and Livingstone 1993). In that case a possible hypothesis is that when dyslexics are confronted with fast moving *auditory* information, in particular with the sounds of speech, they are impeded in their attempts to organize it. In the words of Tallal et al. (1993):

'We conclude that a primary inability to process acoustic information that enters the nervous system in rapid succession (within a time frame of tens of milliseconds) will serve to disrupt or delay the development of phonological processes, and subsequently lead to more global delayed development of receptive language.' (p. 32)

Two further papers (Merzenich et al. 1996; Tallal et al. 1996) have claimed that temporal processing and language comprehension in language learning-impaired children may be ameliorated by suitable training. This claim, however, is not firmly established.

It has long been known that in many cases of dyslexia – though not all – a hereditary factor is at work (DeFries 1991), although mechanisms are not yet fully understood. Galaburda's (1999) suggestion is that dyslexia is a 'multi-level' syndrome: that is to say, anomalies exist at a number of different levels:

'Dyslexia represents a complex interaction of both low-level and high-level deficits affecting language and perhaps visual performance.' (p. 183)

For a suggested model representing the relationship between biological bases, cognitive deficiencies and behavioural manifestations readers are referred to Frith (1997). An overview of the field will be found in Miles and Miles (1999).

## Concluding remarks

The first main section of this chapter contained some informal observations on the behaviour of dyslexic subjects at different ages. In the light of these observations and the evidence reported in the second and third sections it is possible to offer a theory – albeit a tentative one – of how the typical manifestations of dyslexia come about. This theory would run as follows:

> For neurological reasons (including, in some cases, genetic reasons) dyslexics have a weakness in the magnocellular system. As a result of this they are impeded in their ability to process information at speed; and in the case of auditory information the result is a weakness at the phonological level. This weakness creates a wide range of different sequelae (consequences) which vary considerably from one individual to another.

Finally, although some of the suggestions made here are tentative, it must be emphasized that there are certain things in the area of dyslexia which may now be regarded as firmly established. First and foremost we know that dyslexia has a physical basis – which means that *blaming* dyslexics for their struggles over literacy is about as sensible as putting a crippled child in the middle of a rugger scrum and telling him off for not coping. It is also known for certain that in some cases the manifestations of dyslexia have a genetic basis, and in addition it is highly likely that signs of dyslexia are present in late foetal life and early infancy.

This last finding underlines the inappropriateness of blaming parents for being over-anxious or teachers for failing to teach reading properly. Understanding is better than blaming; and in order to achieve such understanding one of the most important skills is to be a good listener.

# Chapter 3
# Visual difficulties with print

SUE MAILLEY

---

Questions addressed in this chapter include:

- What is the nature of visual difficulties with print, their causes and treatment?
- What is the impact of such difficulties on literacy learning?
- How can we build a bridge between multi-discipline specialist research and the classroom?
- What are the implications for policy makers, educational practitioners and the students themselves?

---

## Introduction

An exploratory study involving classroom observation (Mailley 1997) indicated that a surprising number (up to as many as 33%) of pupils in primary schools experience symptoms of visual stress when faced with print. Investigations into studies in this field led to the recognition that many sources of information about such difficulties lie outside the field of education and are rendered inaccessible to parents and teachers because of:

- the terminology used
- the technical nature of much of their content
- their publication in specialist, often medical, journals.

Surveys of teaching staff and parents suggested that there was a general lack of awareness about the nature and extent of visual problems; and that even when there was an awareness of screening procedures such as infant health screening, the school eye test and opticians' vision tests, the assumption that these procedures would provide an adequate assessment of a child's visual status was not questioned. The interview data indicated that if teachers knew that a student had been pronounced visually fit by some or all of these procedures, they would not consider the possibility of visual problems when attempting to delineate the learning difficulties affecting that student. It might thus be suggested that teachers' lack of awareness may lead them to a false sense of security about their students' visual competence (also noted by Holland 1988). The aim of this chapter is to address these issues by:

- raising awareness of the problems that can occur;
- exploring how these problems manifest themselves;
- describing how they can be assessed and treated.

## Limitations of current screening procedures

Tests commonly used in the assessment of vision have proved inadequate for the purposes of identifying all pupils experiencing visual difficulties. Some students who are not routinely identified experience some categories of 'visual stress', a factor not necessarily considered in tests of visual acuity. A diagnosis of 20/20 vision is not enough to rule out visual problems as a cause of difficulties with print. Unlike difficulties with focus, visual discomfort and distortion do not appear to be considered as components of problems with reading and writing, either by teachers and tutors, or by those health professionals responsible for administering routine screening tests. Thus there is a need for widely available information for teachers and parents about the more obvious difficulties.

The symptoms and effects of visual stress will be discussed later in this chapter, but there are two related issues which require prior consideration.

First, it does not appear to be generally appreciated that the smaller, denser print, commonly presented to pupils from the age of approximately seven years, can have anomalous effects (Irlen 1991; Wilkins 1993). From around this age in particular, problems with print may begin to manifest themselves and one would expect that vision testing for these children would be correspondingly rigorous. However, in at least some Health Authority areas, it is policy to refer those children aged seven and older who require vision assessment to opticians, rather than to the orthoptic department of a hospital which would provide a wider, more exhaustive testing procedure. Policies of this nature can therefore deny access to tests which can subsequently only be provided through referral by a child's general practitioner, and often at a crucial stage of literacy development.

Second, methods of screening are in need of refinement. The use of a reading age to determine those 'at risk' is not a reliable indicator. Some pupils can develop coping strategies that may mask their problems and some fluent readers may experience discomfort or difficulty when faced with print.

One 'at risk' group, identified by Wilkins et al. (1984), appears to be those suffering from, or with a family history of, headaches and migraine. It is suggested that the use of health questionnaires on school entry, and their subsequent regular revision, would go some way towards targeting them.

Although reference has been made to quite young children, it will be appreciated that if their difficulties are not adequately assessed, diagnosed or treated, these children are likely to continue to experience problems, which may increase in severity as work becomes more demanding. It is suggested that what begins as a consideration for the teacher at the lower end of the primary school may, in time, become one for the secondary teacher or the tutor in further or higher education.

The kind of information which would be of assistance to teachers and tutors would include:

- which tests have already been carried out, and where;
- an understanding of the test procedures a student has undergone, or is likely to undergo;
- what tests are available, at what ages these might be administered and by whom;
- what those tests are designed to show;
- the specialist personnel whose assistance may be sought;
- the referral procedures required.

## Symptoms of visual difficulties

If screening for problems is undertaken, what symptoms would such procedures be seeking to identify? The symptoms may be considered in two categories:

- the ways in which letters are perceived to appear on the page;
- those which have physical manifestations.

### Ways in which letters are perceived to appear on the page

Letters can appear to move in a variety of ways on the page, making sustained work with print difficult, sometimes impossible, and tiring. These and other reported effects on print include:

- blurring
- letters swirling or flickering

- words squashing up or spreading out
- print running off the edge of the page, or simply disappearing.

**Physical manifestations**

These relate to how an affected reader can feel when faced with print and include:

- dizziness
- nausea
- migraines or headaches
- tiredness
- eyes which itch or sting, water or hurt.

# Other indicators of visual difficulties

The effects on the student can be numerous, and observant teachers or tutors can do much to identify those within a group who are likely to be suffering from vision-related problems. The way in which a student works can be indicative of such difficulties and may include pointers such as:

- skipping words or lines when reading;
- using a marker or a finger to keep their place on the page;
- working very close to the page;
- reading very slowly, using a jerky rhythm, hesitating;
- losing their place on the page;
- repeating words or lines when reading;
- moving the head instead of using eye movement in order to keep their place;
- experiencing difficulty with working from the blackboard;
- losing concentration, being distracted easily;
- sitting awkwardly, curling up over work.

Additionally, some students will find hazy conditions, strong sunlight, bright light or some fluorescent lighting uncomfortable, and some could feel dizzy or agitated when working under such conditions. The page and the print on it may be perceived to compete with each other: the background white of the paper appearing to take over, partially or wholly obliterating the print. Other phenomena such as flashing lights, the appearance of colours on the page, or halos of light around letters have all been reported. Problems with print size, spacing and the amount of print on a page can occur, or letters can be seen to shimmer, move, float up off the page or disappear. Letters can run into other lines, or lines can be perceived to superimpose one another.

It must be stressed that not all those suffering from such symptoms will be dyslexic and, conversely, not all dyslexic subjects will suffer such symptoms. Not all symptoms may be experienced by all sufferers and levels of severity and their effects will vary. Some students will become more adept than others at compensating for their problems with print, rendering themselves more difficult to identify.

## Irlen syndrome

Symptoms such as those listed above were noted by Helen Irlen, an educational psychologist, who clustered them together and described them as 'Scotopic Sensitivity Syndrome' now more commonly known as 'Irlen Syndrome' (Irlen 1991). She defined the syndrome as:

> 'a perceptual dysfunction which is related to difficulties with light source, luminance, intensity, wavelength and color contrast' (Irlen and Lass 1989, p. 414)

and divided the syndrome into five components:

* light sensitivity;
* inadequate background accommodation;
* poor print resolution;
* restricted span of recognition;
* lack of sustained attention.

The same symptoms have been noted independently by Wilkins, a former research psychologist for the Medical Research Council in Cambridge, during his research into the effects of pattern sensitivity on migraine and on dealing with print (Wilkins et al. 1984; Wilkins and Nimmo-Smith 1987; Wilkins et al. 1989; Wilkins et al. 1992; Wilkins 1993; Wilkins et al. 1996). They are also discussed by researchers in the field of optometry (Holland 1986; Kamien 1983).

## The impact of symptoms on literacy

As a consequence of such symptoms, not only those skills at the core of coping with literacy (such as word recognition) are affected but also the development of more advanced skills (such as speed reading, skimming and proofreading) will be difficult, if not impossible, to master. For delineation of the role of eye movements in reading and for an overview of what is involved in reading for understanding, see Underwood and Batt (1996).

For students with visual difficulties with print, spelling will tend to be phonetic through lack of visualization skills, and copying from blackboards, whiteboards and greenboards, and from overhead projectors, can become laborious.

It will be appreciated that the extra effort involved in trying to overcome such problems can be so demanding as to render the tasks of reading, writing and computing very tiring, thus requiring frequent breaks. The longer the task continues, the more demanding it becomes, until some students may have to stop altogether. However a student who looks away more frequently than others from their work, or who takes frequent breaks from work, may be vulnerable also to being punished for behaviour deemed by the teacher as inappropriate in the classroom.

Whilst there have been many studies of visual difficulties with print, opinions still vary about their causes: Irlen refers to the processing of various properties of light; Wilkins to pattern sensitivity, spacing and fluorescent lighting; Holland, an optometrist, to conditions of the eye (such as squints, refractive error and convergence difficulties); and Livingstone et al. (1991), Cornelissen et al. (1995), Stein and Walsh (1997), working in the areas of neurobiology, psychology and physiology, to impaired processing in the magnocellular visual system of the brain.

A variety of testing procedures is recommended. These include the Irlen screening and diagnostic procedures, Wilkins' 'Intuitive Colorimeter', the familiar optician's Snellen chart and the Dunlop Eye Referencing Test, as well as a battery of optometric tests recommended by Holland. Various treatments are advocated: the use of colour, corrective lenses, patching, prisms and exercises (Lehmkuhle et al. 1993; Wilkins et al. 1994; Robinson and Conway 1994; Evans et al. 1996). For the lay person, it represents a bewildering array with few firm conclusions to be drawn. However, whilst the research remains complex and scattered, and access to its findings requires perseverance, it does highlight significant problems – problems which appear to have no single cause, assessment procedure or treatment.

## Implications for health and education policy makers

It is of concern that in some local authority areas little note seems to have been taken of existing research, suggesting that there may be a significant number of students who may be trying to cope unaided with problems that can be crippling. Preliminary studies of 8–10-year-olds in a Lincolnshire school revealed that up to one-third of pupils in each of four classes reported significant symptoms of visual stress, despite all having passed the school eye tests. Not only that, those who had also visited an optician had been pronounced visually fit. Of those children who subsequently underwent more rigorous orthoptic testing, all were found to have problems of a physical nature and were prescribed treatment (Mailley 1997). If those children had lived a few miles away in neighbouring Cambridgeshire, they would have received the support of a specialist vision team, including personnel from the Health, Social Services and Education departments, offering a wide range of services. The implications of such discrepancies in care are far-reaching.

So what can be done to address the problem? Should there be a body which has overall responsibility for the detection and remediation of such difficulties? Should it be made up of medical personnel, educationists or a combination of both?

As long ago as January 1980, the BMA stated:

'It is not basically a medical problem . . . this is something which will be universally recognized by teachers as essentially a problem that does not concern doctors.' (BMA 1980)

and more recently, but still over ten years ago, Holland (1986) noted that:

'Sadly there is generally little contact and liaison between the optometric profession and the education professions.' (p. 21)

and his opinion still appears to be as relevant today.

Given the educational implications of the problems described, it is reasonable to suggest that bodies such as schools and colleges should consider taking on the responsibility of identifying those affected. Since it appears to be the nature and extent of screening which is inadequate at all stages of a pupil's education, and not the medical treatment given once a problem has been identified, it might be suggested that, at school or at college, the purpose of such screening should be to enable teachers/tutors to inform students, parents and concerned medical professionals of the existence and reported nature of problems. Students may then be referred through the appropriate channels for further diagnosis and treatment.

It is recommended that teachers and tutors carry out a general screening of their classes in order to identify those suffering from any combination of the range of symptoms noted in the research in this multi-disciplinary field. The skills required to do this should be within the scope of teachers and the procedure should not require extensive time for carrying out screening and analysis of results, nor expensive equipment. Responsibility for further, more rigorous diagnostic testing should lie jointly with students, parents, education and health professionals, as would any subsequent treatment. Such collaboration between major agencies of family and community, medical and education professionals, would go some way towards avoiding the current problems of the overlooking or the misdiagnosis of some students' visual problems.

# Implications for students, teachers, tutors and parents

### Awareness and identification

The implications for students, teachers and parents are clear, once it is understood that the learning process is very likely to be affected by symptoms of visual stress. There may be an effect on students' self-esteem, discipline and attitude to work. The most important issues for parents, teachers and tutors will be those of recognition and identification. However, seeking to classify the symptoms by a particular procedure in order to label them as a particular syndrome, and then to treat that syndrome by a single, specific approach, should not be the primary aim of assessment. The primary aim of screening for those symptoms should be just that – to identify individual students' possible difficulties across a range of likely related visual difficulties which should then lead to further, more specialized, multi-disciplinary diagnostic assessment.

### Provision of learning support

There are measures which teachers and tutors may take to alleviate some problems. These fall mainly into two categories:

### 1. Measures that modify the working environment

This can be achieved through employing any or several of the following:

- using curtains or blinds to modify the amount of light entering the classroom;
- allowing affected students to work when and where possible by natural daylight, rather than by artificial light;
- changing fluorescent tubes with slower flicker rates to those with faster flicker rates;

- positioning of seating to suit individual needs when possible (nearer to screens, for example, or away from sources of bright light);
- allowing the use of coloured lenses or overlays;
- use of double-spacing and/or larger font size when creating documents such as worksheets or sets of study notes;
- avoiding strong contrast between background and print (by using cream or beige paper instead of bleached white);
- use of reading masks, which would cover potentially distracting print on a page while permitting students to scan two or three lines ahead (Wilkins 1993, p. 442).

*2. Measures that help to create a profile of each student*

This can be achieved through:

- use of medical questionnaires to identify some pupils 'at risk';
- keeping a record of close observation of students' working strategies;
- discussing with students and asking questions pertinent to their perceived difficulties, then noting their responses;
- being aware of the range of assessment procedures already undergone and prior test results, of their significance, and, where appropriate, of avenues of further diagnostic testing.

Older students may note for themselves if they suffer any of the problems described and may be encouraged to self-refer for diagnostic assessment. They can normally arrange their own visit to an optician, but a more detailed diagnostic assessment with a wider range of tests may be made at a hospital orthoptic department, following referral by their general practitioner. It should be made clear that the involvement of the general practitioner is both desirable and facilitatory for further assessment.

# Implications for initial teacher training and continuing education

The above measures could enhance teacher awareness of visual difficulties with print. Inclusion of such issues in initial teacher training and continuing professional development courses would make a significant contribution towards addressing the problems, as would closer liaison between medical and education professionals. The provision of easily accessible information for all involved in the care and education of students, especially for the students themselves and their parents, is both necessary and important, as is the development of assessment techniques.

Work has already begun which will result in a screening procedure for use in schools, colleges and universities, and preliminary trials at primary school level seem promising. Research indicates that the use of coloured overlays can have a sustained beneficial effect on reading ability and further studies are being carried out on the visual problems related to migraine, head injury and epilepsy. Robinson (2000) concludes that:

'There is growing evidence of a biochemical basis for a visual processing sub-type of dyslexia'

While pointing out that there are still many unanswered questions, a need for caution with reference to directions of causality and the complex interactive effect of environmental influences and further investigation is required with particular reference to dictary intervention. It is clear that there remains much work to be done to ensure that those who experience visual difficulties when faced with print receive the help, and ultimately, the education to which they are entitled.

# Chapter 4
# Restructuring the
# structured approach

MORAG HUNTER-CARSCH

Questions addressed in this chapter include:

- Why is it important that teachers know about the historical multi-disciplinary basis of the field of specific learning difficulties?
- What has changed over the years in the use of the terms 'structured teaching' and 'multi-sensory teaching'?
- Should 'relationship structure' be 'rediscovered' and updated in the modern context?
- How can specialist teachers be assisted to develop and maintain a 'hypothesis-testing' approach to their work?

## Introduction

Many educational psychologists' assessment reports recommend that students with SpLDs, especially dyslexia, should be taught by structured multi-sensory teaching methods. However, not all reports indicate exactly what the psychologist intends in making this recommendation. There appears to be a widely held assumption that the term is generally understood among teachers and requires little or no definition or modelling of the intended meaning. This chapter questions that assumption and suggests that there is a need for examining what may actually be involved in this taken for granted central concept in the field of teaching students with SpLDs.

To do this it draws upon the author's experience of teaching within and across primary, secondary and tertiary education in the UK and in North America. This has been invaluable in recognizing the range of learning and behavioural problems, the characteristics of those students who may be considered as borderline cases and are sometimes described as having

49

'dyslexic tendencies' or showing 'dyslexic-like behaviour' and the overlap between normal, dyslexic learners and those students who have other kinds of SpLDs. It has been helpful also in observing the ways in which these issues are addressed through different education systems.

The purpose of the chapter is thus to contextualize the historical determinants of the multi-sensory structured teaching approach. Following the introductory discussion of models of teaching including multisensory and modality emphases, in the first part, the original structured approach is revisited and deconstructed in order to draw attention to the limits of contemporary understanding of its basic tenets and of perceptions about specific learning difficulties. The second part reports a small-scale action-research project designed to explore the place of structured teaching in the perceptions of a sample of specialist SpLD teachers' reports about effective strategies they use in their teaching. The third part relates the structured teaching factors they employed to those discovered through reconstruction and amplification of the original, holistic and characteristically multi-disciplinary perspective of the structured approach to teaching. A revised framework is offered, for relating 'micro-strategies' of structured teaching to 'macro-strategies' concerning the meeting of special needs, teaching literacy across the curriculum and maintaining a research-oriented record of the impact of the structured teaching.

## Models of teaching

A quick survey of current literature in the popular fields of teachers' and schools' effectiveness, and quality assurance, suggests that the structured approach is not recognized among different models for teaching. For example, Joyce et al. (1997) provide a wide overview of models of teaching but do not mention it as a discrete approach. These authors cluster the models of teaching into four main classes:

- **Processing**: seven models in which teachers are concerned with 'helping students to learn how to construct knowledge and are focusing directly on intellectual capability'.
- **Social**: seven models concerned with 'helping students learn how to sharpen their own cognitions through interactions with others' and 'to work with others'.
- **Personal**: five models concerning 'the self-hood of the individual'.
- **Behavioural systems**: five models with a common theoretical base, 'social learning theory – behaviour modification – behaviour therapy – cybernetics'.

Assuming that this classification is accepted as delineating crucial differences in orientation of the models, the processing models may appear to have a greater focus on learning, whereas the social-personal and behavioural systems models may appear to have a greater focus on behaviour. Thus, in the search for the likely location of either the multi-sensory or the structured approach it might be anticipated that both would be found among the learning models and that the structured approach might also be found among the behaviour models.

In the absence of immediate location of either approach as a discretely labelled and recognized approach, the wider questions become:

- In which ways, and to what extent, do the various models explicitly address the structuring of learning and of behaviour?
- What factors (and combinations of factors) are taken into account in the theoretical framework for systematically structuring individual student's learning (including learning about behaviour and how to 'control' behaviour) or the learning of groups of students?

For full answers to these questions, a more substantial investigation would be required than is within the scope of this chapter. Meanwhile, the need for breadth of knowledge on the part of the teachers whose students include some with SpLDs must be recognized: of the range of possible models for teaching, as well as familiarity with selected, preferred models, since it is only through 'meta-cognitive awareness' (revealing their particular conceptual map of methods and their theoretical bases) that it becomes possible to discover how to address some of the more subtle issues of increasing effectiveness of teaching such students. Exploration of the extent of shared understanding of 'the structured multi-sensory approach' and the wider 'structured approach' (encompassing behavioural as well as learning emphases) thus becomes crucial. Here, a preliminary investigation involves, first, a reflective account based on training and experience.

## Structured multi-sensory teaching at present and in the past

In the UK the current context is one of rapid educational change, in particular in the field of literacy and teaching students with literacy difficulties (McClelland 1997; DfE 1998b; BPS 1999 and the current revision of the DfEE (1994) Code of Practice which it is anticipated will be completed by 2002).

The roots of the structured approach are firmly grounded in the past in terms of the history of educational ideas. With reference to teaching students with SpLDs in particular, they may be traced through the past 60 years to pioneering teacher–researchers in the USA who discovered the structured approach to be the defining diagnostic strategy which differentiated students with SpLDs from those with general learning difficulties.

The author's understanding of the concept of the structured approach in relation to specialist teaching in the field of SpLDs is based on her possibly unique series of training experiences with pioneers in the field in the USA, Canada and the UK. At that time, children thought to require this kind of teaching were described as 'brain-injured, hyperactive children', 'perceptually handicapped children' or as 'neurologically impaired'. During the next decade the preferred subgroup title within the wider classification of 'exceptional children' (this included 'able' children and children with English as second language) became 'children with learning disabilities' and this group was then differentiated from the group with 'emotional disabilities'. In North America the medical orientation of terminology in this field persists and there is still a more widely shared and characteristically broader, multi-disciplinary understanding of the structured approach than is currently shared in the UK, where the term has become reduced to little more than a recommendation for use of structured phonic materials and methods for teaching basic literacy.

The term 'multi-sensory', when used along with the recommended approach for teaching dyslexic children, appears to be interpreted in one of two ways:

- presenting information through visual, auditory, kinesthetic and tactile forms (VAKT), with the implication being to offer as many as possible;
- following a 'prescription' emphasizing modalities which are 'diagnosed' to be preferred avenues for learning for the individual student.

## Multi-sensory as VAKT

With reference to the first point (presenting information through visual, auditory, kinesthetic and tactile forms), in the UK mainstream non-specialist primary teachers, including 'early years' teachers, tend to be well aware of the value of providing all young learners with sensory experience and 'multi-sensory immersion in learning through play'. However, not all teachers systematically record young children's responses to different combinations of sensory teaching within the idea of multi-sensory teaching, or indeed, to the totality of the prepared multi-sensory environment including both informal and direct teaching. It is not clear to what extent multi-sensory teaching is explicitly planned to include (for example) the use of speech mirrors for children to observe the operation of their own speaking as well as keenly observing, listening, articulating/modelling the speech sounds of others. It does not seem to be routine procedure in most primary classrooms to relate explicitly e.g. kinesthetic and tactile learning experience to auditory and/or visual experience through the use of speech mirrors in the course of teaching the letters and sounds of the alphabet.

Discussions with teachers and teacher-trainers during visits to Finland, a country with a distinguished record in literacy achievement, suggest that the multi-sensory approach, including the use of speech mirrors, is taught in initial teacher-training and forms a routine part of children's classroom experience. Observation of children on their first day at school at seven years of age, by the author, found this to be the case. There was strong emphasis on music, rhythm, song, visual links with kinesthetic-tactile experience and use of speech mirrors as an integral part of introductory literacy teaching. The use of speech mirrors was as commonplace as the use of visual mind-maps for planning, recording and organizing whole-class work on the large board (no longer black boards but green or white ones!) and for individual use in written work. Many examples of paired work and groups of children were observed practising and checking the experience of saying words slowly and exploring by tracing, touching, feeling and observing movements of lips, tongue and jaw whilst shifting position from one phoneme to the next within words and noticing the operation of breath in making voiced and non-voiced sounds.

This intense exploratory work, much-enjoyed by the youngsters and celebrated in songs and movement to music, constitutes an important part of establishing phonemic awareness which is increasingly recognised to be vital for successful literacy learning. Bearing in mind the limits of experience, the dangers of generalization and that no attempt is being made here to recommend early formal teaching or more direct teaching, one vital observation that might be made in comparing the practices and understanding of 'multi-sensory' in different countries is that the relevant expectations and ages of children may differ.

For Finnish children, starting formal learning to read in school at seven years of age (whether or not they had kindergarten experience) the novelty and excitement of the particular multi-sensory games approach may be quite different from the experience of the child in the UK who comes to school at five years of age, possibly after attending a nursery class or school and for whom there is a greater likelihood of having a 'play-oriented' approach to learning. The degree of 'directness' of the teaching is central to this discussion as it relates to teaching dyslexic children. Clearly, the more thorough the records of children's responses to multi-sensory early literacy experience, the easier it may be to recognize the nature and severity of difficulties which persist.

It is also of central importance to understand both the teacher's and the child's intentions in play and interactive learning-teaching exchanges. As there is now a substantial body of research suggesting that phonemic awareness, rhyming and learning by analogy are vital components to successful early literacy (Treiman, 1987; Snowling and Nation 1997; Goswami 1999, 1999; Seymour et al. 1999; Stuart 1999), the issue becomes one of how best to facilitate development of relevant relationships (e.g. phonemes and graphemes, larger meaning units and morphemes), especially for youngsters who find that relevant awareness, discrimination and connections do not 'register' for them as easily as for other children. They may require focused teaching involving, for example, the relating of kinesthetic experience of making sounds and changing the shape of mouth, tongue movement and direction of breath to the experience of seeing the changes whilst hearing and repeating sounds; also handling letter shapes in two-dimensional materials and relating these to models in three dimensions, and in different materials. This kind of structuring of learning in UK classrooms, within a play context, as well as within more formal learning contexts, is needed for dyslexic children, for youngsters who are learning English as another language, and is essential for children who are both dyslexic and multi-lingual.

In England and Wales the position of inservice training materials concerning the teaching of the Literacy Hour (DfEE 1998) has already done much to provide a shared knowledge base and range of ways of teaching at word-level. However, it may be necessary for teachers to undertake further diagnostically linked training in order to be able to identify dyslexic children at an early age and to support their learning. Even the excellent group teaching support material for teaching dyslexic children within the Literacy Hour (a Multi-sensory Teaching System for Reading (MTSR) (Johnson et al. 1999) may require additional information for teachers to make best use of them in a generally more fully informed and more structured approach to multi-sensory teaching of all children. The MTSR programme (based on Margaret Taylor Smith's MTS approach developed in Texas) which bears some similarity to other well-known and successful multi-sensory approaches for teaching individuals (e.g. the Hickey approach (Augur and Briggs 1993) Alpha to Omega (Hornsby and Shear 1982)), is distinctive in that it has been researched and developed with DfEE support and in collaboration with the BDA for work with a group within the Literacy Hour.

# Preferred modality

With reference to the second point (following a prescription emphasizing those modalities which are 'diagnosed' to be preferred avenues for learning for the individual student), recommendations about learning styles tend to imply that styles are distinctive, static and persistent (for further information on identification and teaching of different cognitive and learning styles see Riding and Rayner 1998; Reid 1998; Zdzienski 2000). There is seldom sufficient information about how to structure teaching to make optimal use of relevant preferences in ways which go beyond the direct teaching model and recommendations may also emphasize one-to-one or individualized teaching. Some prepared programmes tailored to certain styles of presentation offer replacement of traditional pen and paper practice with information and communication technology (ICT), but guidelines with reference to whole-class interactive teaching are hard to find.

# Origins of the structured approach and its multi-disciplinary basis

Terminology in SpLDs research literature in the UK and in North America and elsewhere may differ not only regarding the influences of different disciplines (for example, 'learning difficulties' *educational* emphasis in the UK; 'learning disabilities' *medical* emphasis in the USA) but also in relation to the multi-literacies orientation and expectations which individual teachers bring to their interpretation of the literature (Kress 1997). This is perhaps a sufficient reason for advocating wider sharing of theoretical perspectives as part of promoting increased multi-disciplinary communication in SpLDs.

By suggesting that the frequently recommended 'structured multi-sensory approach' in the UK may differ from 'the structured approach' as originally recommended by pioneers in the USA, the purpose here is to prepare to examine what appear to be gaps between two perspectives and possibly important losses of knowledge with changes over time. The attempt is not so much to delineate historical developments comparatively, nor to refer in particular to pioneering work in the UK. It would require a substantially longer account to do justice to developments on either side of the Atlantic. The purpose of this discussion is to consider what might be useful in connecting the early American strand with current interpretations of structured teaching in the UK.

Historically, it is the educational, not the medical, diagnostic criterion of students' positive response to the structured approach that constitutes the single, unifying factor in the field of SpLDs in the USA. It is the common factor found to differentially identify this subgroup of 'different learners' (i.e. those who responded positively to this approach but did not thrive under normal educational provision). The original structured approach may thus be expected to provide the basic conceptual framework for teaching students with SpLDs. It is this frame of reference which underpins Turner's (1997) position, referred to in the DCEP (1999) report:

> 'Turner (1997) has proposed a rather different distinction suggesting that dyslexia can be considered a subset within the range of different specific learning difficulties that includes autism and ADHD. Only some areas of functioning are affected in each condition.' (DCEP 1999, p. 19)

The perspective can be traced from Strauss et al. (1947) and Cruickshank et al. (1961) in the USA, to Scotland and training of educational psychologists at the University of Strathclyde and elsewhere (Hunter 1969, 1970, 1972, 1981, 1982).

The wider emphases in the American-based early use of the term 'structured approach' may be traced back through the work of Cruickshank and Kephart in the 1960s to Strauss, Werner and Lehtinen in the 1940s at Wayne County Special school, in the USA. This work emphasized the importance of structuring the following factors in the classroom:

- space
- time
- materials
- methods
- relationships.

It may be seen that they include not only structuring teaching methods and materials (familiar to UK teachers) but also structuring other factors (space, time and relationships; Hunter-Carsch 1990, 1993). These workers recognized the impact of secondary factors (such as frustration and inappropriate behavioural responses) as a result of the primary condition of SpLDs. Consequently, structuring interpersonal relationships and affect in the classroom was seen as an integral part of the teaching framework. The structuring was thus planned in response to systematic observation of learning needs, on the basis of tracking the impact of structuring several factors simultaneously, in combinations which were uniquely suited to meeting the individual's needs within a carefully prepared framework for individual group or classwork.

This approach was implicitly psychosocial in its recognition of the impact of social factors in the learning environment and of differences when these factors were altered. Youngsters whom we now describe as having SpLDs were able to thrive in an altered learning environment with an individualized education programme (IEP) in a group context, but they were not able to progress with basic learning (e.g. literacy) in the normal classroom and school context.

Although both Cruickshank and Kephart employed the structured approach, their main foci of attention differed. Cruickshank was particularly concerned with the management of behaviour in children whom we might now describe as having attention deficit hyperactivity disorder (ADHD or ADD). Kephart was interested in teaching children now described as having developmental motor disorder or dyspraxia. However, both researchers employed and developed the structured approach and had some among their students who would (in the UK) now be described as having 'specific learning difficulties, e.g. dyslexia'.

Cruickshank and Kephart shared a broader understanding of SpLDs than is currently considered in 'the discrepancy model' which constitutes the basis for the definition of SpLD in England and Wales (DfEE 1994) and relates to students with average or above levels of general intelligence. Cruickshank and Kephart and their contemporaries were less concerned with intelligence levels than with the dynamics of learning by students of all ability levels. Nor were they greatly occupied with labelling or separately teaching subgroups (for example, according to motor, language and speech or literacy-related areas of difficulty). They viewed learners' differences and difficulties through a teaching and learning framework based on discerning students' learning potential, not in terms of intelligence quotient (IQ) assessed through a battery of subtests administered on a single occasion, in comparison with measured academic achievement, but in terms of 'learning quotient' (LQ), a concept promoted by a contemporary, Myklebust (1971), involving monitoring students' responses to teaching of 'new' learning.

The focus on measuring learning (as a result of teaching intervention) was closely related to measuring speed of perceptual and cognitive processing (see e.g. Birch and Belmont's auditory tapping tests) and to discovery of what was successfully learned, not just the identification of areas of difficulty. Emphasis was on the teacher as well as the learner in the close monitoring of learners' responses to designed (structured) teaching strategies. It was dynamic. It involved close observation of changes as they happened and long-term case studies, not static testing to establish an entry point to a programme and then to retest after a given time as if taking two transverse (unconnected) sections of behaviour. This approach was holistic and essentially multi-disciplinary as it arose from collaborative work with specialists in medicine, psychology and education who shared a keen interest in neurological functioning and learning.

The recent working definition of dyslexia (DCEP 1999) may seem to reflect, to some extent, a return to valuing of monitoring pupils' responses to teaching as an indicator of successful learning or persistence and severity of the relevant learning problems. It may also seem to reflect the earlier perspectives by employing a more inclusive approach with reference to general intellectual ability and, in this sense, it rejects the discrepancy definition. The DCEP (1999) report, however, has a narrower focus, selectively on one kind of SpLD (dyslexia) whilst simultaneously opening up use of the term 'dyslexia' to include the range of reading-related difficulties, regardless of causal factors. It does not appear to recognize fully the importance of monitoring the effect of teaching methods as a key diagnostic factor (that is, the individual pupil's responses to structured multi-sensory teaching) in dyslexia and other SpLDs.

Recent developments in the study of SpLDs are typified by a tendency to specialization within single disciplines, and may neglect the stance which was characterized by the wider, holistic perspectives of the pioneers. The liveliness of their professional dialogue which arose within special education centres was often strongly medically oriented and somewhat separated from discourse in the prevailing mainstream education context.

# Reduction of the structured approach to the multi-sensory approach

### Multi-disciplinary or separate discipline perspectives?

There is now a danger of loss of the holistic and multi-disciplinary perspective with a resultant fragmentation for trainee teachers (and perhaps also for speech and language therapists) of the principles which underpin the holistic stance inherent in the early formulation of the structured approach. If, for example, trainee teachers and therapists are introduced selectively to what has now become the reduced and impoverished view of the multi-sensory approach, even if the emphasis continues to be on systematic, sequential, structured teaching, there is a risk that instead of having an integrated awareness of SpLDs across the areas of motor, language and literacy, trainees may be taught selectively about only one or two of the following:

- a literacy-related emphasis, as developed originally through the work of Orton (1995a, 1995b), Gillingam and Stillman (1940), Fernald (1943) and Hickey (1977);
- a linguistic emphasis (e.g. Kirk et al. 1968) and, recently, the language-focused work by Stackhouse and Wells (1998);

- a motor and behaviour  emphasis (including emotional and behavioural difficulties) by e.g. Kephart (1960), Getman et al. (1964), Gordon and McKinley (1980), Wedell (1984);
- therapeutic/counselling emphasis with a focus on personal, social and emotional education (Redl and Wineman 1952; Bettleheim 1960; Mannoni 1967; and to some extent the developments of Frostig and Horne 1979) within educational therapy.

## Static or dynamic models for assessment and teaching?

There is the further problem of the historical move away from the integrated teaching and testing approach with its sensitivity to the dynamics of factors affecting situational and interpersonal aspects of teaching–learning interactions and towards separation of the assessment process from the teaching–learning process, in particular for school-age students. This separation was speeded up by the drive towards production of 'prescriptive programmes' and the related commercial discoveries of 'programmed learning approaches'. In North America in the late 1960s, this period included the innovatory introduction of a professional layer of diagnosticians whose job included preparing prescriptive teaching programmes for teachers. The 'dial-a-programme' approach reached a peak with the production of compendia of skill definitions and graded exercises for compiling into prescriptive programmes (e.g. Valett 1967).

Although the dangers of separation of the role of diagnosticians were recognized to some extent (e.g. Hunter-Carsch 1980; 1983), emphasis continues on the production of programmed materials with investment in attempts to design packages of assessment and teaching materials which are based on static rather than dynamic (test–teach–re-test–adapt) assessment models.

In North America the 'diagnostician' role was found to be unsatisfactory. This was not only with reference to the static view of assessment (based on a 'once-off' test battery and sometimes not representative of the actual range of performance of the characteristically erratic SpLD group) which contrasted with the educationally based dynamic approaches which had been developing. It was also because it separated the teacher from the process of identification and the related continual hypothesis-testing approach which characterized 'research-based' early work in the field. The trend toward the use of prescribed teaching programmes by teachers, some of whom had a limited grasp of the clinical concepts and were prohibited from using the diagnostic instruments, progressed and is still evident in the UK. It is perhaps also reflected in the tendency for specialist diagnostic work to be undertaken selectively by educational psychologists and speech and language therapists who have professional access to use of certain diagnostic tests which require specialist training which is not open to teachers. It is possible, however, that the new working definition of dyslexia (DCEP 1999) may return some of the work of the diagnostic–exploratory phase to teachers.

Interestingly, special education training in both North America and Germany differs in this respect, where there is some provision for specialist teachers to train to use some tests of 'intelligence'. The role of educational psychologists, however, appears to be one which in England and Wales has recently been constrained by the weight of referrals of students for assessment for a Statement of Special Educational Needs, the legal requirement for access to funded special educational support in schools and, more recently, also in colleges and universities. Educational psychologists thus become testers and gatekeepers of access to funding.

This raises the question of whether the direction of the trend toward educational psychologists becoming the new separate layer of diagnosticians may be altered in the wake of the new working definition of dyslexia (DCEP 1999) which to some extent returns recognition to teachers of their role in identifying and evaluating pupils' responses to teaching. In any event, closer, routine monitoring of pupils' responses to structured teaching is needed, whether carried out by teachers, educational psychologists or both.

For teachers to develop the relevant skills has implications for initial training and for continuing professional development. Training would involve planning to take into account the needs of individual students in relation to structuring their learning experience with regard to space, time, materials, methods and relationships. Clearly, it would also be necessary to study closely the relationship between assessment methods, planning and monitoring of individual teaching and learning programmes and evaluation of their effectiveness and efficiency in meeting students' needs.

These underlying concerns involve the possibility that vital elements in teacher-training are being lost. The larger question concerns the integrity of the whole approach to teaching students with SpLDs, including dyslexia. Over time, and with increased specialization, has there been a gradual drift away from the multi-disciplinary basis with the educational approach at its centre? Are the research and clinical perspectives which characterized the early pioneers' attitudes to collaborative work simply becoming forgotten in all but a few designated multi-disciplinary centres and in exchanges at interdisciplinary conferences?

## SpLDs and/or emotional and behavioural difficulties (EBDs)

The current tendency to split up specialist teaching into separate approaches for those with either learning disabilities/difficulties or those with behaviour disabilities/difficulties (DfEE 1994) not only poses a challenge to anyone wishing to become a specialist teacher with training designed to support the learning of students with SpLDs, EBDs or both, it goes against the integrated basis of the structured approach which was claimed to be helpful for both groups. In particular, the structured approach sought to study the nature of students' attention during learning (its focus and the sustaining of attention), facilitating remembering and ways of increasing self-control. The risk is thus one of potential loss of specialized teaching of students with behavioural difficulties by methods which have been found helpful for them in the past, but which are now likely to be selectively employed with students with SpLDs.

Constellations of problems involving both SpLDs (in particular, literacy difficulties) and EBDs have been drawn to the attention of the public in recent media campaigns, including communications about the high incidence of dyslexia among prison populations. Questions of early diagnosis and teaching intervention are compounded by concerns about prioritizing scarce resources for specialist teaching and routes for access to appropriate learning support.

The diagnostic and provision issues are well-illustrated by Forness (1996) in his discussion of the 'Social and Emotional Dimensions of Learning Disabilities' in the USA. Forness addresses the question of overlap between diagnostic categories of students with learning disabilities (LD) (SpLDs in the UK) and attention deficit disorder (ADD). He notes that 'only 20% of all kids with ADD have LD when properly diagnosed'. In his study of 67 children diagnosed as having 'conduct disorder', almost a third (31%) had mild forms of conduct disorder 'oppositional/defiant disorder' and 27% had a conduct disorder but also qualified as having a learning disability. Forness notes that:

'In essence there were two disorders in the same child, and it was very clear that after psycho-educational testing these kids did indeed qualify as learning disabled in California, but in many other states would not qualify because they had a primary emotional disturbance.' (Forness 1996 p. 74)

He reported that nearly nine per cent of that group received special education through learning disability not under the category of emotional disturbance. Forness (1996) refers to the findings of the work of Weller and Strawser (1987) of literature on more than a dozen studies of the incidence of five subtypes of learning disabilities classified by their underlying cognitive processing disorders. Table 4.1 lists the five subtypes, briefly describes the problems to which they relate and notes the incidence of each subtype across the range of studies.

The first subtype relates to perceptual motor problems. The second relates to what are often subtle language processing problems which can

**Table 4.1** Subtypes of learning disabilities classified by their underlying cognitive processing disorders

| Learning disability type | Problems | Percentage of learning disability |
|---|---|---|
| 1  Non-verbal organization disorders | Visual-spatial-motor deficits Possible social misperception/ withdrawal | 11–15 |
| 2  Verbal organization disorders | Poor understanding/ use of language Possible aggression/acting out | 14–17 |
| 3  Global disorders | Multiple deficits in processing Possible problems in all coping skills | 8–10 |
| 4  Production deficits | Inefficient cognitive strategies Possible inattention/hyperactivity | 22–30 |
| 5  Non-LD pattern | Discrepancy from grade but not IQ Possible frustration, absences | 25–38 |

From Forness 1996, p. 76. Reproduced with permission from Harwood Academic Publications

affect reading, including reading comprehension. The third category involves both the previous problems and is often compounded by impaired social skills. The fourth is described by Forness (1996) as the largest identifiable subtype of learning disability. Forness notes that 'they do not have good impulse control nor good attentional skills. As a consequence they might be at risk for a psychiatric diagnosis such as attention deficit disorders.' The fifth subtype, the largest group, has a discrepancy between IQ and academic achievement, because of having a high IQ and functioning close to their grade levels or a low IQ and functioning below their grade levels but not far enough below to qualify as Learning Disabled. Forness (1996) draws attention to the problems of categorization and to pragmatic factors affecting placement decisions in situations of limited resources.

It may be seen from Table 4.1 that dyslexic students do not all fit easily into the second subtype. Some dyslexic students have difficulty with handwriting, fine motor co-ordination and show visuo-spatial organizational problems. Would they be allocated to Category 1 (what might now be described in the UK as 'developmental motor disorder')? There is also the question of visual stress and how this condition relates to dyslexia (see Chapter 3). Would dyslexics have to be accounted for by a single category? If so, what are the implications for arriving at a single (measured) differentiated diagnostic category? The importance of shared understanding of what constitutes the structured approach becomes even more apparent when it is considered in terms of being part of a legal entitlement concerning provision of a Statement of Special Educational Need.

Briefly summarising the main points thus far, it is argued that there are dimensions of the originally conceptualized structured approach which have become neglected (its holistic, multi-disciplinary and research emphases integrating diagnosis with on-going teaching and the fact that it provides for both learning and behavioural difficulties); that these are vital dimensions of the approach and that there remain advantages in employing the structured approach as a basis for exploring underlying factors which characterize successful teaching of students with SpLDs.

## Do effective specialist SpLD teachers employ the structured approach?

To investigate the extent to which factors associated with the structured approach might become evident in the work of a sample of successful SpLD specialist teachers, a small-scale exploratory survey was carried out with a class of SpLD teachers following a specialist diploma course (diplomates) at the University of Central Lancashire (Hunter-Carsch 1993). The diplomates were all considered to be effective teachers by their specialist tutors who worked with them in primary and secondary schools. It was understood from the outset that this was an exploratory exercise and that the sample of teachers could not be regarded as representative of the entire population of specialist SpLDs teachers in England or further afield. It was also clear that there were neither opportunities nor resources to go to observe the teachers, thus a self-report method of investigation, with all its limitations, had to be employed.

Some 30 diplomates were invited (by post) to respond to a single-page questionnaire which asked them to provide a very brief note describing an effective teaching strategy they had employed with a student, whom they were asked to describe briefly in terms of age, gender and area of SpLD (Figure 4.1). The diplomates were not given any indication of the categories for analysis nor was any mention made of the idea of structuring learning or of the structured approach as such.

A short exemplar was included and there was limited space left for the respondents to complete their answers in brief notes. The diplomates appeared to have no difficulty in completing the questionnaire. Table 4.2 illustrates in summary, the kinds of comments made by the respondents.

Responses from the first 15 replies were analysed on the basis of indications of 'specialist concerns' (e.g. attempts to work in an interdisciplinary manner/collaboratively with non-teacher colleagues). Other concerns which emerged were classified as the 'M' factor (multi-disciplinary) and 'systematic structuring of learning' (the 'S' factor). Additional factors emerged across the returns. Illustrations are drawn from the teachers' responses.

What constitutes 'good teaching' may depend on a range of factors. From your own experience, particularly with reference to teaching reading/basic literacy to pupils with SpLD:

(a)   Please provide one example of what you consider to have
      been an effective teaching strategy in your teaching of a particular pupil*
(b)   What made it successful ('good teaching') in this case?

Please give a brief descriptive profile of the pupil's abilities, interests and SpLD with a summary of test results before and after teaching.

*Pseudonym:
Chronological age:
Test results:

**Figure 4.1** Extract from the single-page questionnaire sent to the specialist SpLD teachers.

## Results of the exploratory survey

The teachers' effective teaching strategies and special qualities which emerged from the analysis of their reports and was evident from all of them included awareness and skill related to the following factors:

- the 'S' factor – employing the structured approach to planning and teaching with attention to the structuring of e.g. time, space, relationships, methods and materials (Cruickshank 1961);
- the 'N' factor – recognition on the part of the teacher, of students' will to be normal(that is, not specially needy) and efforts made by teachers toward facilitating this state for dyslexic students, whether children or adults. This does not imply that individual differences should be ignored, but that cognisance should be taken of them in an informed and sensitive manner so that students feel included not excluded from normal experiences including success in learning;
- the 'C' factor – any means by which the teacher seek to provide the student with a sense of feeling in control; this involves students in making meaning and decision-making about their own learning and also attempts to move the student along a path towards increasingly greater independence in learning (see also: Gerber et al. 1992; Walker 1999, 2000);
- the 'T' factor (teacher/tutor) – signalled by various lively comments, often in parenthesis, added as notes or explanations and usually with an air of lightness and individuality (*'This is the way I usually arrange it.' 'We tend to have a chat first.' 'If he is in a good mood, we start right away.' 'It works better if I sing the words as well as say them.'*). Part of

**Table 4.2** Diplomates' views of what constitutes good teaching of basic literacy with dyslexic children in the mainstream classroom

| Child | M/F | Chronological age | Test results | Difficulties | Strategies |
|---|---|---|---|---|---|
| Laura | F | 11;5 | 7.0–8.2 (RA Acc) 7.1–8.10 (RA Comp) 7.9 SA | Difficulty in reading textbooks, esp. history/geog (books RA 12+) | adapting texts – worksheets/puzzles (collab. with class teacher – use for others also + bright children – rhyme, humour, cartoons) |
| John | M | 11;11 | 5.5–8.1 (RA Acc) 4.10–8.3 (RA Comp) 6.7–7.6 SA | Anxiety about others knowing his literacy difficulties verging on school phobia | Paired reading with teacher and peers; taping own stories (teacher says sentence – pupil repeats onto tape/own voice to practise reading also at home); use of USSR (uninterrupted, sustained silent reading) + self-esteem programme/no pressure |
| Duncan | M | 12;0 | – | Reading, spelling, writing diff. but good oral skills | Three in-class support situations: (1) Science – help with recording, esp. note-taking; (2) English – collab. with class teacher, drama - scriptwriting; (3) Use of pocked-sized dictaphone to record homework – enlist co-operation of all subject class teachers; oral contributions to lessons |

the T factor relates to reading the student's feelings ('emotional literacy', Faupel et al. 1998; O'Neill 1999; meta-affectivity, see Chapter 5).

### Discussion of the results

Perhaps the most striking shared quality of the respondents was the way in which they were all able to respond to and to adapt several factors simultaneously. They all made efforts to recognize students' choices, to promote their confidence in feeling that they were increasingly able to direct their own work and e.g. to choose resources/ICT, to consult/work with peers and to adapt their time schedules in the light of growing self-awareness of their needs and capabilities (the 'C' factor).

The S, N, C and T factors emerged as shared characteristics. The basic framework of structured teaching was being operated so that, within its parameters, flexibility was employed in terms of adapting a range of variables. The limits of the sampling procedure must be remembered. The survey related only to the school context. It did not include designated further or higher education tutors, although some of the respondents had experience of working with adults. Although there may be good reason to suggest that similar characteristics might be found among effective tutors of adults with SpLDs, questions remain as to whether the same factors might feature so prominently and indeed if they might also be evident in a study with a sample of generalist class teachers at any phase of education. Further research is required to illuminate the dynamics of the operation of the N, C and T factors as aspects of the 'S' factor, in all educational phases, to explore evidence to support the 'M' factor and to track any possible developmental shifts of emphasis within the framework of structuring selected factors.

It appears to be the case that there is increasing awareness of the relevance of the S factor in the field of primary education. The value of structured teaching, albeit it on a very general level (and without the dimensions of relationship structure and perhaps with limited attention to structuring of space) may be gaining some recognition in literacy teaching in the course of the Literacy Hour. This may relate to timed subsections of the Hour for different types of presentation and its emphasis on structured teaching at word-level, sentence-level and text-level as part of the government's National Literacy Strategy Framework for Teaching (DfEE 1998).

## Reconstructing or re-structuring the structured approach

In addition to Cruickshank's (1961) original five basic factors for structuring teaching (space, time, methods, materials, relationships) a further two might be suggested: the amount of choice offered to students and the extent of the learning challenge (how hard the task is). The design of what we now refer to as individual educational plans (IEPs) involved management of all seven factors. With further experience of working with students with SpLDs another four factors emerged in relation to task design. These are:

- whole-part learning
- sequencing
- speed
- accuracy.

The resultant framework, based on an earlier representation (Hunter-Carsch 1990), has been further developed in Figure 4.2 and in Table 4.3.

---

Student's name: ——————— Teacher's name: ——————— Date: ———

- Think: What aspects will I structure, to what extent and in what ways?

### STRUCTURE
### S factors

| | |
|---|---|
| (i) | choice (reduce/systematically increase) |
| (ii) | challenge (get the baseline right first and take only small steps with 'guaranteed' success) |
| (iii) | space (adjust for max. concentration e.g. office) |
| (iv) | time (set task times/vary/plenty of rests) |
| (v) | materials (highly motivating/e.g. use IT) |
| (vi) | relationships (keep 'cool', avoid demands) |
| (vii) | methods (multi-sensory, sequential) |

| | PROCESS<br>a b c d | | ORIENTATION<br>C N H T M R |
|---|---|---|---|
| (a) | Whole-part learning | C factor: | student feels in Control |
| (b) | Sequencing | N factor: | student feels 'Normal' not 'specially needy' |
| (c) | Speed | H factor: | teacher maintains an Holistic perspective |
| (d) | Accuracy | T factor: | Teacher's style, ways of directing attention |
| | | M factor: | use of Multi-disciplinary support/consultation |
| | | R factor: | teacher's Research focus/ stating hypothesis |

- Do: Indicate where your priorities lie with reference to the 'S' factors (i-vii) and the 'process' variables (a, b, c and d) and how you propose to take into account the orientation factors (C, N, H, T, M and R).

---

**Figure 4.2** Micro-strategies for structured learning: Planning Priorities.

**Table** 4.3 Framework of macro-strategies for planning and teaching students with SpLDs

---

**Macro-strategy I:** Five steps to meeting special needs

(*Think: Which step am I working on at this moment?*)
1. Describe difficulties
2. Analyse notes
3. State needs (hypothesis)
4. Adapt teaching
5. Record findings

---

**Macro-strategy II:** Supporting literacy, communication and learning across the curriculum

(*Think: What is my stance/view/theory/conceptual map for each of these concepts and how do they relate to each other?*)
Make explicit to self, the nature of expectations built upon awareness of the particular conceptual map of the developmental process involved in each of the following: literacy (reading, writing, handwriting, spelling), communication (listening, speaking, understanding, expressing), learning: SpLDs.

---

**Macro-strategy III:** Evaluating and recording interactions/interventions and their effects

(*Think: How will I keep track of ways in which the learning interactions are affected by my planned structuring? How can I be sure about the direction of cause and effect?*)
Employ a system for observing and recording plans, targets, changes in behaviour and increments in learning (e.g. Kemp 1987).

---

Figure 4.2 represents some of the factors which effective teachers may take into account simultaneously as they plan, teach and record the effects of teaching interactions.

In the mainstream classroom, all these 'micro-strategies' are likely to be operating within the larger context of teaching the national curriculum and providing learning support where necessary in response to the relevant stages of the Code of Practice procedures for identifying students with special educational needs and meeting their needs (DfEE 1994; 2000).

The larger contextual framework might be regarded as providing 'macro-strategy' parameters, within which to employ the 'micro-strategies'. The following macro-strategies might be considered to be necessary:

- recognition of the current location in a notional cycle of steps to meet special educational needs;

- clear conceptualization of the personal conceptual plan of the literacy framework being employed to support communication and learning across the curriculum;
- recording and evaluating plans, progress and problems in response to structuring within teaching–learning sessions.

A brief outline of the main points of consideration for each 'macro-strategy' is given in Table 4.3.

## Macro-strategy I: 5 steps to meeting special needs

### Step 1

This involves exploring interactively, observing and describing the student's learning so that a profile of interests, strengths and abilities as well as difficulties can be noted over a period of time (more than a week). It is important that some estimation of the stability or extent of fluctuation of the characteristics can be made in the light of observation and consultation of previous records and possibly other sources (such as students, parents, other teachers or learning assistants who teach the student).

### Step 2

This requires the collation of information from diverse sources to draw together the main findings about strengths and difficulties, and to organize them in the form of a profile from which to analyse the relationship between areas of relative strengths and weaknesses. For some students it may be necessary to look very keenly to discern strengths; these may merge with 'preferences' and interests.

In norm-referenced terms the student may seem to achieve at a similar level across different school subject areas, but they may have distinctly different attitudes to the kinds of learning experience involved in different areas. These can range from being regarded positively to being regarded negatively (or distinctly less positively). The 'fine-line' decisions in this analysis cannot be made without knowing the student's feelings as well as achievements in norm-referenced measures. In some subject areas they may seem to be struggling, in the sense of taking longer than others, yet in fact, be enjoying the work and engaged in learning in a manner which is relatively stress-free. It is the teacher's awareness of what is 'comfortable' and 'not so comfortable' that can affect judgments about what constitutes learning support and what actually impedes learning.

Analysis of findings in the second step is geared towards achieving a 'working summary' from which it is possible to formulate a hunch (hypothesis; Step 3) as to what is the difficulty (or one of the difficulties) and what aspects of teaching should be structured in order to support the student's learning and overcome or ease the difficulties. Clearly, what constitutes a difficulty in one situation need not do so in another. Recognition of contextual dimensions is vital. Too often in the past the tendency was to treat such matters as absolutes, whereas in fact, they are relative within the dynamics of the human-interactive context. For example, avoidance may be a very sensible adaptive response in some situations. The teacher's underlying assumptions and expectations need to be checked as to the wider relevance and in that sense 'validity' (as well as 'reliability') of the emerging 'concluding statement' about strengths and weaknesses in educational terms.

The formulating and reformulating of the hypothesis to ensure its precision is pivotal to the improvement of professional practice. It should be rendered 'testable' in the light of the 'evidence' derived from the previous step. The educational focus must remain on the proposed action to alleviate the difficulties while sharpening focus on likely causal factors and refining knowledge about relevant factors which appear to interfere with or may even facilitate a particular learning processes. The interest in causal factors necessarily requires teachers to work closely with colleagues from other disciplines. The shared focus, however, is not so much on 'medical' dimensions (in the sense of illness and/or disability) as on well-health and differences in learning. In this sense, education and medicine (with all its specialisms e.g. ophthalmological and hearing specialists, physio and language therapists) are inseparable within the well-health model.

The fact that the kind of specialist teaching which is needed requires a multi-disciplinary approach becomes evident, in particular when working with children with attention difficulties and 'disorders', whether their problems are related to bereavement, depression, boredom, dysphasia, ADHD and/or SpLDs which manifest themselves in disturbances of literacy skills. For such students, the teacher's hypothesis should clarify the rationale for the proposed learning support and indicate all major contributing factors in the proposed IEP. But, the idea of 'the teacher as healer' should not be misunderstood: even in the early days of use of terminology such as 'educational therapy' (Frostig and Horne 1970) there was no confusion in the minds of the pioneers about the primacy of their teaching role. There was, however, recognition that learners whose feelings, self-esteem and self-concept had become so damaged as a result of repeated rejections and the 'crippling' experience of being unable to cope with tasks which seem easy and automatic for others, might be regarded as requiring care of a quality which is analogous to the care required by those who sustain physical 'insults' or trauma as in motor accidents. For the learner experiencing psychic pain it may be that it is not so much the discovery of a seeming or actual inability to learn something which is easy for others, but the fact that this is perceived by others to be a disability that brings with it a sense of broken spirit. For the teacher to ignore that fact and proceed as if it did not exist is calculated to impede, not facilitate, the discovery of an avenue through which (even if neurological healing does not occur) a suitable 're-routing' may be found and an 'educational prophylactic' or 'prosthesis' can be designed to be of support on the journey.

In this sense teachers avoid confusion about their role and its borders with medical specialist support. However, they do need to know how to recognize the differences between *resistance to learning* (for whatever reasons) and *persistent difficulties with any stage of the learning process*, thus also to know when to call for further advice and become aware of diagnostic indicators which relate to biochemical factors requiring intervention at the multi-disciplinary level (see also Haase 2000, Chapter 7). To do this, in addition to being systematic and rigorous, specialist SpLD teachers need to be imaginative, creative and even artistic in designing individually tailored 'appliances' to overcome different aspects of learning difficulties (including, for example, promoting metacognition and meta-affectivity, see Chapter 5).

Perhaps one of the most vital ways in which special educators can simultaneously contribute to their own discipline and make a multi-disciplinary contribution to the welfare of all children is to have the courage to confront simplistic ideas about learning and its relationship to mental health, and to recognize false alignments of lack of learning with lack of will to learn. Too often, substantial numbers of children are relegated to the scrapheap or seen as no good because it is assumed not only that they won't learn but also that they can't learn (see e.g. Summer Literacy School interviews with children, Hunter-Carsch 1998, and children's reasons why they don't learn, Norwich 1999).

The language reflecting values attributed to the 'conditions' which learners share becomes the currency of the new educational economy which increasingly encompasses 'the global village'. The implications of terminology, meanings and associated values relating to what constitutes a difficulty, disability or disorder, and what the support of the learning process involves, include indicators of societies' concern for human dignity. Special education specialists continue to be at the forefront of education in this respect, some not by choice, but by conscription. Yet they are required to carry the banners which identify the values set by the society with which and for which they work (see Hunter 1953 and Warnock 1978).

## Step 3

This step (forming the hypothesis) requires great care so that it contains the rationale for the connection between observed difficulties, assumed needs and plans for intervention (see Step 4). There are many intuitive teachers who are able to facilitate remarkable learning on the part of their students and to whom it may seem not only unnecessary to have to go through a process of trying to reveal the thinking underlying their actions, but to whom it may even seem to be an impediment. For such teachers it may not be necessary to work out all the details in advance and record everything when all goes well. It becomes essential only when learning is not straightforward and as anticipated. In such circumstances i.e of unanticipated challenges or complexities it is the manner in which the teacher proceeds that needs to become the focus of attention. In exploring their particular modes of working, the otherwise unseen dimensions of facilitating pupils' progress may be revealed, and thus clarify the value of carrying out the five-step cycle of documenting students' progress.

When some teachers experience difficulty in finding words to describe their intuitive behaviour, they may be able to seek assistance from more experienced teachers through informal discussions as well as consultations with specialist educators and through advanced training and the relevant literature. The point should be made that records of the 'revelation' (in written words) are not only for teachers who carry out the immediate interactions but are also for communicating to others the critical details of what structuring/learning support resulted in successful learning for the individual student. Inadequate communication of the records may risk discontinuities, impede further learning and may even cause setbacks for students.

It should also be commented that records about more than one student taught by the same teacher may reveal subtle adaptations of teaching strategies. Since casework tends to concern one individual at a time, the focus of refinements to teaching strategies employed differentially by the same expert teacher is seldom documented. An opportunity to observe and read the reports of expert teachers can constitute an experience on a par with 'master class' teaching by celebrated musicians and artists. And like great art, the 'script' (whether in Laban, Benesh, musical notation or other written language forms) remains static until  the dynamics are interpreted by readers making the words come alive.

### Step 4

This involves the delineation of the proposed adaptations to usual teaching (i.e. the IEP). It may be consciously influenced by the principles of the structured approach (Cruickshank 1961), which are broadly that the learning environment and mediation of the curriculum content should be planned in such a manner as to minimize the possibility of failure by removal of distractions and heightening the focus on essential points of carefully structured learning. The micro-strategies described earlier then come into play with different emphases and in different combinations. The prescription is not necessarily repeated in the same form for different students, although it is likely that all may benefit from establishing certain routines which promote trust via predictability and, from a pupil's point of view, consistency, which promotes a sense that the teacher is 'reliable' in conduct and attitude (see Erikson 1968, p. 141 re Basic Virtues which are outcomes of 'favourable ratios' at each of the psycho-social stages of development, see Chapter 1, p. 30).

*Step 5*

The research focus and regular recording of findings necessarily depend on a systematic review of information derived from steps 1–4 above, and lead to an evaluation of the information from the whole cycle, and possibly the reformulation of the relevant hypothesis. To provide an adequate sample of the range of formats for records and to do justice to the exemplification of different kinds of SpLD, diversity of teaching and learning contexts, and of teachers' preferences would clearly require a longer discussion than is possible here. Rather, the immediate purpose of this chapter is to share the rationale for inclusion of detailed consideration of each of the stages involved in such a way as to try to avoid possible miscues. The written account tends to render possible a greater level of professional detachment which makes it easier to check whether the appropriate questions are being raised at each step and, in this way, prevent miscues.

**Macro-strategy II**

Supporting literacy, communication and learning across the curriculum involves teachers in raising their own meta-cognitive awareness of their particular theoretical perspectives with reference to these concepts. The aim is to sharpen focus, at will, on relevant aspects of the conceptual maps which they may have generated with regard to how reading and writing develop, how listening and speaking relate to these aspects of literacy and in what ways they are influenced by different purposes of communication. Included in this is also awareness of the operation of motivation in achieving automaticity of basic literacy skills, their application in different curriculum areas and different kinds of learning (see also Chapter 1).

In the case of teaching reading comprehension, it is only when there seems to be a difference between what the reader *assumed or expected* the content of a passage to be about, and what it *actually transpires* to be about when it is decoded (any sign of 'dissonance') that prompts re-reading and determination of the differences between expected and actual findings. It is in this way that the discovery of 'new' meaning resulting in increased comprehension. The essential component of 'hearing self think' significantly involves an internal dialogue.

Macro-strategy II involves the provision of assurance and rendering explicit the particular concept (the 'normal' development of literacy). This does not necessarily imply 'negligence' on the part of teachers. Rather, it prompts recognition of the possibility that there simply may not yet be available or accessible, sufficient knowledge about the particular question or issue that is to be tackled, and that assumptions are made so often about shared understanding (of images conveyed by words) that they are taken for granted. Individual differences deserve and may demand further questioning.

Too often in the past, current knowledge has been taken as complete when perhaps it was insufficiently understood (see, e.g. the development, operation of  and relationship between the teaching of analytic phonics, so-called 'synthetic' phonics, rhyme, and analogy). A more recent tendency has been to make false polarizations between perspectives of 'phonics researchers' as distinct from 'rhyme and analogy researchers' (Goswami 1999). Such selective emphases can lead to perspectives on teaching which fail to be sufficiently comprehensive to grasp some important relationships (see e.g. Lazo, Pumfrey and Peers 1997 re. metalinguistic awareness in the development of spelling, reading and writing; Scholes 1998 re. 'the case against phonemic awareness'; Stuart and Johnson's response to Scoles 1998; Goswami's 1999 overview of the current confusion, misunderstandings and the need for clarity about the role of rhyme in beginning reading; Stuart's 1999 research with both monolingual and multilingual beginner readers; Rappaport and Hunter-Carsch 1999 re. developmental factors within the process of learning about rhyming).

Further examples are provided by colleagues in the Leicester City Literacy and Numeracy Strategy Consultative Group (Spring 2000). Sue Welford, Numeracy Adviser, suggests that teachers are beginning to observe that it seems to be relatively easier to engage children in progressively deepening and lengthening their utterances (indicating progressively deeper understanding) in the Daily Mathematics Lesson than in the Literacy Hour (see also Dadds 1999; Mroz et al. in press and Hargreaves' and Hislam's current research in guided reading (Leicester University)). As a result of exploring assumptions about what was expected in 'interactive whole-class teaching' and literacy in both the Literacy Hour and the Daily Mathematics Lesson, questions arose as to whether the relevant expectations and assumed parity of importance attributed to different subject areas was perhaps being confused with those learning processes that attend each of them.

That discussion prompted questions such as whether 'interactive whole-class teaching' within the Literacy Hour and the Daily Mathematics Lesson may be fulfilling the same function(s); whether it is the same kind of 'literacy' that is being taught in the Literacy Hour and that is being employed for working within the Daily Mathematics Lesson; are the learning processes different for acquisition and use of the relevant literacy or literacies; how does the necessary 'automaticity' in reading, writing, spelling and numeracy develop; how are these related to learning new vocabulary and concepts?

It might be suggested that discussion about the associated mental images generated in the minds of learners through 'the language of mathematics' may more readily reveal the degree of 'concreteness' or 'abstractness' with which learners are engaged in the course of particular interactions in mathematics lessons than may be revealed in English lessons. In working through language to learn about how language works (language as both the means and the end) the referents may be less 'concrete' and correspondingly less accessible to some. Possibly, the idea or mental picture of the source of an idea or information may become less of a mystery to children who do not readily seem to grasp the connections, if the teacher engages in 'concretizing' by making others' voices (and awareness of 'one's inner voice', i.e. thinking) more accessible by dramatizing (for example, by use of visible puppets and audible voices – teacher's or child's). Yet, curiously, it may be assumed by some teachers that the opposite is the case (i.e., that literacy learning is 'easier' than numeracy or mathematics; that learning about English, in the language of the classroom, is 'easier' to learn, except, perhaps for some children for whom English is another language).

Further questions arising in discussion with Bob Vincent, Literacy Advisor Leicester City LEA, bring to the fore the importance of relating research findings concerning dyslexic learners in association with research in beginning literacy and language teaching for multi-lingual children, whether or not they are dyslexic, in relation to differences in e.g. rate of cognitive processing required in the use of different languages (see e.g. reference to research relating to auditory temporal threshold (Haase 2000; Von Steinbuchel et al. 1999; Lotze et al. 1999; Tallal et al.) and also to visual processing e.g. Tsunoda's work in Japan (reported in Haase 2000) and in neuroscience research, London University and Milan University).

When studying the effect of structuring teaching, it is the designing teaching to direct learners' attention to selected features and experiences that can heighten or lessen their chances of making the relevant mental connections about matters which seldom concern a simple one-to-one relationship, but more often involve sequences of associations, if not simultaneous connections. The directions of the connections are not necessarily from sensory to cognitive but may, in fact, be 'cognitively led', as in the case of basic curiosity (What does this mean? as distinct from What does this feel like or taste like?). The relationship of these two directions may not always be distinguished in evaluations of structured multi-sensory teaching materials, programmes and actual teaching (e.g. when the focus is on letter perception in learning to spell and when it is on 'rules'). In planning structured multi-sensory teaching it becomes important for structuring the learning environment and interaction, to distinguish between drawing out and perhaps dramatizing in a multi-sensory manner, the perceptual foci (in for example, phoneme discrimination and the transition from one phoneme to the next in reading a word) and the cognitive foci on the process of making analogies employing the recognition of the differences in 'sounds'. Both in planning and recording responses to teaching, their integration in the course of their application with new words and non-words, new phrases and stories should be noted.

The value of the structured approach lies in the extent to which it assists teachers to identify and disentangle the direction of cause and effect in relation to operating factors associated with:

- assumed/expected and intended learning;
- factors related to planned structuring of teaching to mediate learning;
- observed and interactive responses which occur in the delivery.

In this sense, the entire structured approach is designed to offer a means of checking the accuracy of the hypothesis which may be formulated initially as a question (recognizing that the answer cannot be assumed but must be tested). Application of the structured approach may throw light on issues affecting the effectiveness of teaching of the entire range of learners, not just those with SpLDs. For example, while it is recognized as necessary for young learners (and possibly also for older learners of English as another language) to be given sufficient opportunity to practise the relevant connections once they have been illustrated and experienced at sensory–perceptual and at cognitive levels of processing, as yet, it is not clear to what extent teachers in mainstream classes and those with SEN specialist training share awareness of the precise nature of their working assumptions and expectations of their pupils, regarding the optimal sequence, pace and manner of presentation and practice required for individual children (or groups) to learn effectively, i.e., to master Phonics 44 (Morris 1984). The tendency is for published materials, programmes and methods to be employed diversely, in part or whole, sometimes taken for granted as reliable, and for teachers' individual differ-

ences in employing them not to be checked rigorously. This is in contra-
diction to the use of certain methods and materials which form integral
parts of systematically developed approaches, such as the Montessori
approach and Reading Recovery (Clay 1979), in which specialist teacher
training aims to ensure continuity in the basic principles while adapting
materials and practices in the light of continuing research. It is in this
more systematic manner, also advocated in the structured approach, of
requiring thorough exploration of assumptions which underpins the
hypotheses being stated in greater detail for teaching children with special
needs, that some 'more general needs' can also be better understood. The
steps which cumulatively lead to the generating of research questions and
clarification of knowledge about the nature of literacy learning and
teaching, are conceptually very closely linked to the implementation of the
next macro-strategy (Macro-strategy III).

**Macro-strategy III**

Maintaining a research focus and evaluating by means of recording interactions and analysing their effects, should not be confused with Step 5 in
the sequence outlined in Macro-strategy I above. At the Macro-strategy III
level, the issue of concern is evaluative thinking about cumulative records
and what may be derived from their analysis. For example, the frequency
of specific kinds of difficulty and the range of difficulties encountered
across students' records can be examined in relation to the range of strategies employed to assist them. In this way, an overview of the effectiveness
and efficiency of the record-keeping system in relation to the intended
purposes of the records prompts questions such as whether findings
about the efficacy of particular kinds of structuring are emerging, which
students seem to benefit most from what kinds of intervention, might
there be more helpful ways of 'translating' the cumulative written records
and rendering them (or possibly selected parts of them) accessible to
colleagues, parents and appropriate others in the wider constellation of
those who are in a position to assist the student. The ethical issues
involved in access to databanks of professional material also constitute
vital and related questions.

In short, the idea of macro- and micro-strategies is intended as an aid
for teachers toward making decisions about priorities in terms of structuring the learning situation and locating the most effective ways of
mediating learning. Since teaching and learning interactions involve, for
the teacher, orchestrating constellations of factors, often simultaneously,
the intention in offering the framework is simply to provide a checklist or
'cue card' for highlighting certain priorities at the planning and reviewing
stages of the routines of teaching. Clearly, it is the teacher's responses to

the student as 'a whole person' (H factor as holistic) not as a set of symptoms or problems, that constitutes a major factor in providing the possibility for facilitating successful learning. To do this at a necessarily sophisticated level of intervention requires the simultaneous maintainance of the research perspective or 'stance' (R factor),which includes keen observation, hypothesis-testing approach, openness to adopt plans in the light of unanticipated responses, flexibility and readiness to engage in shifts of perspective which may be promoted also through other interactions including, for example, collaborative work with colleagues from other disciplines (M multi-disciplinary factor).

This amalgam of H, R and M perspectives facilitates a stance which assists in maintaining a sense of balance between the role of teacher as scientist and the teacher as artist, in addition to sustainance of a readiness to maintain the a researcher's detachment, hence also to try 'to see ourselves as others see us'. This acknowledgement of Robert Burns's oft-quoted line, seeks also to reconnect it for readers who do not have the opportunity to see it in its original context, with the social commentary Burns was able to make through his poem, in which the lines are included:

'O wad some Pow'r the giftie gie us, to see oursels as others see us!'

Burns's messages through songs and poetry reflect a psycho-social perspective with a powerful capacity to operate simultaneously engagement and detachment (deep-centred and de-centred in Jackson's idiom in Jackson and Michael (1985)) from human interactive learning. Burns illuminates the process and, in this example, points the direction of his vision towards heightened awareness of the need for that kind of humanity which manifests itself in humour and shared laughter – **with**, not **at**, ourselves! (See also chapters 1 re. perspectives and 5 re. meta-affective awareness.)

## Discussion

### The historical multi-disciplinary basis

Returning to the questions posed at the beginning of the chapter, this discussion will consider each in turn. The first asks why it is important for teachers to be familiar with the historical multi-disciplinary basis of the field of SpLDs since trends over the past 60 years in both the UK and North America suggest that, with diversification, it is less easy to retain the key perspectives of the pioneers, especially their view of priorities in structuring learning within the classroom. This entails the risk of losing both the multi-disciplinary approach and the holistic perspectives that integrate assessment and teaching as related modes of exploring the nature of SpLDs. There is a further danger of separately produced packages of static materials being employed without adequate understanding of the principles of the structured approach. Finally, this entails the danger of forgetting the value of structured teaching for a wider group with learning difficulties, not only those with SpLDs related to literacy, speech and communication or motor control but also those showing social, emotional and behavioural difficulties, some of which may be secondary rather than primary indicators.

Some illustrative evidence has been presented to support the idea that vital components of the original structured approach can be traced among characteristics of a small sample of contemporary specialist SpLD teachers, although there are few classrooms which follow the strictly clinical patterns of the original structured approach. However, questions arise as to the extent of shared awareness on the part of contemporary curriculum subject teachers, specialist SEN teachers in primary and secondary schools, and lecturers and learning support staff in colleges and universities, about the nature and place of planning and recording the systematic structuring of teaching-learning interactions in terms of selected factors which include those delineated by the pioneers. An attempt has been made to rediscover the basic five factors (space, time, methods, materials and relationships) to render explicit the need also to plan for and record the structuring affecting the following aspects of learning processing:

- whole-part learning
- sequencing
- speed
- accuracy.

These are required in addition to awareness of the perspectives relating to shared characteristics emerging from analysis of self-reported work from a sample of effective specialist SpLD teachers, which generated the following factors:

- C  aiming to assist the student to feel 'in Control';
- N  assisting students to feel 'Normal' rather than 'specially needy';
- H  maintaining a Holistic perspective;
- T  being aware of bringing an individual style and how that tends to affect the direction of attention within the Teaching-learning interactions;
- M  aiming to seek Multi-disciplinary support where relevant;
- R  maintaining a Research and recording focus so that systematic recording of efforts to structure teaching can be rendered poten-

tially communicable to colleagues while the findings about the
teacher's successes and limitations or difficulties (as well as those of
students) may be drawn upon for professional development and
possibly for sharing through contributions to the literature in the
field, so that educational and multi-disciplinary understanding may
be extended.

## Changes over the years

The question of what has changed over the years in the use of the terms
'structured teaching' and 'multi-sensory teaching', has been further
explored with reference to the fact that it is students' responses to the
structured multi-sensory approach as conceptualized by Werner, Strauss
and Lehtinen (Strauss et al. 1947) which constituted the single unifying
factor underpinning this complex field of SpLDs. The delineation of the
approach by Cruickshank et al. (1961) and the subsequent specialization
of teaching of subgroups, separating those with what were considered to
be mainly learning problems from those with behavioural and emotional
problems, may have contributed not only to valuable diversification of
teaching methods but also to the loss of sharing between teachers, of
dimensions and details of conscious planning designed to emphasize
different aspects of the multi-sensory approach. The resultant assumed
shared understanding of the term, and an increased tendency to introduce
published packages relating to structured teaching *materials*, has further
disengaged their use from its contextualisation within the wider perspective of structuring teaching *methods*.

## Rediscovering relationship structuring

Among the casualties of diversification and the passage of time are the
seeming diminution of awareness of the potential efficacy of structuring
spatial factors and the virtual loss of recognition of relationship structuring as a factor. In response to the question posed at the beginning of
the Chapter, it is the author's view that the very purpose of structuring
relationships seems to have been neglected or misunderstood. It was
intended primarily as a means of decreasing students' distraction from
emotional uncertainties and removal of their anxieties in response to their
perceptions of the 'demands of pleasing the teacher', whom they necessarily see as in a position of authority, whilst simultaneously increasing the
students' freedom to concentrate their attention on the learning task in
hand. Like the establishment of calm routines as a means of building trust
and avoiding apprehensions about the unknown and potentially
unpleasant learning experience, the structured approach has become

misunderstood and misrepresented as 'boring', even becoming associated with particular published 'structured materials' which have been cut off from contextual settings that ensured an appropriate balance of stimulation and relaxation, active engagement and reflection.

However, there appears to have been a simultaneous increased awareness of the potential value of structuring materials, and only limited recognition of what the pioneers actually meant by 'structured teaching methods'. Perhaps this is inevitable in the absence of the establishment of designated teacher-training building regular revision of the principles of structured teaching (e.g. in the manner of the internationally recognised 'Reading Recovery' teacher training by Dame Marie Clay and her qualified specialist teachers, or Montessori Teacher training by an organisation supporting trained Montessori teachers). It may be wise also to take into account that over-rigid adherence to *methods* as distinct from *principles* might render the entire approach vulnerable to abuse. The aim here has been to rekindle the fire that warmed the hearts of the early team and to share the spirit and direction of their quest.

## Developing and maintaining a hypothesis-testing approach

With reference to the fourth question the development of a research-based 'hypothesis testing approach' is particularly important for specialist SEN teachers whose major task is to discover how best to assist students to become independent learners and, in the light of their findings, to share relevant information with their mainstream colleagues. While there is sympathetic recognition of the increased amount of record-keeping that is required at all levels, questions remain as to the extent to which, as a professional group, specialist SEN and SpLD teachers in particular are able to maintain both the rigour of research-based investigatory work on a daily basis with the sense of quest which attended the pioneers' work, and to maintain the enthusiasm to communicate their classroom-based findings through collaborative work across the related disciplines.

The implications for practice include the necessity of making time for essential detailed planning and record-keeping. Assuming that this simply cannot be done in addition to the already overburdened teacher' schedules, there is a way in which teachers can adapt their timetabling to include a designated time for planning, and for review and analysis of findings within every lesson. This can be done by training their students to relax for up to 10 minutes at the beginning and end of each lesson. Such training can include e.g. 'brain gym': breathing and relaxation exercises while drawing upon strategies related to visualization, such as those developed by neurolinguistic specialists. The increased efforts which are able to be concentrated during the reduced lesson time more than make up for the time allocated for 'tuning in' and 'tuning out' and will be recognized by other teachers during subsequent lessons to have a beneficial effect on students.

The general plan (allowing introductory/transition and final rest and relaxation time) has been found to be effective in the provision of timetabled learning support sessions for groups as well as individuals in primary and secondary schools. It is particularly helpful for freeing the teacher to undertake essential record-keeping associated with research and during 'write-up' moments immediately after a shorter teaching session, it becomes possible to note plans and make links with parents, colleagues and, possibly in the future e.g. by 'e' mail and classroom computer access, to include instant contact with education colleagues and multi-discipline specialists.

## Conclusion

Many of the points made in the pursuit of the argument in support of revisiting the early approaches, deconstructing and reconstructing them, are based on qualitative analysis (classroom observation, dialogues with teachers and students and reflection, including analysis of teachers' responses). Not surprisingly, perhaps, some of the strongest influences in the author's attempts to promote greater understanding of what constitutes structured teaching are the voices of her own teachers. It is a privilege to recall amongst them Professor William Cruickshank who shared his personal memories of working with Strauss, Werner and Lehtinen; Marianne Frostig who had amongst her followers fellow psychologists and teachers some who also knew Beth Slingerland and who respected, as does the author, the remarkable contributions of both educators to assessment and teaching. It might be suggested that Slingerland's cross curricular application of what was later termed 'miscues' (Goodman 1973) and her focus on multisensory teaching for 'preventative' purposes rather than 'cure' have not yet become sufficiently assimilated into commom practice. Reading their published writings, however illuminating of aspects of their contribution, cannot fully reflect the impact of observing their teaching styles, their interactions with pupils and hearing their commentary on their own work. The author feels an obligation to try to communicate their recognition of the need for continuously developing their own multi-disciplinary knowledge and classroom experience. These great educators presented a sense of professional stature not only in their presence but, perhaps most memorably, in the intensity of their interest as active listeners, observers and contributors to conversation with their students and colleagues. They were alert and always ready to share their thoughts in ways which revealed their own internal professional dialogue, including their hypotheses, doubts and responses to new ideas. Observing these master teachers at work brought increased levels of awareness, deepened understanding and potential for increasing the relevant professional skills.

However, they differed strikingly in their channelling of the affective aspects of their personality in the teaching context with children with SpLDs. Marianne Frostig emanated a cheerful and smiling energy and mobility which carried learners along with it, whereas William Cruickshank emanated a calmness which contrasted markedly with his speed of mind and readiness to provide the precisely needed and quietly articulated words in dealing with a hyperactive child who needed reassurance. It is only as a result of watching them in action that the author carries a mental image of their voices, actions, 'stance' and vision so that these contribute additionally to reading their published work, and can be brought to bear in current analysis of learning interactions between teachers and students. Both Cruickshank and Frostig employed observation and interaction with students, in addition to standardized assessment procedures when compiling student profiles*. Both continued to add to profiles and modify them in the light of students' responses to systematic structuring of teaching in a manner which was individually tailored. Both continued to test their working hypotheses and refine them in the light of further information. Their research focus, traced through their routine records, did not separate for teaching purposes the emphasis on learning and behavioural difficulties. Their teaching through structuring students' experiences was designed to bring greater control of both learning and behaviour within the framework of the structured approach.

Slingerland's contribution was perhaps most vital in her emphasis on developing and updating local norms, having all class teachers involved in a full understanding of multi-sensory teaching, and trained to observe, note and classify errors in a manner which rendered visible to them the range of severity of difficulties, subtle patterns of difficulty and misunderstandings which could be identified as early as possible and corrected. Her preventative approach (to avoid dyslexia) and inclination to an inclusive education and 'well-health' perspective rather than 'disability' was inspiring.

Finally, there is still much that we do not know about how exactly certain teaching–learning interactions bring about effective learning, how to avoid errors and how to chart the most direct routes. The question of

---

* Frostig's profile components included representation in graph form of the related results of sub-tests including the following: Wechsler (WISC), Kirk and Kirk's Illinois Test of Psycholinguistic Abilities (ITPA), Wepman's Auditory Discrimination Test, and Frostig's Developmental Test of Visual Perception (DTVP).

the contribution made historically by structured teaching may be best understood if it is addressed in the recent and still current terminology of 'differentiation'. It then becomes one of how to employ what we already know about structured teaching for the purposes of differentiating in order to meet the range of learning needs in a class of students. To move towards answering that question, teachers will need to have a keen awareness of their conceptual map of the learning process, literacy learning and SpLDs, e.g. dyslexia. In addition, they will need heightened awareness of where their preferences about learning and their own styles differ from those of their students. This awareness is necessary for recognition of the extent to which they can (or cannot) empathize with, and understand, the experiences of the dyslexic learner across the range of curricular content and process, matters which constitute the exchanges designed to facilitate the learning for the student. An appreciation of such matters can affect positively the manner in which the principles of the structured approach can be effectively translated into practice in the current context.

## Acknowledgements

Thanks to Judy Dunning and the Leicester City Local Education Authority Advisers in particular Sue Welland and Bob Vincent for helpful discussions; the Lancashire SpLD teachers who gave their vital discretionary time to complete the exploratory questionnaire; to colleagues in the Assessment Centre, Beechgrove, in Kingston, Ontario, and in the Dumbartonshire and Leicestershire schools who shared an interest in increasing understanding of structured teaching, and to all the students and teachers with whom I have had the privilege of working. With appreciation, in recognition, to Professor Margaret Clark of the manner in which she promoted a multi-disciplinary approach to teaching educational psychologists in the 1970s at the University of Strathclyde. Her courses included shared sessions with teachers, parents and doctors working together through discussions about children with SpLDs.

# Chapter 5
# Beyond meta-cognition: the integration of meta-affectivity as a component of meta-comprehension

MORAG HUNTER-CARSCH

Questions addressed in this chapter include:

- What is the relationship between cognition and affectivity in the context of the learning experience for dyslexic and non-dyslexic learners?
- Can a single theoretical model for the development of meta-comprehension adequately take into account the different forms of reasoning and levels of thinking and experiencing for both groups of learners?
- How could such a model affect teachers' attitudes and methods of teaching?

'The unexamined life is not worth living.'
Socrates

## Introduction

This chapter explores the quality of the learning experience and its evaluation for dyslexic and non-dyslexic students. The chapter has three sections. The first discusses cognition and affectivity in the learning experience. It indicates the advantages derived from meta-cognition and meta-affectivity and their proposed synthesis as meta-comprehension. The second attempts to relate this to the effects of students' use of distinct forms of reasoning and to generate a model which explores the dynamics of the learning experience in terms of diverse levels. The concluding section discusses the tentative model in relation to motivation to learn and understanding of subtle psychosocial factors possibly compounding the learning difficulties experienced by some dyslexic students.

# The learning experience and the need for a theory of meta-comprehension

Healthy young children characteristically have a curiosity to understand how the world works and how they function in it. Optimally, learning in school can sustain this curiosity and promote comprehension, not only factual learning of curriculum content. However, comprehending, in that sense, seems to present many dyslexic students in school and college with a particular challenge which involves the satisfaction of a prerequisite need to feel in control of both the content and the context (that is, to have the structuring of learning needed in order to address the 'C factor' discussed in Chapter 4).

We may speculate that this perceived need may relate to students' prior experience of not finding certain kinds of learning (such as literacy) to be either easy or automatic; possibly also anticipating that if and when they reveal their experience of these kinds of learning being different from those of others, they may not be understood by teachers and/or peers; also, seemingly in contrast, feeling that they have a right to expect their teachers to understand their specific learning difficulties (mobilize their capacity for empathy) and to be able to offer practical assistance to cope with the impact of these difficulties. The frequency of such reported experiences on the part of students suggests that, in short, their expectation of teachers is that they should 'comprehend comprehension'. This, it may be suggested, may involve both the relevant *cognitive* and *affective* aspects, i.e. 'meta-comprehension'.

The teacher's conceptual model of meta-comprehension would thus require to include along with their understanding of the learning process in general, understanding, in particular, about how specific learning difficulties affect students' learning and relatedly, what part motivation, attitude and interpersonal factors play in this process (see also chapters 1, 2, 6, 7 and 14). This requires an understanding of the following three issues:

(i)   how cognition and affectivity are related to motivation;
(ii)  how diminished motivation to learn can be explained in terms of cognition, meta-cognition, affectivity and meta-affectivity;
(iii) how the dynamics of the learning process can be explored in the classroom with reference to depth of penetration and synthesis of learning experience, or arrest beyond which point the learning experience becomes dysfunctional.

Since the literature on these three issues spans several fields and crosses disciplines, a search for information about models of teaching and of learning in both mainstream and special education is required, as is an investigation of the literature on both cognitive and social psychology. Study of substantial bodies of material on different aspects of these issues (Bindra and Stewart 1968; Maslow 1968; Riding and Taylor 1976; Burton and Radford 1978; Roth and Frisby 1986; Dunn et al. 1989; Vauras et al. 1992; Adey and Shayer 1994; Gardner and Alexander 1994; Reid 1994; Singer et al. 1994; Sotto 1994; Gardner 1995; Leong and Joshi 1995; Hewstone et al. 1996; Underwood and Batt 1996; Vauras 1996; Ashton and Conway 1997; Cassidy 1997; Crozier 1997; Joyce et al. 1997; Kress 1997; Topping 1997; Turner 1997; Biesta 1998; Claxton 1998a, 1998b; Duffield 1998; Howe 1998; Riding and Raynor 1998; Yzerbyt et al. 1998; Gleitmann et al. 1999) revealed gaps in the explanation of the dynamics of learning in terms of relating motivational, affective and cognitive dimensions of 'normal learning' as well as the learning experience of students with SpLDs e.g. dyslexia. Investigations of literature on SpLDs included neuro-psychological models and pointed to a need to take into account the findings of modern brain research employing techniques such as Magnetic Resonance Imagery (MRI) and the tracking of cerebral hemisphere activity (see Chapter 2).

The considerable challenge facing teachers involves synthesizing the information into a multi-disciplinary model. But, the starting point remains the clarification of meanings of descriptors they employ in everyday discourse in schools and the community. To appreciate the importance of these 'meanings', the following discussion of terminology seeks to illuminate some of the central concepts in the process of addressing issue (i) above concerning the relationship between motivation, cognition and affectivity. Some of the etymological investigations then lead to the generation of a tentative model which addresses issues (ii) and (iii), the dynamics of the learning process. The model is then described.

## Terminology and the relationship of cognition to affectivity and motivation

Drever's (1952) definition of cognition contrasts it with affectivity.* The notion of the contrast becomes increasingly evident in subsequent litera-

---

*Cognition is defined as 'a general term covering all the various models of knowing - perceiving, remembering, imagining, conceiving, judging, reasoning'; affectivity as 'the tendency to react with feeling or emotion' ('affect' being defined as 'any kind of feeling or emotion attached to ideas or idea-complexes'; 'motivation' is defined as 'the term employed generally for the phenomena involved in the operation of incentives, drives and motives' (Drever 1952)). What is perhaps vital to the discussion of the position adopted in this chapter is the further definitive comment made by Drever, with reference to cognition, i.e. 'The cognitive function, as an ultimate mode or aspect of the conscious life, is contrasted with the affective and connative – feeling and willing'.

ture in which there is separation of consideration of cognition from that of affectivity. The progressive dissociation of the two concepts is facilitated by adoption of a range of terms used in preference to affectivity or in association with that concept, (as distinct from cognition) for example physiological, personality and social factors (Hayes 1991; Drew and Watkins 1998).** Perhaps this progression is unfortunate as there seems to be a close relationship between operation of both cognition and affectivity in interactive learning in the classroom. What is perhaps even more unfortunate is the further separate consideration of the idea of motivation, as if in a field of its own rather than in an integral relationship with affectivity and cognition. It is as if the border between motivation and affectivity was perhaps acknowledged but their joint proximity to cognition neglected. In the literature therefore the relationship between these areas becomes the poor relative, rather than the separated fields, each of which is substantial. The following paragraphs consider aspects of the *components* and their associated terminology, and seeks to reconnect some of the strands.

## Cognition and meta-cognition

Hayes (1991) refers to five cognitive processes: perception, attention, thinking, memory and language, indicating that these processes underlie reading, social understanding and shared beliefs. Merry (1994) provides a practical tabular overview (Table 5.1) intended to assist teachers with the process of generating ideas for activities in the classroom.

Not being intended as a detailed model of cognitive processes, the table omits specific mention of a number of factors, such as attention and short-term memory, which it is particularly important for teachers of dyslexic students to consider in the course of their classroom interactions. However, Merry (1994) helpfully reminds us that:

> The ultimate aim of interactive teaching is for the child to develop meta-cognitive skills to be able to 'interact' with their own thinking.

Such skills including e.g. study skills (see Edgar 2001) need to be developed in and beyond the primary school. For example, Wray (1995) points out that reading for meaning inevitably involves the meta-cognitive activity of comprehension monitoring. Wray explains the concept of meta-cognition in relation to cognition by referring to Vygotsy's (1962) distinction between two stages in the development of knowledge: first, the automatic,

---

**Drew and Watkins (1998) refer to 'affective variables' in the title of their article. The term is not directly employed but reference is made to 'personality variables' and in particular to 'motivation' and 'self-concept', 'locus of control'. With reference to the 'locus of control' dimension, they draw upon the work of Jonassen and Grabowski (1993).

**Table 5.1** Merry's (1994) Practical classroom model of cognition (reproduced with permission)

The cognitive process

| Inputs/stimuli (first-hand experience) | Processes (invisible) | Outputs/products (observable) |
|---|---|---|
| real objects | recognizing | moving/arranging |
| models | remembering | completing |
| video/audiotape | matching | highlighting |
| pictures | comparing | connecting |
| other people | finding/selecting | drawing |
| maps/diagrams | synthesizing | constructing |
| words/text | transforming tables (e.g. words into images or vice versa) | identifying |
| speech | predicting | answering/asking questions |
|  | applying | telling |
|  | inferencing | acting |
|  | imagining | writing etc. |
|  | hypothesizing |  |
|  | evaluating etc. |  |

unconscious acquisition (not knowing that we know); second, what Wray (1995) describes as:

> a gradual increase in active conscious control over knowledge – we begin to know that we know and that there is more that we do not know.

Wray (1995) goes on to refer to Brown's (1980) use of the term meta-cognition to refer to:

> the deliberate conscious control of one's own cognitive actions – i.e. thinking about thinking - and applying to knowledge about cognition in general.

suggesting, perhaps, that generalization of such learning is dependent on meta-cognitive activity. Its dependence on abstraction and the nature of mental imagery are discussed elsewhere (Donaldson 1992; Brook 1997; Ohlsson and Lehtinen 1997).

To a large extent, understanding what is involved in the operation of cognition (as distinct from meta-cognition) must be inferred, although through studies of reading comprehension, analysis of observed eye movements and with the learner's discussion of the process, some closer match may be approximated between what is considered to be the meaning of a text and that of its reader. It is in instances of mismatch that the reader discovers the need to resolve the perceived differences (that is, to try to comprehend) (Vauras et al. 1992; see also Chapter 13).

## Reading comprehension as creating and re-creating meaning

Hall and Myens (1997), studying children's meta-cognitive awareness of the reading comprehension process, reported that:

> because teachers rarely make explicit the processes involved in reading, emphasizing instead the influence of time and practice they may be contributing to children's somewhat naive beliefs about the **role of effort in correcting reading problems.** (p. 8) (author's emphasis)

An important link may be made between young learners' grasp of the relationship between printed text and its purpose, but perhaps more vitally, between their will to learn, their feelings about the learning and the intensity of their investment in building the relevant relationships between the process and the hoped-for outcome. The work of Hall (1997; 1998) highlights the active component in learning to read and, through reading, harnessing of motivation to comprehend.

Experience of helping learners to become aware of how to direct their own effort into grasping processes such as reading (understanding that it involves not only decoding but also actively creating meaning and re-creating the writer's intended meaning) led to the recognition that meta-affectivity not only meta-cognition comes into play, not only when reading printed texts but in wider interpretations of the idea of reading, including reading of paintings, music, dance, facial expressions and body-language (Hunter-Carsch 1989; Leong 1989; see also Chapter 1). Meta-affectivity draws upon experience at different levels of association and employs different kinds of imagery. It includes imagination to reach out into the process of communication in directions which are both inter- and intra-personal. This wider sense of the concept of reading, including reading music, can refer to both translating (e.g. of musical notation) mentally and responding (e.g. to hearing music). Interactive in character, meta-affectivity may also relate to empathy, which may require insight into one's own dynamics and those of others (that is, possibly both meta-cognitive and meta-affective, as well as potentially meta-comprehensive in nature).

The development of empathy (beyond sympathy) may have its early roots in imaginative play (Kitson 1994; Moyles 1995; Slade 1992) and be fostered by creative teachers. Its continuing successful development through adolescence, a time of particularly intense exploration of images and of identity, may require special insights and skills on the part of secondary school teachers and the continuity of models of inspiring teachers into college experience, teachers who continue to engage their students' imagination.

## Reading comprehension, reasoning and the dyslexic student

The 're-creation of meaning' through reading takes personal effort and the employment of imagination. Underwood and Batt (1996) note that reading has been described by Neisser (1967) as 'externally guided thinking' and suggest that in this sense reading is equivalent to reasoning. They discuss the reading comprehension process in terms of three levels. The first involves word identification. The second and third levels involve mental representations; words collected into ideas or propositions, then 'beyond the meanings in this propositional textbase to form a mental model or situational model in which the text is interpreted.' (Underwood and Batt 1996, p. 216). They conclude their definitive text on reading and understanding with the statement that 'For skilled readers, comprehension can be said to require the construction of a mental model in which the formation of inferences acts to link the individual propositions in a unified representation.' (p. 217).

Dyslexic students generally have difficulty at the word level in both decoding and encoding. It has been suggested that their problems relate to phonological factors including awareness of fine discriminations between phonemes within the flow of the word (BPS 1999; Herrington 2001c; see also chapters 2, 7, 8 and 10). It has also been suggested that dyslexic students have characteristic learning styles and that some show strengths in visuo-spatial thinking (West 1991). What is somewhat unclear as yet is the manner in which the comprehension of printed texts beyond the word level and the creation of written text by dyslexic students is affected by matters of motivation, cognitive processing patterns (some of which may be learned and some of which may be influenced by neurologically predetermined 'preferences', 'problems' or 'limitations') and affective factors.

The reading comprehension process is one which presents reading as an avenue through which intensive exposure to another's thinking can lead not only to meta-cognitive experience but perhaps also, to meta-affective activity which may in this way extend the individual's potential achievement of meta-comprehension.

## Towards a developmental model of meta-comprehension

This tentative theoretical model includes two main components. The first concerns two forms of reasoning and the second explores levels of experience.

### Forms of reasoning

Reasoning, in this sense as both the driving force and process (both cognitive and affective) is, in the English vernacular, broadly recognized as a single line of associated meanings, one which relates to drawing inferences from premisses, ways of persuading, trying to reach conclusions by connected thought, 'thinking out' . However, in other languages (such as German) distinctions are made between two kinds of reasoning which determine and mobilize cognitive and affective factors which can be applied to the learning experience.*

Two such forms of reasoning appear to be relevant:

- an OBJECTIVE/transcendental/contemplative/reflective/universalistic form
- a SUBJECTIVE/instrumental/calculative/practical/particularistic form.

The first of these extends, transcendentally, the individual's direct and specific interests. It is guided and informed more or less objectively by, ultimately, critical considerations such as awareness of and perhaps emphasis on the maintenance of relative harmony in society and, in its widest sense, the testing of the 'reasonableness of aspects of human effort'. The relative prepotence or one of the other form is culturally determined, but varies between cultures and in complex societies may vary further between subcultures or in terms of situation specificity. It is the relationship between these forms of reason which constitutes the

---

*Donaldson (1992, p. 90) asserts that 'all thinking involves abstraction'. Her model of mind is perhaps exceptional in its scope and depth. It integrates dimensions, including both time and space, and a notional continuum of contextual dependence (i.e. support of experience or of inner imagery or recall) to independence. She discusses the manner in which we deal with abstractions in the operations carried out towards the disembedded extreme of this continuum. (For the dyslexic learner, in particular, this involves awareness of the kinds of internal images which assist in dealing with relations between the concrete and the progressively more abstract, or, in reverse, the translation of the abstraction into concrete examples in the flow of thinking and in directions of thinking/experiencing which may be 'taken for granted' by others.) Donaldson's model contains elements of both emotion and thought at different developmental levels towards ultimately 'transcendent thought'. She draws attention to the need for better understanding of the manner in which the core modes of mind relate to the advanced modes 'and how within the latter category, the intellectual and the value-sensing varieties of experience relate to one another' (p. 266). Ohlsson and Lehtinen (1997) view abstraction as 'our ability to go beyond the stimulus, to act and think in ways that are not dictated by the perceptual input'. Rather than viewing abstraction in the classical sense in which learning moves from the concrete towards the general, they consider abstraction to be a 'prerequisite for learning because ideas have to be abstract in order to be assembled'. The prerequisites for dealing with abstractions are discussed by Kant (1787) who is referred to by Brook (1997) as insisting that 'cognition requires both concepts and percepts, where concepts (as he perceived them) were linguistic or at least propositional .' Brook (1997) goes on to comment that ' what we now need is an account of how the two are linked' (p. 86).

parameters of 'permissable degrees of freedom' which underlie the specific ethos of societies and which constitute the subject matter of ethics.

The second form of reason involves, individuals' and institutions' direct specific interests and focuses on the instrumental and perhaps calculative testing of implicit potentials of the content. Both forms may be universal. The preponderance of one or other form may be situation-specific and/or subject to subcultural variation.**

In possibly most societies the instrumental form is expected to be subordinated to the transcendental form. In such cases, individual expediencies are tested before implementation of instrumental considerations.

For teachers, recognition of which form of reasoning is being adopted by individual students can facilitate adjustments to the presentation of information so that attempts can be made to connect the content to the direction of the student's motivation. It is generally taken as axiomatic that teachers' perspectives tend to be guided by the objective form of reason and that they tend to interpret their remit in terms of their realization that they are part of humankind and that their efforts are consequently dedicated to the integration of their students into the larger, if not total human context. The same cannot be said of all students, some of whom may incline to consider only what they perceive to be useful to them and to connect with their personal experiences and expectations. In the course of such selectivities they may be assisted, if not guided by extra-curricular, counter-academic influences competing with those of schools and colleges. Thus, it becomes possible that entire groups of students may adopt the subjective form of reason to the exclusion of the objective. More usually, a mix of the two forms prevails, with variation in the selection of one or other influenced by the composition of the school's (or college's) population arising out of demographic variables.

---

**Horkheimer may have followed Aristotle's distinction between the contemplative and the calculative forms of reasoning, the latter being equated with practical wisdom or 'phronesis', which he saw as being exercised 'for the attainment of truth in things that are humanly good or bad.' (McKeon 1941: The Works of Aristotle, NY, Random House, p. 913; Thomson 1955, The Ethics of Aristotle, Harmondsworth, Penguin Books, pp. 176–180).

In English this polarisation of forms of reasoning is rarely made. In German they lead logically to a differentiation between the two relevant forms of reason itself, i.e. Verstand deriving from the objective/trancendental/contemplative form of reasoning, and Vernuft deriving from the subjective investigations of this relating to numerically small nomadic groups with relatively low levels of material culture, but it may, perhaps, be safely assumed that such a distinction may have evolved by the Neolithic as indicated by Hamurabi's code (c. 1700 BC). (Mumford 1961, The City in History, NY: Harcourt Brace and World, pp. 50–108).

'Personality' (including affective) factors may play an important part in students' responses to the teacher and affect their attitudes to the content of what is being taught (particularly in the compulsory education sector). A related acceptance and possible identification with the teacher may be contrasted with a rejection of both the teacher and teaching content.

In some instances, some students may reject both forms of reasoning, resulting in their alienation from the learning process. This contingency may be concealed or rationalized by platitudinous allegations that school (or the curricular subject area) is 'boring' and perhaps the suggestion that it requires 'more effort than it is worth' (that is, it interferes with other usually subjective interests); in short that it is irrelevant to the student's current or anticipated experiences. It is, of course, difficult to generalize about the extent to which such expressions are based on free will or affected by prior or accompanying forms of interpersonal influence.

### Diagnostic issues: dyslexia and the impact of conflicting forms of reasoning

Teachers quickly become aware of the ranges of achievement in their classes and can draw upon various measures to indicate how individual students rank in relation to the class as a whole. They can ascertain which students are at the lower end of the achievement range and can relate this information to the individual student's profile of achievement across the curriculum. They may also have access to diagnostic assessment reports, including profiles of cognitive strengths and areas of relative weakness, for some students with identified special educational needs (e.g. SpLD/dyslexia). Such profiles may include static descriptors of measured positions on notional dimensional polarities, such as 'visualizer–verbalizer', (not to be confused with forms of reasoning). However, it is unlikely that these profile measures provide information about the vulnerability of individual students or groups to rejection of objective or both forms of reason, prior to the onset of serious learning difficulties, nor are they likely to provide guidance on dealing with the impact of filtering systems on the part of subjective reasoners' responses, or to the social context of learning as well as to their dyslexia. Moreover, the existing forms of assessment seem to neglect this particular kind of information in the case of students who without discernible cause have seemingly sustained a distinguished academic record and who diminish in the quality of their performance.

For the teacher with one (or more) dyslexic students in the class who observes that they are having difficulty with an aspect of classwork, there may be a tendency to consider that dyslexia is the primary causal factor. However, compounding difficulties in progressing with the relevant learning may involve a lack of engagement of either form of reason – more often the negative attitudinal impact guided by the subjective form of reason – whether experienced by the individual and/or intensified by (or causally related to) the group's preference. It would be helpful for the teacher to discern the forms of reasoning of the students concerned, together with the range of the group's relevant preferences over sufficient time to reach a general sense of their normal response patterns.

The diagnostic challenge, however, includes not only a differentiation between primary and secondary influences at work in particular learning/teaching interactions but also their relative intensity and the direction of impact. It may be further compounded in the case of dyslexic learners by the fact that they frequently report experiencing acute affective awareness in the pursuit of learning (for example, 'knowing it feels right', 'gut feelings' about the direction to pursue; 'global feelings about the answer'; keen 'feelings'/recall of characters' movements and voice patterns by learner actors; 'just knowing' what to do 'because it feels right'). This tendency to filter experience through a seemingly generalized sensing or feeling may generate a perceptible attitudinal predisposition towards or against continuing engagement with learning experiences. It may also extend towards subsequent potential learning experiences.

This may occur particularly in students who are generally guided by the objective form of reasoning and may include many dyslexic students. Such students may find it difficult to integrate particularistic information into their personal pre-existing frame of reference (until and unless they can locate quickly the starting point for the experience on their internal cognitive map of prior experience/knowledge). They may seem to regard information which is presented in atomistic manner as fragments, unconnected to a more universal perspective. Attempts on their part to integrate information may be (a) unsuccessful and hence, (b) frustrating. The consequences of such experiences and their resultant frustration may be that (c) the student feels inhibited from appreciating the relevance of the materials involved. The difficulties are therefore not due to adoption of a subjective exclusive form of reasoning but precisely because the particular information remains separate from their relatively universalistically-oriented cognitive perspectives which are rooted in objective reason.*

---

*This is particularly important with regard to the arrival at (c) the state of feeling inhibited from appreciating the relevance of what is involved since it is not a conscious decision that is being made to reject these materials but a non-engagement with the potential experience which they afford (i.e. it is at the level of 'pre-experience' and thus only 'orientation towards the possibility' – perhaps similar to not happening to 'look in the right direction' as distinct from having the potential to see, if given the appropriate cue to 'turn round' – which would require active adjustment but can conceptually be separated from the outcome of the adjustment, that is, did not move, as distinct from 'chose not to move' or 'cannot move').

On the other hand, it seems possible (especially if integration has not taken place) that such contingencies tempt students, perhaps in the hope of more effective learning, to abandon partially or otherwise, the objective form of reasoning in favour of aspects of the subjective idiom. As a result, some dyslexic students may develop a progressively negative disposition towards aspects of the curriculum and hence limit their personal engagement with those forms of motivation which underlie certain levels of the learning experience, levels which may be related to deepening the experience.**

## A closer look at the (a)-(b)-(c) sequence (unsuccessful-frustrating-not recognised as relevant)

With respect to teaching strategies, the above contingencies present the teacher with a considerable challenge. For instance, if a teacher limits a presentation to the 'facts' of the materials involved, the majority of students may follow the exposition with more or less ease, with those given to subjective forms of reasoning selecting whatever items they deem to be relevant. Dyslexic students may behave rather differently from non-dyslexic students. However, in such a situation non-dyslexic students may hope, if so inclined, for the moment of integration to arrive presently, and thus may remain content to allow fragments of information to remain suspended in a state of relative decontextualization.

Dyslexic students (not experiencing sufficient contextualizing), may balk at the struggle to integrate material (often compounded by simultaneous efforts to make notes, which they may find difficult to do at speed), their initial experience of failure being followed by a compulsion to engage in a 'fishing' venture in an effort to find a niche or context of meaning and value into which relevant items may be introduced. It is at this point that concentration risks being lost, focus and attention being engaged in 'fishing' may wander off-topic (that is, away from the teacher's intended direction of argument). Consequently, much material which follows in the course of the teacher's expositions is most likely to be lost, together with its internal logic and conclusion.

For the dyslexic student, the learning experience seems to be disrupted, perhaps even halted at that particular stage, inhibited and prevented from following the teacher's discourse until the desired niche is located, by which time it may be too late for the student to catch up, or the teacher may have proceeded further before the student became fully aware of, and able to formulate, the kind of question that was needed. But, even if the question were raised at a later time, in both contingencies its

---

**This concerns the ease with which students can adapt from visuo-spatial information processing (location of place on their cognitive map) to temporal-linguistic processing (which may be influenced by, and influence timing, pace, flow, rhythm and sequence).

content can serve as an indicator of the nature of the student's problem because it demonstrates an instance in which the dynamics of the student's learning experience was not only diverted, but it also signals the precise juncture at which such an event took place. Once this has been located, the secondary consequences arising out of the student's seeming 'inattention' to the teacher's presentation become more apparent and may be addressed.

Further implications for teachers include the need to go beyond (or look behind) the student's response (i.e. to follow-up with another question). With respect to such situations it should be noted that if the teacher questions the student about the lesson (perhaps as a result of noticing signs that suggest that the student is not 'on track'), the student's response may seem to be not directly connected to the antici-pated content-related answer and seemingly irrelevant answers may be dismissed. If however, the teacher follows up the interaction with at least one further exploratory question, the connections may be revealed (e.g., *'Can you tell me more?' 'Well, can you explain how that links up with what I was saying?'*). But time is seldom taken to follow up exchanges in class beyond the single response so students quickly learn how to avoid asking questions, explaining their problems or trying to provide extended answers, for fear of repeating the experiencing of a sense of failure which is both personal and public.

## Levels of learning experience

The term, 'learning experience' is intended here to take into account the complexity of learning and its penetrating effects on the learner. The expectation is that the dynamics of this kind of experience will yield increasing levels of cognition.*

In this connection it is perhaps unfortunate that the term 'experience' tends to be employed unidimensionally, as if it were not subject to variety and as if it were qualitatively identical for all. For students, such contin-gencies may strongly influence learning responses and, with that, changes in the relevant levels of cognition. Such variations may include the inten-sity, impact and duration, magnitude of penetration (depth, breadth) and its amenability for integration into the context of preceding, simultaneous (or even fantasized) content.

Although the vernacular does provide descriptors for such distinctions, they are used separately, i.e. not in conjunction with the concept of experi-

*Experience: from the Latin, *ex* 'from', *piriri* 'going through'. Mannheim (1964) refers to 'forms of experience which characterize the cognitive mode'. Beqiraj and Carsch, and independently, Moor have made reference to these forms of experience (Hunter-Carsch 1993).

ence. It may therefore be useful to delineate five distinct levels of experience which may be regarded as components of cognition and are prerequisites to awareness at the meta-cognitive level. These distinctions are not,
unfortunately, made in English. The levels are, however, rendered explicit
in German. They are:

- sensing/feeling (*empfinden*)
- becoming aware (*erfahren*)
- going through (*erleben*)
- grasping (*erfassen*)
- comprehending (*erkennen*).

### Sensing/feeling

This relates to sensing or feeling that is experienced or perhaps even
precedes first encounters with an idea or concept. For the individual student
in the classroom/lecture room context, it is mobilized by contextual associations (including prior knowledge) which seem to signal what is coming next
logically in the teacher's presentation. This requires an initial, perhaps very
brief, cognitive experience followed by an affective response which may
become dominant, increasing the intensity of the impact and perhaps deter-
mining its duration. In this manner it sets the stage for whether and how it is
apprehended at subsequent level(s) into which it may be guided by the
teacher's next contribution to the (interactive) learning experience. It is
tentatively generalistic (rather than particularistic) and sometimes described
as 'vibes' or 'ambiances', but its existence cannot be tested empirically.

### Becoming aware

Whereas the preceding level is tentatively aware, this level begins to focus on
the particular, especially if it follows the first level. Its impact is one of
gradual penetration of the new learning experience which brings about a
sense of discovery, eliciting a relatively durable impact. It may involve
stirrings of specific sensory awareness, focusing attention on auditory,
visual, kinaesthetic, tactile or gustatory stimuli, but it does not yet come into
association with other identifiable experiences and conscious awarenesses.

### Going through

This level of 'going on with', 'going through' or 'living through' is closely
related to and often follows the above two levels.* Notably, it is at this level
that prevailing cultural configurations, both pre-existing and on-going,
make their most poignant impact on the learner while simultaneously

---

*The German noun *erleben* ('living through it') is derived from *Leben* ('life' or 'living'),
the prefix 'er-' suggesting an absence of choice.

positing parameters on the teacher. As such it may involve a varying sense of engagement with the experience but not as a consciously decided choice to do so. It may simply be 'endured', either positively or negatively, as the speed of the interactive teaching process does not permit fully conscious definitions. The intensity of the experience at this level, its impact, duration and penetration with cognitive and affective investment may vary considerably between individuals and groups. Yet it is precisely these factors which determine to a large extent the efficacy of subsequent learning. By definition universalistic, if approached in objective reasoning mode, and without affectively based inhibitions, this level promotes the momentum for further/deeper experiencing. In contrast, the beginning of the subjective reasoning mode's filtering tendencies can be found at this level.**

### Grasping

In contrast to the preceding level, this level is essentially particularistic.*** It resembles the level of 'becoming aware' in as much as both forms of experience involve a sudden appreciation of pre-existing material, albeit the two levels are distinct as the experience of 'becoming aware' derives from previously internalized matters indicated in the student's conceptual map, whereas at this level what is being grasped is external. It (the purpose of grasping) resembles its kinesthetic form in the sense that it is usually a prerequisite for the next step in a sequence. It may follow a period of difficulty; it may reflect a sudden penetration, the impact of which may be felt to be an accomplishment thus eliciting the requisite affective response at the appropriate level of intensity followed by cognitive investment. The duration of the experience may be brief, its ultimate impact depending on its significance in the relevant learning sequence. Being particularistic, subjective reasoners may wonder where grasping fits into their conceptual map and may initially resist it as relatively trivial. (It resembles the follow-up of the preceding kinesthetic form of 'grasping' in

---

**The dynamic relationship of these three levels of experience is illustrated in Mannheim's (1964) suggestion that 'the initial levels of experience (of this kind) tend to establish themselves as a "natural" world view, while subsequent ones may be sensed (*empfinden*) as their confirmation, or satiation as their negation and antithesis, reflecting an inward dialectic which is decisive for the formation of consciousness' (pp 536, 538) and that 'past experiences (of this kind) may be rendered conscious and serve as organizing principles for their selective assessment.' (pp 532–3); and also that 'significantly the meanings of this form of experience involves a range from the purely cognitive to the affective.'

***The German verb *fassen* ('to grasp') is modified by the prefix *er-* which limits its denotation to mental phenomena in *erfassen*. This development parallels that of the French verb *apprendre* ('to learn'), itself derived from the Latin *apprehendere* ('to seize'). This parallels the meaning of the English verb 'to grasp', involving both manual and mental phenomena.

the sense that it prompts taking action to 'put something into gear' in order 'to go on' experiencing.)

*Comprehending*

[From Latin *com* ('together with') *prehendere* ('to grasp'), that is, 'to grasp together']. The penultimate level of learning experience, comprehending, optimally synthesizes the experience of becoming aware and going through, and integrates in the conceptual map the experience of grasping.* It is necessarily universalistic and predominantly cognitive. In a sense, on this level, the cognitive dimension incorporates the affectivity mobilized in the course of the preceding levels, and provides its impact with additional intensity for decisive penetration. For subjective reasoners the benefits of this are selective. For users of the objective mode, they accrue.

### Meta-cognition, meta-affectivity and their synthesis into meta-comprehension

Although comprehending is represented in Figure 5.1 as the most complex (seemingly 'highest') of the levels, it is nevertheless the most

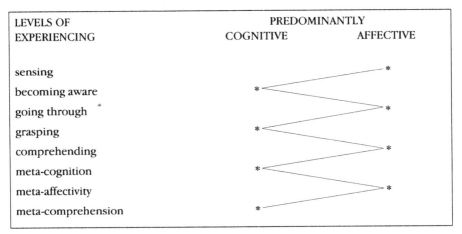

**Figure 5.1** Levels of experiencing and their dynamics

---

*The German noun *Erkennen* is translated almost literally as 're-cognition'. It is derived from the Latin *cognisere* ('to know again'). This double knowledge implies that the process of cognition is taking place on a variety of levels. Mannheim uses the word *Erkennen* in the following two contexts: 'the peculiarity of historical perspectives involves the RECOGNITION of the dynamic nature of historical facts' (p. 399); and also 'as distinct from the exact natural sciences, the methods of the social sciences RECOG-NIZE hierarchies of relative depths of interpretations', p. 293, (author's capitals).

basic of levels at which meta-cognitive experience appears to become accessible. At this level, learners are likely to be able to recognize, label and deal with experience(s) internally. If, however, meta-cognitive aware-ness is not yet (or not readily) accessible, students may not find it easy to explain their mental images or 'how they know'. This relates to all learners, not selectively to those who may be described as dyslexic or those with other areas of special educational needs.

### Dynamics of levels of experiencing

It is not intended that the model encompassing the levels is regarded as representing a series or somehow discrete stages or phases of cognitive development. Rather, the model attempts to represent differing emphases within what can be a fluid or sequential system of experiencing; one which includes affective components. The relationship between the levels is not so much hierarchical as explanatory of a rhythmic and perhaps wave-like relationship between cognitive-affective polarities.*

It is not age-specific, nor does it suggest a particular developmental sequence within experiences for all learners. It might be possible to 'log in' at any level. However, it does appear that it is not until the experience reaches the 'comprehending' level that meta-cognition (awareness of the understanding) comes into play. The previous four levels are thus not yet consciously discriminated in the same manner as the fifth level of experi-encing (see Figure 5.1).

## Apprehending the dynamics of interactive teaching and learning

It cannot be taken as axiomatic that:

- the processes involved in interactive teaching and learning are not easily apprehended, or that;
- the skilled teachers' learned patterns may conduce to the illusion that these processes are easy or it may seem to be 'luck', or;
- that we cannot directly observe the teacher's expectations of the student or the teacher's intentions in the course of an interaction.

We are dependent for our understanding not only on the existence of definitions of such conceptualizations but also on the extent to which we

---

*The longer-term experiencing of time should also be taken into account: the scale of different rhythms of experience (e.g. Whitehead 1932, 'Aims of Education' reference to 'the rhythm of education' as involving phases of 'romance, precision and generalisation').

share assumptions which our particular conceptual maps employ. Increasingly, we are acquiring information through the coming together of researchers across different fields of research (e.g. artificial intelligence and human cognitive studies) which may endorse the importance not only of 'checking our bearings' in terms of our particular field of reference (e.g. to SpLDs) but also of looking at the scene from a different stance. Without confident sharing of our meta-cognitive journeys (including, where relevant, meta-affective) experiences, we may miss whole dimensions, not just events, in our communications.

It is when there occurs the recognition of a mismatch between perceptions, mental images, or what is intended and what happens that, for the teacher, there is an opportunity to examine the process. It may be helpful to label such events as 'potential learning hurdles' (PLHs). They constitute experiences which present a hurdle which may seem to be 'too high to leap over' at first attempt and which requires recognition of the fact, i.e., a re-assessment of the situation. This can relate to either the teacher's perceptions about the student's difficulties or the teacher's own recognition of their own professional potential learning hurdles (PPLHs). This might require mentally (meta-cognitively), standing back to judge 'the height of the required jump', then perhaps a concerted effort concentrated into a 're-run and higher leap', followed perhaps by even further substantial training before making another attempt.

Such opportunities leading to recognition of the student's hurdle may be suggested to be occurring within the parameters of the student's 'Zone of Proximal Development' (ZPD) (Vygotsky 1962; Wood 1998).

## Contributions of the proposed model

These are four main areas to which the proposed model makes a contribution. These are discussed below. They involve the provision of an operational vocabulary, a diagnostic framework, a recognition of the role of affectivity, and the coincidence of factors affecting learning.

First the provision of the theoretical model contributes by its creation of an operational vocabulary for making distinctions between critical aspects of learning which affect decisions about teaching, together with proposals of criteria for assessing efficacy of the student's learning process which simultaneously prompts teachers to re-examine their personal cognitive maps relating to the dynamics of the student's learning experience, particularly that of dyslexic students.

Secondly, it contributes by providing a framework for designing an exploratory and diagnostic procedure for systematic understanding of students' learning experiences, especially with respect to variables which are not immediately apparent. The proposed model does this by distinguishing between forms of reasoning and their relationship to various levels of cognition. Such diagnostic strategies may be useful in the identification of individual students or groups who are vulnerable to exclusion from access to potentially useful forms of reason, which as a result, may compound their specific learning difficulties.

Thirdly, it places emphasis on the appreciation of the role of affectivity in the learning experience. In this sense, affectivity is seen as a facilitator of the student's approach to learning, as shown through the extent of their interest (penetration) and readiness to engage their attention towards harnessing their memory (duration) and willingness to integrate aspects of learning into their personal conceptual map (locating/contextualizing learning content). The impact the student allows teaching/learning and mental experience to make is thus ultimately related to their motivation.

Fourthly, it contributes by drawing attention to the dynamics of a series of factors associated with the learning experience, and to the dangers of measuring components separately.

In summary, the contribution of the proposed model is thus to indicate the manner in which it is likely that meta-cognitive activity, without the relevant accompanying meta-affective awareness, may preclude progressive integration of understanding towards the synthesis which, it has been suggested, needs a conceptually discrete descriptor, such as 'meta-comprehension'.

For specialist teacher-training purposes it might be further suggested that, the model may provide a useful framework for professional discussion of PLHs and PPLHs in a manner which, like the Reading Recovery Specialist Training observation and analysis, as employed by Clay (1993), provides opportunities for 'micro-teaching'.

## Limitations of the model and implications for further research

The model is both tentative and exploratory in nature. It does not provide detailed teaching prescriptions for the specific event. Evidence generated by research employing other theoretical models' implications for practice needs to be more fully explored in comparison to materials which may be provided through the application of this model in order to test the extent of its 'best fit' in the quest to explain the relevant dynamics. Such investigations might include Donaldson's (1992) model which provides an epigenetic table suggesting the progressive integration of thought and emotion to the most advanced modes which she describes as 'intellectual transcendent' and 'value-sensing transcendent'. There are also other models from meta-cognitive social psychology which explore attitudinal factors (Nelson et al. 1998) and studies of social influences on memory (e.g. Bless and Strack 1998) which may shed light on some facets of the model and also raise issues about reliability of self-reports which are factors of importance to be taken into account in any investigative work involved in social contexts.

Taken in conjunction with some of the materials from social meta-cognicists' investigations, and along with research emerging from neuropsychological studies employing MRI technology, future work may turn to further exploration of the subtle psychosocial factors which are anticipated to be illuminated by employing the proposed model. Future studies might include exploration of the high incidence of dyslexia in the prison population, with a view to exploring the vulnerability of this particular subgroup in terms of their reflective accounts of their educational experience and current examination of their characteristic forms of reasoning and meta-cognitive awareness of their own levels of experiencing of particular learning events.

Additionally, there are currently fashionable models of cognitive style some of which refer to 'left hemisphere and right hemisphere' preferences (e.g. Riding and Raynor 1998; Given and Reid 1999). These might prompt the suggestion that with reference to the illustration of the proposed model (see Figure 5.1) the columns representing 'predominantly cognitive' and 'predominantly affective' can be regarded as directly comparable to left and right hemisphere preferences (i.e. that the cognitive may be linked with 'particularistic' and affective with 'universalistic') and that the further association can be made between the 'analytical–synthesizing' dimension.

However, it may not be so simple. The proposed model addresses issues of the direction of the dynamic, not only its origins and impetus, or even strength, but seeks to understand how it propels the engagement with experience. For example, it may not be particularly helpful to describe an individual dyslexic (or non-dyslexic) learner as a synthesist rather than an analyst without also describing/appreciating what makes possible the activation of the relevant directional shift when it is required and how readily the appropriate shifts can be made, as well as the quality under optimal conditions, of the relevant kind of 'thinking'. Thus it is a directional dynamic that is vital to understand and that may contribute to explaining cause and effect.

It is perhaps in the sense of illuminating the dynamics of motivation that the model may be of assistance. The levels of experience can more readily be appreciated when the forms of reasoning are seen as motivational directors of the experience. If, for example, the student is motivated to engage in the subjective form rather than the objective form of reasoning, it is likely that at the level of 'going through' there may be a 'block' in response to certain experiences intended by the teacher. The 'invisible wall' remains invisible to both student and teacher unless, somehow, the teacher recognizes the signs of its existence and the student can be brought to 'see through' or 'go through' somehow to 'grasp onto' some facet of the experience and recognize the potential of the experience. There may then be some chance that the teacher (operating in objective mode and at the 'comprehending' level and beyond, with both affective and cognitive sensitivities) may, in recognizing the student's dilemma, exercise greater tolerance of this seeming impasse, on the part of the student, be able to formulate some idea and 'communication avenue' through which it may become clear to the student that engaging with the learning experience will be worthwhile. This constitutes 'the scaffolding of learning within the ZPD'. This kind of scaffolding relies on the use of affective as well as cognitive building bricks. In teaching emergent adults and adults, as distinct from young children, the scaffolding comes to rely more and more upon verbal interaction as a means of mobilizing meta-cognitive (and meta-affective) activity. The 'qualitatively rich data' (e.g. from conversation with the learner) may provide evidence of both meta-affective and meta-cognitive awareness and the use to which such awarenesses are put (i.e. the directional development towards metacomprehension).

It has been mentioned earlier that to come to a judgment about the student's level of experiencing on the basis of a conversational interaction, the teacher may require to listen carefully to more than a single response to a question. It may take reflective analysis of several exchanges before the teacher can gain a sense of the student's attitude and extent of interest in the point under discussion and begin to discern the extent of the student's awareness of both personal and contextual factors affecting understanding of the content of the discussion.

In conclusion, the model provides a diagnostic framework for exploring PLHs and PPLHs. It illustrates ways in which it is likely that reduced motivation to learn certain kinds of curriculum content may have a compounding impact on some dyslexic students' potential to deepen their learning experience sufficiently to begin to engage both meta-cognitive and meta-affective awareness in the process of trying to make learning meaningful (i.e. the direction towards meta-comprehension). By understanding the dynamics of the impact of the suggested subtle psychosocial factors leading to the restricted use of certain forms of reasoning which thus impede the individual's further development, the teacher has a means of more readily coming to informed decisions about how to assist the student.

Clearly, engagement in reflective conversational exchanges even in the relatively discreet environment of the individual tutorial, requires considerable trust and self-confidence on the part of the learner, and sensitivity as well as professional skill on the part of the teacher/diagnostician (see also McLoughlin 2001; Herrington 2001a; Chappell and Walker 2001). There is much to be studied and researched in practice on the part of teachers before generalizations can safely be made about the implications of findings based on work with this tentative model, for different kinds of teaching, learning contexts, and for different age groups. It remains likely that the road to increasing 'understanding of understanding' will be one on which the student's contributions in classroom interactions can inspire the teacher sometimes to risk taking 'the less travelled road' (Frost 1955) and together, they may find perhaps unanticipated routes to effective learning.

# Chapter 6
# A social interactive model of Specific Learning Difficulties, e.g. Dyslexia

MARGARET HERRINGTON AND MORAG HUNTER-CARSCH

---

Questions addressed in this chapter include:

- What are the most frequently raised questions in the field of SpLDs, e.g. dyslexia?
- What are the authors' responses to these questions?
- How might learning support for dyslexic learners be integrated into a framework of support for all?
- What are the implications for teachers?

---

## Introduction

In the course of working together on the editing of a separate publication, (Hunter-Carsch and Herrington 2001) we were privileged to have the opportunity of corresponding and conversing with contributing authors. In this way we were able to relate our own conversation about research and practice in the field to the range of contributors' perspectives. We discovered not only that we each shared certain perspectives but also that we brought different emphases and experiences to the conversation. The similarities and differences which we were discovering in our own views, along with our discussions about the various writers' contributions, brought into focus the different ways in which researchers and practitioners think and talk about dyslexia. For example, some discussed 'in-person' characteristics of dyslexic learners; others addressed contextual factors; some engaged with particular theoretical questions and others were more concerned with practical responses to the realities facing learners. The nature and complexity of issues of theory and practice and their interrelationships became increasingly evident in our shared quest for clarity.

We deepened our appreciation of the range of questions which continue to be debated in this field and found ourselves having to organize the questions for our own purposes. We classified them broadly into five categories:

- the nature of dyslexia;
- assessment issues;
- teaching and learning methods and approaches (and whether these differ from those used for non-dyslexic students);
- training and professional development of staff;
- the research agenda.

(See also the Appendix which refers to all the above categories).

Our conversation necessarily addressed issues which underpin the provision of effective learning support for dyslexic students in the compulsory education sector, as well as in further and higher education. As one of us worked mainly with teachers of young children and adolescents and the other with adult students and teachers of adults, we were in a position to discuss areas of overlap and differences in our perceptions and priorities, our professional experience, the stance we each held and what we believed to be the characteristic interests and concerns among our colleagues across the sectors. We are grateful to the students, teachers and researchers who have contributed both directly and indirectly to the conversation which we now invite readers to share.

In the first section we attempt to draw together the questions raised most frequently and to make our own responses to them. The obligation to go further on the journey of 'bridging the secondary–tertiary education divide', which we undertook for a separate publication, (Hunter-Carsch and Herrington 2001) led us to attempt to create a shared framework to support the learning of dyslexic students. We outline this framework – which seeks to re-integrate support for dyslexic learners with broader notions of learning support for all.

In the second section a wider integrative model, which takes the framework into account is presented, and its implications for teachers are discussed.

## The nature of dyslexia

The question which still puzzles many educators, learners and members of the public concerns the actual nature of dyslexia. The problems of definition remain and are discussed more fully elsewhere (see chapters 2 and 7; also DECP 1999). Snippets of information which reach busy practitioners from snatched reading and media information present a confusing mix:

reading and spelling problems, genes are responsible, brain waves are different, dyslexics are right-brained three-dimensional thinkers, artists, engineers, architects, etc.

Although there is agreement in much of the literature about some of the identifying features of dyslexia, there is no single 'story' about dyslexia which convinces at all levels and in all sectors. Some dyslexia activists (and parents of dyslexic children) hold the view that it is an inherited disorder and seek early identification and treatment. Primary school teachers face increased pressure to identify early, but their level of knowledge is not always well-developed and the implications for teaching are not always clear to them. In so far as secondary teachers are aware of dyslexia issues (and this is still a very mixed picture) many are still puzzled by the problems at the heart of the debate and remain anxious about unfairly allocating resources to one group with learning difficulties at the expense of others. Such concerns can impede and even effectively paralyse teachers in terms of identifying and responding to dyslexia.

In higher education many teachers are prepared to acknowledge a disability but are unclear about the significance of the uncertainties about definition and assessment. Even educational psychologists who, by virtue of the Code of Practice (DfEE 1994), have become the official identifiers of this 'condition' hold very different views about the validity of the syndrome (Pumfrey and Reason 1991, 1996; DECP 1999). The mantra of 'early diagnosis and treatment' does not take adequate account of this complexity.

Given these uncertainties, there remains a central dilemma across all sectors about how to communicate about dyslexia in ways which others understand. Even when teachers do attempt to develop their understanding, professional development courses do not always encourage a critical stance. Course participants may be trained with a deficit model of SpLDs, without adequate consideration of interesting questions about enhanced skills or without a sufficiently critical understanding of ways in which literacies are perceived and valued. They do not, therefore, always derive from their training a conceptual and linguistic framework for SpLDs of sufficient breadth and depth to inform their discussions with parents, colleagues and other professionals.

Learners, who have most to gain from being able to describe their dyslexia to non-dyslexic people, often have to rely on the use of reports from educational psychologists which may make little sense to them. Relief at diagnosis is often followed by *'But what does this mean? I haven't quite got hold of this'*. These data rarely give learners the vocabulary to describe their dyslexia and so dyslexic students themselves often find it difficult to describe to each other as well as to non-dyslexic people what it means for them. Often, they are restricted to listing their *difficulties* and *problems*.

Even more profoundly, the dynamics of learning processes and language problems still present major challenges for researchers and practitioners. Perhaps this is not surprising as there is considerable variation, even among professionals, in vocabulary and frames of reference for describing normal language, literacy and learning development (see chapters 1 and 5), not to mention diversity of learning difficulties, including SpLDs.

In our view, although it is perfectly reasonable to feel confused and uncertain, given the present state of knowledge and the gaps between the disciplines, it is not justifiable to use such uncertainties as a reason for not exploring further. We therefore offer our own thoughts to illustrate our way of attempting to resolve some of them for ourselves. The following discussion is organized under six subheadings:

- dyslexia, literacy and non-literacy parameters;
- assumed connections;
- an 'including' framework;
- using the framework;
- implications for identification of dyslexia;
- implications for teaching and learning support.

### Dyslexia, literacy and non-literacy parameters

Many accounts of dyslexia start with the notion of 'difficulty with words' and identify areas of language and literacy with which dyslexic learners usually have difficulty. The recent tautologous working definition offered by the Working Party of the British Psychological Society (DCEP 1999), for example, focuses entirely on literacy difficulties. There are clear advantages in this approach. Literacy difficulties are often the first to be noticed in the education system and it is the challenge that dyslexic learners pose to conventional ideas about the relationship between literacy and intellectual ability which often results in such problems for them. It is also useful because whilst others may debate endlessly about whether there is a 'condition/syndrome', the reality is that it is the literacy difficulties which must be addressed if learners are to succeed in educational settings.

However, there are also profound weaknesses in this position. First, there is a tendency to view literacy difficulties through a school-based literacy rather than a 'New Literacy Studies' lens. Dyslexic learners are viewed as having problems with literacy because they have problems with *doing* the literacy which school and college requires and within the timescales set. The notion that it may be possible to have such a difficulty and yet be able to produce publishable literature or be able to engage successfully with literacy activities outside school or college tends not to be entertained. A lack of any serious questioning about the rationale for linking literacy and time in the way it occurs in school and colleges, is common. This fundamental matter of the power issues embedded in the 'schooling of literacy' dominance (Street and Street 1991) cannot be side-stepped in this way.

A second weakness is that if primary and secondary causal factors are not distinguished, inappropriate teaching approaches may be produced; strategies may be devised to impact on secondary factors and fail to address primary factors. For example, the dilemma of dyslexia coexisting with attention deficit hyperactivity disorder (ADHD) may present teachers with conflicts about priorities with reference to structured teaching versus therapeutic counselling approaches.

A third weakness is that in side-stepping the question of distinguishing between causal factors and their effects, it becomes difficult to answer the common question of whether all those with persistent literacy difficulties are dyslexic. There is a tendency by dyslexic learners to view their difficulties with literacy as essentially different from others. But we do not know that this is the case for all aspects of literacy for 'undiagnosed' learners. Dyslexia may be more obvious in the absence of other causal factors, but it may also be present alongside such factors.

Perhaps a key word here is 'persistent'. Many factors have been cited as contributing to difficulties with literacy: lack of opportunity, lack of home support, poverty, moderate learning difficulties etc. and whilst there are some obvious senses in which such claims may be valid, it is not completely clear why they should necessarily produce persistent difficulties with literacy in school; and individual and institutional perceptions may vary in this respect. However, in our view, the presence of such factors should not be used as a reason for avoiding consideration of SpLDs or of persistent weakness in teaching methods. In our view, any persistence of literacy difficulty after years of regular schooling could be a signal for some degree of dyslexia.

Finally, the literacy focus encourages a view of dyslexia as solely a literacy problem rather than as a phenomenon involving a range of literacy and non-literacy parameters. This side-steps a whole raft of insights and evidence about patterns of perceiving, thinking and learning which are now associated with dyslexia (West 1991; Davis 1994; Hetherington 1996; Hunter 1981; 1982). Yet professional educators need to explore these so that they can be sure of developing appropriate responses to dyslexic learners and also to alert themselves in general to the variations in learning approaches within their classrooms. Dyslexia involves more than difficulties with literacy and, though we do not have very much statistical evidence about the range and incidence of the suggested broader dyslexic parameters, it would be remarkably incurious to ignore or refuse to explore them. Such a position would inhibit the development of understanding about the kind of curriculum required by dyslexic learners or about enrichment of the curriculum for all which dyslexic learners may bring.

## Assumed connections

Before discussing these broader parameters, it is important to reiterate that we view with some caution the loose assertions about the links between biological bases, processing factors and observed literacy outcomes. Morton and Frith's (1995) framework for showing these different levels of explanation for dyslexia (identified also by the Leicester University Adult Dyslexia Research Group in 1988) allows an interesting classification of research findings but is often used to suggest links which are not yet proven. We always appear to be looking backwards from a range of literacy/numeracy difficulties to the processing weaknesses profile which could account for these to their likely biological bases. There is a subsequent tendency to think quite simply in terms of a physiological condition/neural structures et al . . . leading to certain processing weaknesses which, in turn, lead to literacy difficulties. Most recently, the same biological and processing linking is evident in discussions about possible strengths of dyslexia: certain parts of the brain are often identified as working well for dyslexic thinkers and artists.

This is not to rule out biological bases for dyslexia. At a reductionist level there must be a biological base for this cerebral functioning anomaly/ phenomenon/difference and there is growing evidence regarding heritability. Of more practical help, however, is the fact that evidence from dyslexic adults in particular suggests a 'physicality' in their experience of handling words in the brain (Herrington 2001a). Powerful descriptions are available about 'blockages', 'too few channels for information in and out of memory', 'overgrown pathways', 'sudden shutdowns' etc. It is not known whether non-dyslexic learners use similar imagery given the opportunity to describe their literacy processes, but the fact that physical descriptions are used suggests at the very least that neuro-anatomical evidence may be able to provide some evidence to explain such sensations.

However, we do not yet have unequivocal evidence that these relationships between biological bases, processing and literacy/numeracy and other features are uni-directional, stable, causal relationships. The examples below may clarify:

• The classification of stable, transient and late emergers among dyslexic school students suggests at least that these relationships do not exist equally for all dyslexics. We know that literacy indicators change over time which may be attributable to different degrees of phonological difficulty/developmental factors and/or different contexts. Clearly, the relationship between processing weaknesses and literacy outcomes is not a simple one.

- There are also differences/inconsistencies, not just over time but within and between days. Whatever the proposed connections, they must account for quite sudden variations in handling language and literacy. Dyslexia does not appear to be a 'once and for all' weakness, unchanging in its manifestations. Changes in biochemistry appear to be implicated.

- We cannot be sure whether we face a scenario in which one main deficit (central nervous system dysfunction, working memory inefficiency or automaticity deficit etc.) accounts for all observed behaviours (which may go beyond literacy and include time management, motor skills and numeracy) or whether these behaviours involve strengths/weaknesses in a range of neurological sites and processes.

- We cannot be certain about how literacy and other dyslexic characteristics are connected. We are only just beginning to understand how a phonological deficit could be related to perceptions of time and thence possibly to time management problems (Miller and Tallal 1995; von Steinbuchel et al. 1996 in Haase 2000). We do not know how this relates to the experience of time as a separate dimension (Herrington 2001b) nor the implications with reference to cognitive style (see Chapter 5; also Zdzienski 2001). It is therefore not easy always to make sense of variations within dyslexia. It seems most unsatisfactory when discussions start and end with, 'Well, everyone is different'. This is obviously true but it does not help us to determine the outer limits of the syndrome, nor who should be included in the syndrome and who should not.

- We cannot be confident that a single processing deficit (phonological) is the defining feature of what we think of as dyslexia. A great deal of useful work has been done on this issue which helps us to understand the phonological processes involved. And we recognize that such problems are experienced by many dyslexic learners and appear to persist into adulthood, irrespective of so-called compensation. However, there are some dangers: links between auditory difficulties associated with dyslexia and literacy difficulties are not completely clear. Goulandris et al. (2001) and Poussu-Olli (see Chapter 8) indicate that there are some degrees of phonological difficulty which are not sufficient to prevent improvements in literacy skills. Further, emphasis on the auditory (including phonological processing) should not distract from investigations of visual, kinaesthetic (and possibly also cerebellar processing) and other possible causal factors such as subtle metabolic and general health issues, nor about possible relationships between these. Nor should it mask the cumulative effects on learners of mild difficulties in several areas. Further, whilst phonological features may seem particularly marked in children, presenting features among adults are a complex mixture and it seems simplistic to consider this selectively as a phonological deficit problem. Finally, the reality for some learners is one of multiple difficulties (dyslexia, ADHD) shading into general health issues, 'supersensitivities', problems with allergies, depression and other vulnerabilities. Clearly, if dyslexia is defined as involving a single deficit then we have to seek alternative descriptors for learners who seem to fall outside this category, but who clearly have specific learning difficulties involving literacy. We would prefer to maintain a more open position in which phonological weaknesses are understood to play an important part for many dyslexic learners but which cannot be seen as a core identifier.

• We do not yet know fully the effect of an intervening variable, such as teaching effectiveness, on literacy outcomes. This argument is that 'if the teaching is good enough then literacy difficulties disappear'. If a school curriculum is sufficiently differentiated or an adult curriculum sufficiently in the hands of adults themselves then an identified set of special methods is not required. There are sufficient models and methods to respond to all. Our experience in tertiary education tends to suggest that whilst this may be true to some extent, and that literacy difficulties do recede, some re-tooling of the staff's focus in the light of dyslexia and its implications in the environment is usually necessary if dyslexic learners are to feel acknowledgement and response.

Frith (1995) and others (DECP 1999) recognized the importance of environment in shaping these processes at all levels, but there does not appear to be a broad-based attempt to integrate models of dyslexia with either radical perspectives of literacy or social models of disability. The dominant paradigm is still one of 'in-person' weaknesses rather than one which shows quite clearly that it is the specific values which are attached to particular concepts and standards of literacy and numeracy which largely shape the way in which dyslexia is perceived and experienced. It is substantially these perspectives which make dyslexia disabling. Those in other cultural contexts, with different concepts of literacies and different expectations of individuals, would not necessarily regard such people as 'impaired' and learners would not be made to feel disabled.

This 'disabling' framework also tends to focus on cognitive matters to the neglect of affect. Adults have already identified some direct connections between lack of understanding from those around them (family, peers, educators and members of the public) and their consequent emotional difficulties. Fawcett (1996) described the pressure on dyslexic learners of simply trying to keep going, and a range of stress factors has been identified. However, we suspect that the relationship between cognition and affect in dyslexia is more profound than has yet been formally investigated (Moore 1995; and Chapter 5) and consider that understanding this relationship is probably key to the generation of effective learning. We suspect that hypersensitivities are involved in many cases and that these can contribute to blocks in cognition. Lack of perceived warmth (open, responsive, interested, unjudgemental) in the tutor may be interpreted as opposition or even attack and a full 'flight' response may be activated.

## A framework

We would prefer a research/assessment/teaching framework in which the multi-faceted, dynamic nature of dyslexia is recognized and explored. This broader framework be understood as:

- including more than literacy difficulties;
- involving more than the characteristic cognitive profile;
- including whole-person factors and the developing dynamics of the cognitive-affective constellation with 'personality' aspects;
- including how interaction with values and practices with regard to literacy and to disability occurs.

It reflects a move from the known to the relatively unknown in an attempt to get closer to the actual characteristics of dyslexic learners in non-test situations.

This preference for broader parameters has emerged as a result of close listening to the voices of learners. Adult learners, in particular, have articulated clear messages for all teachers in relation to dyslexia and there should now be more explicit recognition of the creative contribution of adult learners to this field and the significance of links between their evidence and more formally collected experimental data. As adults, they rediscover their mix of talents (often through success in vocational settings) and begin to challenge the narrow learning focus of some types of schooling. They are often parents and are the first to see dyslexia in their children. Increasingly, they are writing about what dyslexia is actually like from the inside. They have shown us from their experience the limitations of current assessment methods, the value of particular kinds of description and the need for a power-sharing approach in the development of effective practice. Without their contributions, primary sources of evidence about any particular cluster of SpLDs are simply not accessed.

We also believe that this broader framework allows us to make some kind of sense of different clusters of difficulties and strengths within the dyslexia syndrome and the overlap with other types of SpLDs. However, we recognize the problems which this can involve in relation to current funding arrangements in some sectors. There is some pressure for the identification of more and more discrete categories of difficulty with associated 'pathologies' so that monies will only be allocated to those designated as 'in need'. Those who do not quite fit within existing dyslexia profiles, but who do have some specific learning difficulties, are often excluded or are included only by stretching the definition.

However as educators, our challenge is to learn more about how people learn, and if these categories focus on deficits rather than strengths, without having essential and related investigations of ways of supporting learners then the value of employing them is unclear. There may be potential advantages when categories produce particular insights (e.g. non-verbal learning difficulties Mellanby et al. 1996; Hartas 1998), but these still tend to focus on labels and descriptors which are insufficient to explain the dynamics of what may be idiosyncratic patterns of learning. It appears to us therefore that the priority is to devote research resources to allowing learners and tutors to lead the way in establishing demonstrably effective learning and then to explore the implications of their methods for general group teaching situations, rather than to seek to identify further subgroups within SpLDs.

This preference for a broader framework and, ultimately, for wider appreciation of learning differences rather than focusing on difficulties and disability does not allow us to side-step the challenge of saying where dyslexia ends and where non-dyslexia begins. However, we prefer to consider dyslexia in terms of 'continua' and our preferred image is a series of multi-dimensional continua, which include all the characteristics associated with dyslexia. This allows us not only to consider relationships between characteristics but also to consider relationships between dyslexia and other SpLDs. This reduces the danger of single-factor descriptors which may inhibit exploration (see Appendix A, Hunter's 1981, 1982, multidisciplinary matrix for profiling abilities and difficulties across psycho-neurological, psycho-dynamic and psycho-educational factors).

The 'in-person' characteristics associated with dyslexia are listed and a continuum of severity is attached to each, relating to the entire population. Most of these are considered as areas of difficulty, but they should not be deemed to be discrete. The starred items represent areas of potential strength or even outstanding ability. A second dimension is that of time

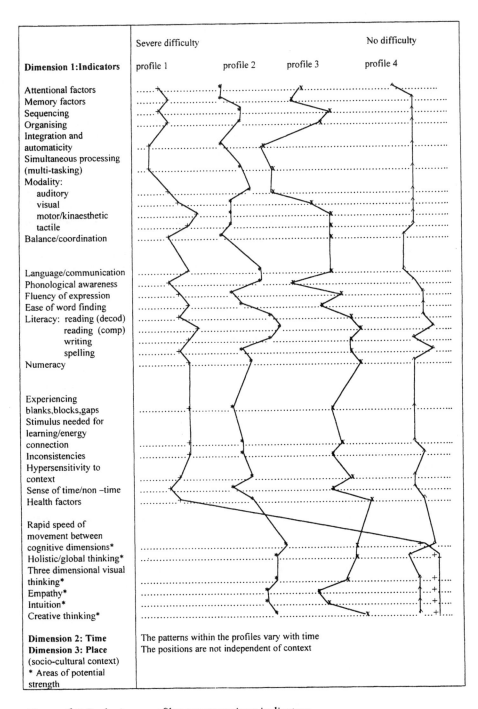

**Figure 6.1** Dyslexia as profiles across various indicators

and these variables are represented as moving in relation to time. A third dimension involves educational and socio-cultural contexts. The 'in-person' characteristics are not deemed to be independent of context.

## Using the framework

Figure 6.1 suggests that when all characteristic difficulties are experienced to a severe degree (1), the condition may look discrete. When these are accompanied by exceptional strengths in the starred categories, the impression of a discrete condition may be reinforced. It is also possible to construct what looks like a non-dyslexic profile (4) (i.e. with no recorded evidence in any areas of difficulty). Such a profile may or may not be accompanied by the strengths starred in the above Figure. Certainly, the presence of such strengths does not necessarily suggest a dyslexia profile. It is possible to have high literacy skills and these other skills.

The main challenge for diagnosis/description lies in the middle ground and in deciding what constitutes significant strength or weakness and perhaps indicators of subgroup patterns. With reference to the middle ground we prefer to view this through a SpLDs lens and consider a severe degree of difficulty (whether consistent or varying from day to day) in any of the unstarred items to be worthy of recognition and exploration of the implications in individuals' particular circumstances. A profile such as (3) which involves two frequently co-existent areas of dyslexic difficulty could be described as involving only two specific difficulties and not amounting to a full profile, or as a residual full dyslexic profile in which many areas of weakness had been overcome. Within the population at large it is not uncommon to find individuals with only one or two of these characteristics, but without longitudinal evidence or evidence which suggests 'compensation', it is not possible to make a judgement about the presence of dyslexia.

It is important, in our view, to be as clear as possible here about the use of the term 'compensation'. There are dangers in considering that it is a once and for all process in all cases. Our experience suggests that at least for some learners, the term 'compensating' should be used because it is an ongoing process and it often has to be actively sustained. This can involve considerable expenditure of energy and so does not entirely remove the burdens. More profoundly, we think it necessary to explore:

- the actual quality of experience of writing from a 'compensating' perspective and whether certain elements become automatic, or whether there are always stages and strategies to go through?
- the neurology of compensation? Are new pathways being created or new uses for existing pathways being found?
- the extent to which individuals are conscious of their own developments;

- the dynamics of the relationship between strengths and weaknesses, e.g. ways in which strengths are employed to avoid or circumnavigate the implications of the difficulties and the directional dynamics of cause and effect. This will enable us to establish whether or not compensation becomes sufficiently reliable in all relevant situations.

The final profile to be considered is (2). This involves a pattern of strengths and weaknesses which presents less extreme variations but yet in which many or all of the characteristics are included. This raises the question of how significantly different the pattern of strengths and weaknesses needs to be from that of the rest of the population for a declaration as 'dyslexic'.

This representation of dyslexia makes no claim to special insights. Rather, it is an organizational device with which newcomers to the field can see the kind of factors which cluster, to differing degrees, over time. It helps in dealing with a problem, which many people have, of making sense of variations in clusters and degrees of what they are told is a 'neurological disorder' in relation to what they know of their own learning style. A frequently heard response is, *'Well, we all have bits of that'*.

## Implications for identifying dyslexia

To argue for 'continua' does not allow us to escape the question of the location on the continua at which the dyslexia 'cut-off' line is drawn. It seems to us that this is fairly arbitrary and the use of discrepancy measures from agreed descriptors of 'normality' rests on the assumption that relevant norms (reliable and valid) are well-established for all the characteristics. This is not the case for adults. However, it may be possible to identify a profile which shows no characteristic dyslexic weaknesses at all, and for less clear-cut cases, decisions for funding purposes should be made by assessing the cluster and degree in relation to the demands of context. This is particularly important in higher education where relatively mild degrees of difficulty can be experienced but which have major consequences for studying at that level. In 1999, personnel in one university were placed in the invidious position of challenging local education authorities' (LEAs') decisions about disabled students' allowances because LEAs considered that students were not 'dyslexic enough' on the basis of WAIS scores etc. to require support, and yet university tutors could see that their students were struggling with the higher education context. Clearly, the dynamics of specific areas of functioning, rather than just global measures, must be considered when deciding where boundaries lie.

It is also important to reaffirm that measures of estimated general intelligence cannot be an essential part of the decision about the whereabouts of dyslexia boundaries since dyslexic characteristics are found across the ability range. So, to be seeking to focus attention and resources for dyslexia only upon those with average or above-average intelligence scores seems odd. It is understandable when the battle has been to persuade educators to recognize that 'low' school literacy skills did not mean low intelligence, but to replace one unfairness with another is not helpful. Continued identification of SpLDs by 'the discrepancy method of assessment' (by comparing achievement levels with levels of measured general intelligence) produces some odd results, and these are especially noticeable among higher education students. It is not unheard of to find students in higher education with a raft of positive dyslexia indicators (and reasonable A-Level grades) who are coping with degree-level study and whose intelligence test results suggest below-average intelligence. They have been deemed not to be dyslexic by official assessors.

Given these complexities it is important to reiterate the rationale for seeking to draw the line at all. This is twofold:

• Within the current educational contexts some cognitive-affective constellations make management of the academic curriculum extremely hard. Students have made clear that they need recognition by their teachers about the nature of their struggle.
• The revelatory insight which such recognition can afford both learners and tutors is essential for the success of some students and for the ongoing development of their teachers.

## Implications for teaching and learning support

It is evident from the above that different concepts of dyslexia can lead to different approaches to assessment and teaching. Those for whom 'dyslexia' is the preferred term, rather than 'SpLDs', may also consider that it is a distinctive neurological disorder, involving problems with some kinds of phonological processing; it should be identified as early as possible by an educational psychologist and treated with a multi-sensory approach by a specialist teacher. Research is driven by professionals within several major disciplines. Whilst this approach is not without merit in terms of some learner outcomes, other writers question this view at each level: 'disorder'?, discrete?, single parameter?, existing 'tests'?, the precise nature of 'the multi-sensory approach'?, type of specialist training?, generalist educator roles?, research focus too narrow?

As noted, funding pressures push staff into seeking quick identification methods and providing a remedial response. The more limited paradigm has advantages in this situation, but in schools this can lead to assessments which focus on what is deemed to be the main disabling component, to the subsequent allocation to one of three categories of difficulty (speech, language and communication; SpLDs, e.g. dyslexia; motor and co-ordination difficulties) and to provision which risks failure to address other areas of need. Two dangers in all education sectors are that the deficit view may continue to dominate as assessors look for key weaknesses and that there is an assumption that what needs to be done by way of remediation is both well-known and relatively simple (the 'structured multi-sensory approach').

It has already been noted that the first of these approaches (the deficit view) is proving less and less helpful as a way of viewing dyslexia. However, this broader framework requires more open-ended and dynamic methods of assessment. Strengths as well as weaknesses need to be identified, questions need to be raised about the unusual descriptions which learners provide and assessment in relation to context is key. It is not difficult to spot the classic characteristics as a minimal position, but the challenge of assessment lies in all the grey areas, in all the different spiky profiles, and across all literacy and learning situations.

The second assumption is an oversimplified one. 'Structured multi-sensory teaching' may be helpful as a genre label but is an insufficiently precise descriptor of what is required for individuals in particular contexts (see Chapter 4). We know that learner development and the building of learners' self-knowledge, self-esteem, confidence, control and balance are at the heart of effective learning support. To this end we know about the need to make learning structures and contexts explicit; the avoidance of short-term memory overload and the value of exploring which mix of sensory inputs may be generally more effective with individual students. Yet, there is much that we do not know and which we can only know through more research with and by dyslexic learners and there are signs within this volume (and in Hunter-Carsch and Herrington 2001) of practitioners seeking a broader framework within which SpLDs can be addressed.

In summary, we consider that it is not helpful to view dyslexia through a narrow lens of 'in-person' weakness. We prefer a broader framework which:

- draws on research from many disciplines and traditions;
- reflects an integrated holistic view of the learners and deeper models of the mind;
- takes full account of the disabling effects of some ideas embedded in the culture about literacy and intelligence/educability;
- adopts a more open-minded and exploratory approach to unravelling the broader parameters of thinking and learning styles of this kind.

Given that the main problem appears to lie in the way these 'differences' are viewed by those who do not demonstrate difficulties of this kind, a social model of disability would be an effective basis on which to build policy. Given that some of the common ideas about 'literacy standards' are the dominant force in manufacturing the 'disability', a more 'radical literacies' perspective would be appropriate. This would involve the explicit recognition of the language and power issues at the heart of notions about literacy standards, which are too often side-stepped in areas of multi-literacies and multi-lingualism.

There are live issues, questions and challenges here for professional educators. More searching questions must be asked about failure to learn; and the easy dismissal of dyslexia as 'a middle-class disease', or maintaining a blindness to patterns of learning difference, are not serious professional positions. Teachers can avoid simplistic descriptions of dyslexia (bizarre spellings, letters and words the wrong way round) and can confidently take the lead in inviting learners to explore and describe how they learn best. Given the relative powerlessness of some dyslexic learners in many educational contexts, the effectiveness of learner support depends heavily on the professionalism of teachers:

* on the depth of their 'focus';
* on their ability to engage in explorations with learners;
* on their ability to understand and manage 'difference';
* on their ability to deal with matters of sharing power of certain kinds with learners.

## An integrative model

In the light of these conclusions, we propose a general social interactionist model of learning support for dyslexic students in all sectors which explicitly locates personal and individual issues within a broad matrix of contexts.

We suggest that the direction of focus of all tutors/teachers can usefully be informed by an understanding of the functional relationship Herrington represents this as follows:

$$Ls\ req = f\ (L, P, PC, D, EC, PSC)$$

where: Ls req = learning support required by any dyslexic learner; L = learners themselves (personality, qualities etc.); P = past experience of the student (education, personal etc.); PC = current personal context; D = dyslexic cluster of characteristics; EC = educational context in which they have to operate; PSC = political, social, cultural context.

**Figure 6.2** Learning Support: functional relationships (Herrington 2001).

This represents the view that any learning support required will be governed by the interplay of specific dyslexic clusters, learners' personalities, personal context, professional norms dominating in the educational context and a whole raft of cultural (especially social/political) factors governing our ideas about disability, about intelligence and literacies (Herrington 2001b). Figure 6.3 provides a simple diagram which encompasses these elements.

The social interactive model was presented and discussed at the Fourth World Congress on Dyslexia in Macedonia (Hunter-Carsch 1997a). The visual representation of the overlapping areas proved to be helpful to those who later participated in further discussions about the idea of teachers' stance (i.e. a location on a personal mental map and on a shared 'map') as well as the need to prioritize issues for research and professional development.

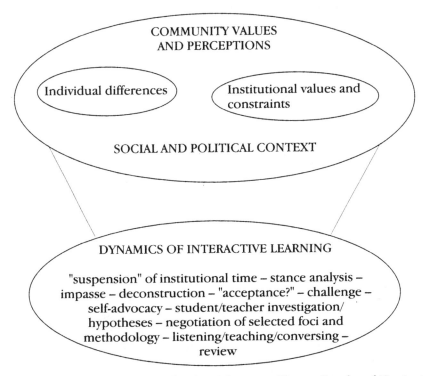

**Figure 6.3** Individual, institutional and social context (Hunter-Carsch and Herrington 1997a) (A Social Interactive Model of Specific Learning Difficuties).

A number of factors emerged through the writers' continuing conversation about the interactions between the individual, institutions and society. We conclude that as tutors or teachers, we should take the following into account.

## The position of the teacher within the dynamics of institutional and social values

We should be aware of ourselves and our own positions within this institutional and societal framework. Limited understanding of our own relative position risks limiting our understanding of the cumulative, negative build-up in some students as they are undermined on all fronts. We may neglect to explain to students that one of the reasons for learned low self-esteem is the unrelenting set of messages from the contexts around them: the personal, the institutional and from the culture in general. It is important to remind ourselves that values and practices which have affirmed tutors are often those which have 'oppressed' learners.

## The historical and developmental factors affecting 'literacy'

We should develop certain kinds of knowledge and skill which allow us to work with this broader view. If, for example, tutors do not know about the contextual factors such as the historical development of language and literacy conventions, or about ways in which literacy is used to grade, exclude and control, then we remain locked into an uncritical servicing of existing systems which may be excluding individuals largely as a result of ignorance. This is not always made clear in the domestic context of Western education systems but in the field of international literacy, the 'hanging on' to inappropriate models of literacy (Herrington 2001a) has resulted in the failure of some literacy programmes.

Similarly, to continue to promote certain forms of literacy above others without understanding their origins and functions, without understanding how they can exclude those from different class, cultural or national backgrounds, and without teaching them explicitly before assessing, can mean that a tutor is simply affirming the status quo. In the case of some academic literacies, teachers may consider that the status quo represents the 'best' in terms of writing and should be preserved. This stance does not readily lead to recognition of the learner as having the potential to lead the professional group to a different position and yet literacies are actually dynamic and ideas about 'best standards' are a matter of dialogue, contest and change.

It is reasonable, in our view, to expect all teacher training for all sectors to include focused critical work on contextualizing and making explicit school and college literacies and on the differences in thinking and learning stances which will face any teacher in any class/group.

Similarly it is important for teachers to develop skills which include being able to 'tune in' to where students are starting from and to be able to relieve stress. These may involve counselling, but such skills are not a sufficient descriptor of what is involved nor are they realistic in many teaching situations. However it is perfectly possible for teachers to be able to ask the right questions to help students 'tune in' to or to relieve their stress simply by making the kind of suggestion which students find supportive, for example, *'What can you see on the page when you read?'* (Herrington 2001a) and e.g. in the higher education context, *'I will make copies of my overhead projector outlines* [lecture notes] *available to you'*.

### Effective and up-to-date assessment and teaching skills

We need to develop good assessment and teaching skills which take account of dyslexia and should in particular:

- be able to explain issues in a clear and succinct way and avoid undue reliance on a teaching style which is very demanding in terms of the auditory memory of learners;
- use models which incorporate visual representations, kinds of 'story', imagery, analogy and metaphor;
- teach about reading and writing in ways which acknowledge differences in processing text, the more profound connections between, for example, writing and identity, and the fundamental dynamic about forms of literacy in different disciplines or contexts. This task is open to all of us, irrespective of subject area or sector;
- acknowledge the particular interface between time and the curriculum when assessment is being considered.

### The necessity of a research stance (hypothesis formulation and testing)

We should have flexible attitudes and an openness in stance. In general, we consider that in this field of SpLDs, it is especially important to be open, to be prepared to operate with a spirit of enquiry and always to consider the question of why learners are not learning (and ask directly in some circumstances). It is essential to be willing to have one's perceptions challenged and to learn from learners themselves.

### Maintaining a multi-disciplinary perspective and a readiness to engage in continuing professional development

Although there are pressures of subject curriculum delivery, particularly in secondary and tertiary education, it should be at least possible to make explicit the language, literacy and cognitive paradigms in use in each discipline. Whenever possible, subtexts, too, should be made explicit for dyslexic learners in all sectors.

Our experience suggests that whenever these practices are in place in higher education (and students report when they are) the pressures on learning support specialists are reduced. However, in the present circumstances we believe that specialist tutors in all education sectors require some additional skills if they are to discharge their functions effectively; as co-explorers with students, they need to engage in a particular kind of informal but structured and structuring 'conversation' (re. higher education see Herrington 2001b and 2001c). This flexible and comfortable 'space' allows the teacher/tutor to listen to what is being said (and what is not said); to analyse the presenting situation with the learner; to bring insights from the broader framework to the appropriate moments within the session and to deconstruct contexts in order to reframe the past. Sometimes this can involve 'challenging' the dyslexic learner to see the impact of some ways of thinking about literacy and learning in relation to others. It also allows the tutor to learn a 'language' for describing these difficulties and listen to the language being used to describe strengths; to structure the process (time, space and content) and offer structures for addressing particular difficulties. The learners recognize that their own questions, insights and cognitive leaps are not only valid, but that their expression may facilitate development of the way forward for them (Herrington 2000b) and can contribute to the tutor's understanding about dyslexia in greater depth than is currently available in text books. For example, one of the most important challenges provided to the deficit way of thinking about dyslexia lies in the sharp contrast learners describe between experiencing the process of creative writing from the inside and the reported processing and organization of other people's information. The common perception of dyslexia as a language/literacy disorder appears odd to dyslexic students who produce fluent, creative writing. This kind of example allows the tutor to 're-tool' in relation to dyslexia.

Students' responses suggest, additionally, that valued qualities in learning support tutors are:

- showing basic personal warmth and interest;
- deconstructing past experience of education if necessary;
- making context and its demands explicit (especially literacy requirements). Explaining about literacies and their conventions; how these have developed over time and in whose interests. Developing exemplars (see RAPAL journal summer 1999);
- explaining how reading, writing and numeracy are experienced by many and describing literacy continua which we all inhabit;

- encouraging meta-cognition and meta-affectivity in relation to dyslexia, as part of raising awareness/exploration of strengths;
- listening and learning from learners about use of visual methods, metaphor and simile as part of teaching;
- structuring the curriculum with learners (encouraging learners to deal with one issue at a time);
- capitalizing on the student's problem-solving skills. Teaching how to analyse, shaping of options and engaging with students in hypothesis-testing in relation to dyslexia;
- investigating and identifying with the student the particular mix of sensory inputs which work for learning and memory;
- being aware of the importance of the learning 'environment' for some dyslexic learners. Sound/noise, colour, atmosphere, material objects may all be important considerations;
- being prepared to explore literacy practices and discipline paradigms in students' individual subject areas.

### Recognition, where relevant, of the need for change

In addition to adopting a research stance, effective tutors may need to see themselves not only as researchers, including 'action researchers' but also, where relevant, as 'change agents' in the contexts. They need to assist with promoting awareness, where relevant, of the limitations of the contexts and what is required in order to make them welcoming and accepting of difference among learners and, where necessary, to enable students to operate effectively as self-advocates.

## Implications for institutions

The need for institutional policies and practices which support dyslexic learners is beginning to be acknowledged in various institutions in all education sectors. The successful drive towards 'dyslexia friendly schools' (Warwick 1999; Rule 1999; Chapter 9) is heightening awareness that formulating a written policy statement is only one step in the direction towards achieving the desired effectiveness of practices and of communication within and beyond the institution.

The following issues emerge as vital for inclusion in the development of both policies and practices about teaching and learning support:

- the recognition of learning diversity in policies about teaching and learning.
- the organization of the curriculum to involve broader discussions among students about the learning process.

- the allocation of continuing professional development/training time to allow teachers to advance their professional knowledge and skills in relation to learning in general and to learning difference in particular.

# Implications for transition

The points of transition from primary to secondary and from secondary to tertiary education present particular challenges for students with SpLDs, e.g. dyslexia. The costs of the absence of continuities for students can be relatively high in terms of emotional distress as well as the price of attempting to 'build bridges' after the time they were first needed. Practices in the provision of continuity of learning support between the phases are, as yet, diverse and, too often, absent. There are many questions about advantages and disadvantages of a 'fresh start' (see further discussion below, Hunter-Carsch 2001) and considerable confusion about who should take responsibility for decision-making about the nature and extent of communications about students' progress and problems.

In so far as learning support is being offered, it seems that it occurs separately within each phase and that it requires students to start to fail in order for it to be activated. Evidence for transitional arrangements about learning support, in particular between secondary and tertiary education, is thin. However, there are some initiatives operating between further and higher education.

When trying to determine the nature of a desirable model of supportive transition, it is important to raise some questions about one particular ideal pattern in relation to transition. It involves:

- early identification of dyslexia and adaptation of the primary curriculum;
- passing updated written reports about students at each transition point, into secondary and then into tertiary education; adapting the curriculum as necessary at each stage;
- staff preparing students explicitly for the next phase at each transition point. In the case of Access Course students, for example, in tertiary education, staff work with higher education staff to clarify explicitly the details and rationale of higher education practices.

Our cautionary note about this model would say, first, that this is not the only possible model. Similar transition practices for dyslexic and non-dyslexic learners could be incorporated in general transition arrangements for all learners. Ultimately, if all learners were considered from a learning approaches and profile perspective and the curriculum differentiated accordingly, such information could be passed between the sectors. However, whilst this removes the need for separate arrangements, some would argue that this was not really necessary or practicable for all learners.

Second, it should be noted that whilst the costs of the present system are high in terms of 'lost knowledge' between sectors, of need to re-test and re-assess at each stage, and of the burden of explanation always remaining with the student, there are some advantages to this situation. Students are not dogged by reports from teachers throughout their careers. They can actually start again in each sector and re-articulate their needs in relation to the new context. These advantages may be more clearly appreciated between the secondary and tertiary rather than between primary and secondary stages. We are not advocating this lack of communication but we are alert to the fact that needs and circumstances vary.

Third, it may be important to distinguish between information about students passing between sectors and arrangements for staff to meet across sectors both to keep themselves informed about what is available and to create transition mechanisms which encourage students to be better informed about the next stage. Finally, even if completely satisfactory arrangements cannot be devised we can at least make a priority of minimizing re-testing at each stage.

## Conclusion

In conclusion, it seems that, at the heart of the matter, dyslexia appears to represent patterns of thinking and experiencing (involving learning strengths and weaknesses), the full contours of which are not yet known. Nor are its links and boundaries with the rest of the population fully appreciated. There are a number of working hypotheses about defining characteristics, and adult learners themselves have started to describe and publish their own first-hand accounts. In general, the dominant paradigm is one of a processing deficit, though dyslexic adults are beginning to lead us away from this. Patterns of strengths as well as weakness are being suggested and a more holistic stance is now emerging.

We know that the 'disability' associated with dyslexia is largely constructed from the perceptions and social practices of others. The nature of learning and assessment systems which encompass particular ideas about literacy standards and timing which have been designed without the diversity of learners in mind, produce most of the disabling effects. The cultural expectations of speed in processing language and certain types of information can exacerbate difficulties experienced by some dyslexic students and it is only by changing contexts (including attitudes and practices) that the disabling effects can be lessened.

As a result of this extended conversation we now have a clearer idea of what is required both within institutions and in the process of teaching in order to support the dyslexic learners and to change the contexts to make possible equality of opportunity. We have heightened awareness of the fact that teachers need to recognize the value of their personal and professional contributions (dyslexic adults always acknowledge the significance of those teachers who were curious and who 'did not give up on them'). Teachers should not feel daunted by the complexities and subtleties involved in the continuing multi-disciplinary exploration in this field. They have the valuable opportunity of discovering with learners how dyslexia is experienced by each individual. This does not just apply to specialist tutors. By asking basic questions about how students learn best and how teaching styles can be selected to cater for them, teachers in all sectors may contribute through their own investigations into learning. The freedoms and opportunities to do so may vary substantially between primary, secondary and tertiary education but relatively short conversations with students in which fundamental questions are discussed are accessible to many staff in all sectors.

Essentially, we consider that what we are proposing is not something different for a particular group, but something qualitatively different for all which will, eventually, provide a more enhancing kind of learning environment for dyslexic learners. One indicator of such change would be evidence in all sectors of students being confident and relaxed enough to discuss their individual differences in learning and to seek alternative representations of knowledge when one approach is not effective. Another would be educational practices which were fully informed by awareness of the range of learning differences. Ultimately, only when 'learning difference' is perceived as 'normal' and literacy practices accessible for all, can we be confident about effective learning for all.

## Appendix A

A three dimensional framework for teacher–psychologist discussion in relation to diagnosing inappropriate learning strategies (adapted from Figure 1 page 146 Reading and learning difficulties: relationships and responsibilities by CM Hunter. In Hendry, A 1982 (Ed.) Teaching Reading: The Key Issues, London, Heinemann).

| DIMENSION II: PSYCHO NEUROLOGICAL (LEARNING DIFFICULTIES) | DIMENSION I: PSYCHO – EDUCATIONAL. (SCHOOL WORK) READING/VERBAL COMMUNICATION/VISUO-MOTOR | | | | | | | | | | | |
|---|---|---|---|---|---|---|---|---|---|---|---|---|
| | 1. Oral | 2. Silent | 3. Listening comp. | 4. Word recog. | 5. Word analysis | 6. Categor. sounds | 7. Visual spelling | 8. Phonic spelling | 9. Hand-writing | 10. Written language | 11. Vocab. | etc. |
| 1. ATTENTION | | | | | | | | | | | | |
| 2. MEMORY | | | | | | | | | | | | |
| 3. SEQUENCING | | | | | | | | | | | | |
| 4. PATTERNS | | | | | | | | | | | | |
| 5. RHYTHM | | | | | | | | | | | | |
| 6. TRANSFER | | | | | | | | | | | | |
| 7. INCONSISTENCY | | | | | | | | | | | | |
| 8. CONTEXT | | | | | | | | | | | | |

DIMENSION III: PSYCHO-DYNAMIC

1. ROSENBERG (1968) — characteristic reaction to problem
- rigid-inhibited
- undisciplined
- acceptance-anxious
- creative

2. STOTT (1978)
- afraid to begin or to commit himself
- assumes role of dull child
- solitary peculiar ways
- ways of evading
- doesn't care
- relies on charm
- seems not aware
- insists on own way

3. GALTON (et al 1980) — work style
- intermittent workers
- solitary workers
- attention seekers
- quiet collaborators

4. HEWITT (1964) — T-P relationship (LEARNING STYLE)
- primary task level
- order task level
- exploratory task level
- relationship task level
- mastery task level
- achievement task level

5. ERIKSON (1950) — Attitude
- hope
- willpower
- purpose
- competence

6. FREUD — Self-perception
- play
- art
- drama
- introjection
- projection and other defence patterns

# Appendix B

## Areas of debate in the support of students with SpLDs

*Conceptualization and nature of dyslexia*

- which terminology: SDD versus LD versus SpLDs versus Dyslexia; acquired and developmental dyslexia, related or distinct conditions?
- which definitions/incidence?
- conceptualization: medical or social models of disability; autonomous versus ideological notions of literacy?
- heritability or not; the nature of the mechanisms?
- determinism versus cure?
- connections with versus separate from hearing and speech problems?
- a type of phonological deficit or broader parameters?
- discrete or overlapping with other 'conditions': dyspraxia, attention deficit hyperactivity disorder (ADHD), DCD, non-verbal learning difficulties (NVLDs), Asperger's syndrome?
- separate versus continuum in relation to the whole population?
- changing or unchanging over time (stability/nature and neurology of compensation)?
- delays in all language-based information processing or some delays, but very fast information processing in some respects?
- deficit versus 'different' thinking and learning styles?

*Identification/assessment (what, how, why and by whom)*

- identify formally or not?
- seeking discrepancy versus positive indicators?
- using minimally defining characteristics or broad parameters?
- single testing event versus ongoing assessment?
- analogies e.g. metaphors to describe the difference versus processing scores?
- who is qualified to do this: educational psychologists or specialist teachers; single- or multi-disciplinary assessment?
- learners as co-explorers versus 'objectified subject' of the test?
- voice of the learner? Voice of the professional?
- holistic dimensions (seeing dyslexia mediated through personality, affect versus identification of specific deficits)?

*Teaching and learning support (what should be done, when, where and by whom?)*

- always do something? Sometimes do nothing?
- one professional group versus contributions from many (educators/

psychologists/optometrists/counsellors/parents/peers/learners/speech therapists/ICT specialists)?
- roles of specialist tutors and general teachers?
- types of specialist intervention: the mantra of 'structured multi-sensory teaching' versus interactive dynamic co-exploration; selective multi-sensory work? A study and thinking skills approach?
- pharmacological intervention; sometimes versus never?
- nature of the specialist role: technicist versus releasing the power of learners through recognition of broader contextual factors?
- early intervention versus recognition that many dyslexic learners learn later rather than sooner (sometimes in vocational rather than educational settings) relative priorities: practical support with ICT/coloured lenses etc.; support from a person?
- separate support groups for SpLDs/inclusive whole-group support?
- responsibility of individual tutors? Whole institution model?
- essentially different teaching methods required versus good-quality teaching will suit all (the relationship between dyslexic learners and others has to be addressed)?
- heavy emphasis on cognitive versus meta-cognitive/meta-affective?
- leaving students with a 'diagnosis' versus helping with levels of awareness and ability to describe/explain their dyslexia to others?
- appropriate learning environments?

*Professional development (who trains whom, and for what?)*

- skills-based training based on deficit models of dyslexia? Training for an enhanced sense of the learner's potential, and awareness of different learning and thinking styles? Training which is informed by a radical literacies stance.
- separate specialist training courses versus modules embedded within all teacher training?
- contribution of dyslexic learners to teacher training versus their exclusion from this process?

*Research*

- whose evidence, questions, methods and perceptions? Professional researchers? Dyslexics themselves?
- what constitutes evidence? Respect for different research traditions versus dominance of some methodologies and disciplines?
- learners' voice versus analysis of pieces of processing?

# Part II
# Roots and branches

# Chapter 7
# Specific developmental dyslexia (SDD): 'Basics to back' in 2000 and beyond?

PETER PUMFREY

---

Questions addressed in this chapter include:

- Does specific developmental dyslexia (SDD) exist? If so:
- What is the nature of SDD?
- How may SDD be identified?
- What is the incidence of SDD?
- How might SDD be prevented? and
- How may SDD be alleviated?

---

## Preamble

In the Summer of 1998, an American clinical psychologist with extensive experience in the teaching of reading, published in the UK a book (McGuinness 1998) that had appeared in 1997 in the USA. It contains many challenging statements. For example:

> There is no diagnosis and no evidence for any special type of reading disorder like 'dyslexia' (p. 165); . . . overwhelming evidence that there is no such thing as 'dyslexia' or 'learning difficulty' (p. 220)

and

> Clear your minds of notions like 'dyslexia' and `learning difficulties'. The research data are overwhelming that these terms are invalid. (p. 226)

The foreword to the book was written by an eminent neuropsychologist, Steven Pinker, Director of the Centre for Cognitive Neuroscience at the Massachusetts Institute of Technology.

In the Autumn of 1998, the Department for Education and Employment (DfEE) issued a pamphlet entitled 'How can I tell if my child may be dyslexic?' (DfEE 1998b). This was intended to sensitize primary school teachers and inform their practice. Inevitably, its brevity meant that it did not help greatly in improving educational decision-making concerning the literacy difficulties faced by individual children. (As an aside, a spelling mistake on the front page did not inspire confidence in the care with which the document was initially produced and distributed). Fortunately, more adequate information is available from various of the publications included in this chapter in which the questions with which this chapter began are addressed. The chapter is an abridged and updated version of the 15th Vernon Wall Lecture given at the British Psychological Society's Education Section Annual Conference in 1995. The full 1995 publication is available from the British Psychological Society (Pumfrey, 1996).

## Introduction

In the year 2000, the concept 'dyslexia' has a widespread and increasing currency. Etymologically, the word derives from both Latin and Greek. The Latin root is *dis* (difficulty) plus *legere* (to read); the Greek *dys* plus *lexis* (words). In the broadest sense, the term includes acquired dyslexia (AD) resulting from injuries to (and illnesses affecting) the brain, and also ostensibly idiopathic conditions collectively known as specific developmental dyslexia (SDD). This chapter is concerned with SDD and its aims are as follows:

- To identify tensions deriving from a paradox concerning the concept of SDD.
- To specify some basic professional skills pertinent to the resolution of the tensions identified.
- To illustrate the promise and the pitfalls of these basic professional skills in current work on SDD.
- To provide information enabling readers to continue their own professional development thereby improving institutional and individual decision-making in relation to SDD.

Dyslexia comprises distinctive difficulties with various aspects of receptive and expressive language in textual and/or oral modalities (reading, writing/spelling, listening, talking). Some theorists include other symbolic systems, such as mathematics and music. The concept includes both acquired dyslexia (AD) and specific developmental dyslexia (SDD). It is important to distinguish between them.

Here, we are concerned only with the latter. Nowadays, the words 'specific' and 'developmental' are frequently omitted, even in official documents. The adjectives 'specific ' and 'developmental' are important in considering the nature of the syndrome. The appealing convenience of contracting SDD to 'dyslexia', rather than the use of SDD, leads to conceptual confusions, avoidable ambiguities and unnecessary disagreements. Not all pupils with receptive and/or expressive language difficulties have SDD.

## Multi-disciplinary context

The medical profession has had a longstanding involvement in the diagnosis and treatment of the aphasias. Identification of a specific aphasic loss of the ability to read, 'word blindness', despite the powers of sight, the intellect and speech remaining intact, is usually credited to a German physician Kussmaul in 1878. He also introduced the concept of 'word deafness'. Such patients are not genuinely deaf and can express themselves in words, but use many words in the wrong places and often distort them (Miles and Miles 1999). In 1887, Berlin, a German ophthalmologist, used the word 'dyslexia' to refer to a group of patients experiencing problems in reading because of cerebral disease. The condition was an *acquired* one and was viewed as one of the aphasias.

One hundred years ago, the first recorded individual case of congenital word blindness in a schoolboy was reported by a medical practitioner in the *British Medical Journal* (Morgan 1896). The one-page note describes a 14-year-old boy, Percy F. He is perceived as one of the brightest pupils in the class. In the opinion of his teachers, if all the teaching and assessments had been oral, Percy would have been the top of the class in his achievements. As it was he was struggling at the bottom. To account for this disability, Morgan suggested that the brain region suspected of being structurally damaged by disease/injury in acquired dyslexia was underdeveloped in this adolescent. Morgan also noted that 'the condition is unique so far as I know, in that it follows no injury or illness, but is evidently congenital'. The full text of this article was reprinted in the British Dyslexia Association's 1996 Handbook (Crisfield, 1996).

From an epidemiological standpoint, it is interesting to note that the annual report of the Medical Officer of Health, Dr James Kerr, in the City of Bradford in Yorkshire, England, was published some weeks before the appearance of Morgan's paper. Kerr reported the existence in local schools of some pupils who appeared to show what he described as 'congenital word-blindness'. Kerr was awarded the Howard Medal by the Royal Statistical Society in the same year for an essay based on his work in Bradford. Included in it was the observation that reading and writing difficulties could be found in children having no other apparent cognitive difficulties. The involvement and interest of the medical profession in certain cases of unexpected difficulties in literacy difficulties represents a longstanding and continuing involvement (Pumfrey and Reason 1992; Hulme and Snowling 1994, 1997; Chase et al. 1996; Stein and Walsh 1997; Klein and McMullen 1999; Miles and Miles 1999).

As professionals working with children mainly in educational settings, educational psychologists and teachers are concerned with both theory and practice. The school, the classroom and the clinic are laboratories within which a wide variety of ongoing and scientifically imprecise 'action research' takes place each day. This research can focus on individuals, small groups, classes, schools, local education authorities (LEAs) and the whole state educational system. Increasingly, technologically sophisticated and systematic studies of the myriad questions raised by SDD are taking place. To date the evidence is that these studies reveal ever-greater complexities, rather than simple answers, concerning SDD.

SDD has been described as 'the hidden handicap'. In its pre-school stages, it is typically *unseen*. Its subsequent early manifestations in difficulties in the acquisition of the skills of literacy, are *unexpected*. The difficulties also prove to be *unusual* in both degree and type and *unremitting* in character. Their cognitive, affective and motivational consequences for the individual can be disastrous (Edwards 1994; Riddick 1996). Is such a group of children distinguishable from other pupils who also experience difficulties in becoming literate? Is the concept of SDD valid?

The unexpected intrigues. Explanations are sought. Despite the considerable progress that has been made over the last century, SDD continues to be a controversial topic (Sampson 1975a, 1976; Pumfrey and Reason 1992; Hulme and Snowling 1994, 1997; Miles and Miles 1999). We remain intrigued, we seek explanations, we discuss and investigate their respective merits, we produce and consider evidence. Agreement, compromise or disagreement concerning the interpretation of evidence occurs. Investigations continue.

Life is filled with paradoxes. A paradox is a statement, seemingly self-contradictory or absurd, though possibly well-founded or essentially true. SDD presents many paradoxes. In an interview given in 1995, Stephen Hawking demonstrated the value of the proposition that 'One of the best places to look for new ideas in theoretical work is in the apparent paradoxes that occur in the existing theory'. With reference to SDD, the following paradoxical statement causes tensions, 'All children are the same: all children are different'.

Put in terms of the tensions between individuals and groups: 'Value and understand my child's uniqueness, but ensure that my child becomes literate at about the same time as his/her peers'.

## Tensions

Setting the scene: values, priorities and resources:

* How important is literacy to you?
* How much is literacy worth to our children and to society?
* How much is literacy worth to the individual pupil with SDD?

In our society, literacy enriches both culturally and economically. Whatever its causes, illiteracy isolates and impoverishes. In principle, there is general agreement that illiteracy, irrespective of its causes, should be minimized. In practice, there are many barriers. They may be summarized as:

* Resources finite.
* Priorities contentious.
* Knowledge partial.
* Demands infinite.

Three of these are largely socio-political in nature. One is scientific.

Disagreements within (and between) disciplines provide the challenge of finding resolutions. Hypothesis and antithesis can either identify mistaken ideas or stimulate syntheses. For example, in education, deriving from the earlier 'Top-down' versus 'Bottom-up' positions concerning the development of literacy, its learning and teaching, have emerged more comprehensive interactive formulations (Adams 1990; Ruddell and Ruddell 1994; Lazo et al. 1997; Reitsma and Verhoeven 1998; Klein and McMullen 1999).

In general, it is constructive to remember that no single profession has a freehold on validity. Similarly, no single research methodology can address adequately all questions concerning SDD. Both qualitative and quantitative approaches have their respective strengths and weaknesses (Hammersley 1995; Neuman and McCormick 1995; Pumfrey 1995a). In their various fields, all professions share equivalent responsibilities to their respective clients and disciplines. **Continuing professional development of one's knowledge, skills and understanding is essential**. [Editor's emphasis.]

## Basics to back?

In clarifying contentious areas of theory and practice, it is typically the asking of challenging questions which advances understanding. Productive questions frequently arise when predictions based on one theory are falsified; or when contradictory predictions derived from competing theoretical positions are tested. We have extensive yet still limited and fragmentary understandings of the initial six questions posed.

Distinguishing socio-political barriers from scientific ones is essential. Paradoxically, the wide range of insights from various disciplines into these complex questions, coupled with professional tunnel vision, can restrict the development of more adequate scientific answers. It is difficult enough to keep abreast of developments within even a single field. **The biggest danger to progress is becoming immured in the conceptual concrete of one's own profession. No one profession has sole claim to expertise concerning the nature, identification, prevention and alleviation of SDD.** [Editor's emphasis.] The perspectives of educational, psychological, sociological, medical and ophthalmological professions are complementary.

The six questions cited at the beginning of this chapter are being actively explored by different professions, using distinctive and often highly specialized methodologies and materials, in a variety of contexts, often working from complementary or even contrasting theoretical positions (Ruddell et al. 1994; Gough 1995). Syntheses of complementary perspective are being sought (Frith 1995, 1997; DECP 1999).

In combination with an appreciation of theories of child development in general and human communication in particular, two 'basics' could help a larger proportion of professionals address more constructively, and thus advance understanding of, the questions concerning SDD posed earlier. These 'basics' are the application of research methods and test theory. Through the generation and testing of hypotheses concerning the nature of SDD (its identification incidence, prognosis and alleviation in individuals or groups) knowledge is advanced. The scientific basis of individual and institutional decision-making can be improved. The miseries of avoidable educational failure and its concomitant effects on motivation and self-concept can be reduced (Turner 1997).

## Q1 Does SDD exist?

Is SDD a legitimate professional concern for teachers and psychologists (among other professionals)? Does SDD exist or is it a conceptual blind alley? (Figure 7.1).

Specific developmental dyslexia (SDD):

Differentiation and labelling

> Differences
> Deviations
> Difficulties
> Disabilities
> Deficits
> Defects

The slippery path from Differences to Defects can lead to the pathologizing of normality

**Figure 7.1** SDD – differentiation and labelling.

Acceptance of inter and intra-individual differences on virtually any structural or functional aspect of development is essential if one assumes that children do not all learn to become literate in the same way. There is a slippery path from the recognition of such differences to the identification of defects.

Does the label SDD lead to the pathologizing of normality? An informed minority of professionals doubt the validity and thus the educational utility of the concept (Tizard 1972; Young and Tyre 1983; Presland 1991; Anon. 1994; Stanovich and Siegel 1994; Stanovich et al. 1997; McGuinness 1998). Others, who are equally well-informed, consider SDD an exciting challenge whereby our understanding of the acquisition of literacy and our ability to alleviate children's difficulties will be enhanced (Bakker 1990, 1994; Miles 1993; Fawcett and Nicolson 1994; Bakker et al. 1994; Hulme and Snowling 1994, 1997; Seymour 1994; Licht and Spyer 1995; Nicolson and Fawcett 1995; Turner 1997; Pumfrey et al. 1998; Miles and Miles 1999).

With Mary Warnock as Chair, the Committee of Enquiry on the Education of Handicapped Children and Young People [England and Wales], argued for the abolition of categories of disabilities and the development of the concept of special educational needs (Committee of Enquiry 1978). This move was reflected in the Education Act 1981. Ten years later, in a House of Lords Debate held in December 1991, Baroness Warnock publicly renounced her earlier position concerning the value of categories of disabilities and in 1994 became President of the British Dyslexia Association.

There are many definitions of SDD. The following represent the views of the Orton Dyslexia Society (ODS), now the International Dyslexia

Association (IDA). These demonstrate a difference in emphasis between the Council and the Research Committee of the ODS appointed to consider a definition based on current scientific evidence.

**Definitions: Orton Dyslexia Society 1994**

Committee of the Orton Dyslexia Society (ODS) Members Definition (ODS 1994a):

> Dyslexia is a neurologically based, often familial disorder which interferes with the acquisition of language. Varying in degrees of severity, it is manifested by difficulties in receptive and expressive language, including phonological processing, in reading writing, spelling handwriting and sometimes in arithmetic. Dyslexia is not a result of lack of motivation, sensory impairment, inadequate instructional or environmental opportunities, but may occur together with these conditions. Although dyslexia is life-long, individuals with dyslexia frequently respond successfully to timely and appropriate intervention.

ODS Research Committee Definition (ODS 1994b):

> Dyslexia is one of several distinct learning disabilities. It is a specific language-based disorder of constitutional origin characterised by difficulties in single word decoding, usually reflecting insufficient phonological processing abilities. These difficulties in single word decoding are often unexpected in relation to age and other cognitive and academic abilities: they are not the result of generalised developmental disability or sensory impairment. Dyslexia is manifest by variable difficulty with different forms of language, often including, in addition to problems of reading, a conspicuous problem with acquiring proficiency in writing and spelling.

Following a detailed study of available research evidence and professional consultations, a Working Party of the Division of Educational and Child Psychology (DECP) of the British Psychological Society reached the following definition:

> Dyslexia is evident when accurate and fluent word reading and/or spelling develops very incompletely or with great difficulty. This focuses on literacy learning at the 'word level' and implies that the problem is severe and persistent despite appropriate learning opportunities. It provides the basis for a staged process of assessment through teaching (DECP 1999, p. 18).

Unlike the ODS Research Committee's definition, that of the DECP makes no mention of dyslexia being 'unexpected in relation to age and other cognitive and academic abilities'.

When Rome ruled the world, the saying 'All roads lead to Rome' underlined the then power of the Empire. In the new century, the 'Royal Road' towards specifying a major cause of SDD is increasingly pointing towards phonological processing abilities. Even at the level of single-word decoding, it is unlikely that all workers would agree that this represents a comprehensive analysis of the situation (Fawcett and Nicholson 1994; Nicolson and Fawcett 1995; Stein and Walsh 1997; Jeanes et al. 1997; Scholes 1998; Robertson 1999; Coles 2000). The fact that profoundly deaf children can be taught to read and spell is relevant.

At least one of the following conditions must be demonstrated if the claim for the conceptual coherence and existence of SDD is to be seen as well-founded. There must be a distinctive:

• aetiology
• pattern of presenting symptoms
• prognosis, or
• response to particular interventions.

Data from studies of twins (DeFries 1991; DeFries et al. 1997), from behavioural genetics (Olson et al. 1999), psychoneurology (Duane 1991; Klein and McMullen 1999), vision science and psycho-ophthalmology (Pumfrey 1993; Willows et al. 1993; Wilkins et al. 1996) provide important but not conclusive evidence supporting the first three requirements for the existence of SDD. Geneticists are exploring genetic linkages to SDD. Chromosomes 6 and 15 have been the focus of recent work. SDD is unlikely to involve the presence of a single gene defect with the inevitable occurrence of SDD, but a genetically linked susceptibility that may be minimized (or maximized) by environmental contingencies (Olson et al. 1999). On completion of the human genome project, it is likely that the diagnosis of a range of genetically transmitted conditions will be able to be made on the basis of single-cell biopsy.

The following non-genetic but biological processes have been implicated as possible causes of dyslexia: the effects of testosterone being released into the developing foetus during pregnancy; the transference from the mother to the foetus of immune-antibodies; and a wide range of perinatal risk factors.

Even if evidence exists for the first three of the above requirements, it does not follow that unequivocally effective interventions are either known or can be developed. In this field, assertions are easy. Evidence concerning the efficacy of a wide range of interventions is less readily available and more contentious (Pumfrey 1991, 1993; Pumfrey and Reason 1992; Wilkins et al. 1994; Rack 1995; Reid 1996a, 1996b; Otto 1997; Turner 1997; McGuinness 1998; DECP 1999; Miles and Miles 1999).

Increasingly, SDD is being described as 'a variable syndrome'. This highlights the distinction between those who argue that SDD has a single underlying cause, but that this can be manifest in different ways, and other workers who argue that there are qualitatively different subtypes of SDD. This controversy is likely to run for a considerable time (Miles 1993; Bakker 1994; Fawcett and Nicolson 1994; Seymour 1994; Stanovich and Siegel 1994; Snowling 1995, 1999; DECP 1999). Arguably, considerations of both 'trait' and 'type' are required in a more adequate formulation of SDD.

## Q2 What is the nature of SDD?

To address this question, it is essential to clarify our uses of the term SDD. The relationships between a *concept* such as SDD (an abstraction that can never be directly measured)(SDD 'A'), the *observable behaviours* in everyday life from which the existence of the concept is inferred (for example, particular patterns of literacy-related behaviours)(SDD 'B') and *tests/assessments* (techniques that systematically sample defined aspects of such behaviours)(SDD 'C') are essential considerations. If the level at which discussion is taking place is not specified, misunderstandings can readily multiply. SDD 'A', 'B' and 'C' must be differentiated. They must also be considered simultaneously if apparent paradoxes concerning the nature, identification and alleviation of SDD as a complex and variable developmental syndrome are to be addressed. Their formulations vary across disciplines.

As noted earlier, a key issue is whether SDD is a unitary condition. If the former holds, pupils' inter-individual differences in the information-processing abilities required for literacy would vary quantitatively. They would be likely to require help in developing the same skills. Some would require more assistance than others. The concept of SDD would, in effect, become redundant. If common crucial skills underpinned all surface failures in reading and spelling, all children can be helped and in similar ways. Currently, the importance of phonemic awareness is receiving considerable attention (Frederickson and Reason 1995b; Snowling 1995; Hulme and Joshi 1998; Scholes 1998; Stuart 1998; DECP 1999).

Other workers point to qualitative differences between pupils' information-processing strengths and weaknesses. If there are qualitative differences between pupils' abilities, pupils are likely to require different teaching and to use different learning techniques (Gjessing and Karlson 1989; Bakker 1990; Tyler 1990; Bakker 1994; Ellis et al. 1997a, 1997b; Robertson 1999). Is a shared theoretical framework possible? (Frith 1995, 1997; DECP 1999).

# Q3 How may SDD be identified? (potential versus attainments)

The cry 'Could do better' continues to reverberate through the educational system. The concept of 'underachievement' is a powerful one. It underpinned the pioneer work of the Remedial Education Centre at the University of Birmingham (Schonell and Wall 1949; Sampson 1975). When the Americans were considering how 'Learning Disabilities' (their equivalent to SpLDs) could be operationally defined, the only consensus was that it resulted in a major discrepancy between what, on the basis of pupils' aptitudes, you would *expect* academically of learning-disabled children and the level at which they were *actually* achieving (Reynolds 1984). In the UK, 80% of educational psychologists considered that some kind of discrepancy was a central attribute of SDD (Pumfrey and Reason 1992). The DfE also considers discrepancies between abilities and attainment as central to identification (DfE 1994a). The same is true of the advice given by the DfEE to primary school teachers in a pamphlet issued during the autumn of 1998 on the identification of dyslexic children (DfEE 1998b).

In general, intellectually able pupils become literate more rapidly than less intellectually able pupils. The ability-attainment discrepancy had a considerable appeal as an initial step in defining underachievement. The selection of particular tests to provide measures of intellectual ability and attainments in literacy is not straightforward (Elliott 1990, 1994; Stanovich 1991; McNab 1994a; Stanovich and Siegel 1994; Turner 1997; Pumfrey et al 1998).

There are also many ways of operationally defining discrepancies (Reynolds 1984; Frederickson and Reason 1995a; DECP 1999). The features of a psychometrically satisfactory method are as follows:

- Age-corrected standard scores are essential to the calculations required to calculate and evaluate differences.
- Account must be taken of the correlation between ability and attainment scores in order to allow for the effects of regression to the mean.
- It is essential to evaluate whether the differences between the ability and attainment scores are significantly larger than could happen by chance.
- The frequency of a difference in the *population of differences as large as the one under consideration* must be estimated.

This definition of underachievement does not necessarily identify SDD (Dobbins 1994). Where the cut-off lines indicating 'unusualness' in the discrepancy are drawn, is an arbitrary decision. How severe is a 'severe' discrepancy? (McNab 1994b). Despite this problem, such an explicit, public, replicable first stage in both institutional and individual decision-making has much to commend it. However, a second consideration is the qualitative characteristics of the pattern of pupils' strengths and weaknesses. Different professionals will bring varying perspectives. The final judgement should be made by a multi-disciplinary team. Probability rules. Professional judgement is central.

Stanovich (1991, 1994) has suggested that discrepancy definitions of reading disability, using conventionally measured intelligence as an aptitude benchmark, hide untenable assumptions concerning the concept of potential. He has argued for the use of listening comprehension as a more educationally relevant aptitude measure. Interestingly, a variant of this strategy was introduced in the 1950s by the late J McNally, when he was Principal Educational Psychologist for the City of Manchester. Over a period of years, it proved increasingly effective in raising teachers' expectations of primary school pupils and the pupils' educational achievements. The approach was particularly effective in raising the reading attainments and success in the 11-plus selection examination used at that time to decide the type of secondary school education for each child within a tripartite school system. The mean reading standards and examination successes of pupils from socio-economically deprived areas of the city increased markedly to approximate the overall levels for the city's schools. The system was not intended to identify SDD but aimed to reduce under-achievement, irrespective of its causes. A Remedial Education Service provided support to schools. The system of testing oral comprehension and reading attainment in Junior School Year 2 was later abandoned as the educational system became comprehensive and pupil selection at the age of 11 did not take place. Currently, in the UK, concern about under-achievement by pupils and schools is, once again, a government priority. SDD is perceived as one facet of this political and educational challenge.

By use of a regression approach, Stanovich's subsequent work enabled him to test the phonological skills of older poor readers with and without (somewhat small) IQ achievement discrepancies. No significant mean differences in phonological skills were identified (Stanovich and Siegel 1994). The phonological-core variable-difference hypothesis was also tested across a range of discrepancy criteria by workers in England by use of the *Phonological Assessment Battery* (PhAB) (Gallagher 1995). Comparison of the differences between normal, poor readers, SDD and 'garden-variety' poor readers were made. The effects of reading age was partialled out for each of the ten tests in the PhAB. The total sample comprised 244 subjects at three age levels 6, 8 and 10 years. In summary, it is suggested that the findings of Stanovich and Siegel (1994) 'may be premature, particularly in relation to pupils with the more severe and complex difficulties' (Gallagher and Frederickson 1995, p. 66). A later publication at the Fourth International Conference of the British Dyslexia Association presents Stanovich's case more fully (Stanovich et al. 1997). The case is not accepted by all workers (Elbrow 1998).

Within the context of child development and educational psychology, an understanding of both research design and test theory is central to appreciating the technicalities of such approaches:

> No other contribution of psychology has had the social impact equal to that created by the psychological test. No other body of theory in psychology has been so fully rationalised from the mathematical point of view. (Guilford 1952)

Guilford's concern was with what is currently known as 'normative test theory'. Its limitations in education are considerable, but it remains an important approach to the assessment of children's relative attainments and progress. The increasing popularity of a method of test construction known as Rasch scaling, based on item response theory, demands that users of tests developed in this way are aware of the technical strengths and weaknesses of the approach (Pumfrey 1987). Item response theory also underpins two diagnostic batteries developed by Elliott and colleagues. These are widely used by British and American psychologists respectively: the *British Ability Scales* and the *Differential Ability Scales*.

Much has happened since then in the area of assessment and its links with both instruction and motivation (Elliott and Figg 1993). Increasing importance is accorded to direct observation of the literacy-related behaviours of pupils with SDD, to domain-referenced assessment, diagnostic batteries based on item response theory and informal inventories which include miscue or error analysis (Pumfrey 1985, 1987, 1991, 1995b, 1999; Blythe and Faulkner 1994; Turner 1994, 1995). A greater awareness of the respective strengths and weaknesses of these approaches to assessment would have helped avoid some of the unnecessary and expensive mistakes made with the introduction of the National Curriculum English Standard Assessment Tasks and Teacher Assessments (Pumfrey 1995e). To use unreliable, and therefore invalid, instruments for such a profile-based decision-making procedure would be likely to result in a very high numbers of false negative and false positive classifications. Albeit belatedly, Her Majesty's Chief Inspector of Schools has acknowledged the unreliability of the Standard Assessment Tasks used by the Qualifications and Curriculum Authority to monitor standards and progress (Cassidy 1998). This calls into question the validity of use of the results of SATs to determine educationally important discrepancies that may be indicative of dyslexia.

Considerable concern has been expressed about the misuse of published tests in education. Problems arise largely because many users do not have the knowledge to make informed judgements about the strengths and weaknesses for particular decision-making purposes of the published tests that they are using. Many test users have not been trained in test administration, scoring and interpretation (Pumfrey 1990). There are also indications that poorly designed tests are being produced.

In order to provide a qualification in psychological aspects of educational testing for professionals wishing to use psychological tests, but not having a background in psychology, the British Psychological Society (BPS) Steering Committee on Test Standards has been developing a certification procedure (BPS 1992; Boyle et al. 1995). The aim is to ensure that users of published tests do so at an acceptable level of competence and hence have the ability to look more critically at SDD screening tests and assessment procedures that are currently in use.

More recent arrivals meriting consideration, but not necessarily adoption, include the 1994 *Dyslexia Screening Instrument* (DSI) from the USA. It is intended to cover the age range 6-21 years. The DSI is based on a rating scale of 33 items to be completed by the student's teacher. Each item is scored on a five-point scale. Using a computer, the ratings are analysed via the *Scoring Programme* software. DSI capitalizes on the potential of 'expert systems' and information technology (Coon et al. 1994). The use of a four-category classification of pupils as 'Passed' (not SDD), 'Failed' (possible SDD) 'Inconclusive' and 'Cannot be scored' is not particularly illuminating. Information concerning the psychometric characteristics of the individual items is not available in the manual. Currently the validity of the DSI is being investigated in a small-scale study in Manchester.

Available English instruments include the *Phonological Assessment Battery* (PhAB) (Gallagher and Frederickson 1995), the *Dyslexia Early Screening Test* and the *Dyslexia Screening Test* (6;6 to 16;5 years) (Nicolson and Fawcett 1996a, 1996b). Additionally, the *Cognitive Profiling System* (CoPS) (Singleton et al. 1996), a *Graded Nonword Reading Test* (Snowling et al. 1996), Wilkins's *Rate of Reading Test* (Wilkins et al. 1996), the *Phonological Abilities Test* (Mutter et al. 1997) and the *Phonological Assessment Battery* (PhAB)(Frederickson et al. 1997) are available and in use.

*Intelligent Testing with the WISC III* is the challenging title of an important book on diagnostic assessment (Kaufman 1994). It is extremely helpful in terms of both the psychometric and psychological evaluation of profiles and discrepancies.

The theoretical assumptions on which all such screening and diagnostic tests are based must be made explicit. Evidence of content, concurrent, predictive and construct validities is important. Its psychometric 'Siamese twin', test reliability, also comes in at least four forms in conventional test theory. These are known as internal consistency, stability (test–retest), equivalence (parallel forms) and stability and equivalence. Reliability is a necessary but not sufficient condition for test validity (Pumfrey 1977, 1985).

Tests are selected to enable hypotheses to be investigated (Pumfrey 1999). Despite the limitations of psychological tests, the identification of SDD demands that exceptionality be quantified as a necessary but not sufficient condition for diagnosis.

The validity of a sophisticated psychometric approach in clinical work with dyslexic pupils has been well-demonstrated by the Principal Psychologist of the Dyslexia Institute's Psychological Service. He has published information describing and commenting on basic tools used in testing pupils' reading and spelling that has been well-received by many teachers (Turner 1993, 1994, 1995). For psychologists, he has made challenging contributions concerning the improvement of professional practice in the assessment of SDD in particular (Turner 1997). The Dyslexia Index that he has developed is an interesting idea based on individualized objective testing. Both his rationale and methodology are explicit. Whether his seven-point scale of dyslexic severity will be seen as fair depends on the validity of the assumptions on which the diagnostic procedures is based (Turner 1997, pp 310-20).

In the USA, State criteria and procedures used in the identification of children with learning disabilities vary markedly (Frankenberger and Fronzaglio 1991). The same is true in relation to the identification of pupils with SDD in LEAs in the UK. Considering the following question indicates why this is likely to remain the case for some time.

## Q4 What is the incidence of SDD?

Exploring the links between SDD 'A', 'B' and 'C', is dependent on quantification. The assertion made by the late RL Thorndike merits restating: 'Whatever exists, exists in some quantity and can, in principle, be measured'.

Never forget the 'in principle'. Some aspects of assessment are more soundly based than others. An understanding of the various levels of measurement is pertinent. The strengths and weaknesses of nominal, ordinal, interval and ratio scale-based instruments for particular decision-making purposes needs to be understood by test constructors and users.

The challenges of conceptualizing SDD and of operationalizing the concept, remain crucial concerns (Connor 1994; Turner 1997; Rispens et al. 1998). As the former Chief Inspector of Schools for England and Wales, Professor Stuart Sutherland, remarked at an interview held in 1992 concerning education in general, *'If you can't measure it, you can't manage it'*. So, too, with SDD. Herein lies a central dilemma related to the establishment of educational priorities and the provision of resources from the public purse (including professional expertise). How can this be achieved in a way accepted as 'fair' to all pupils?

The incidence of SDD is either 4% (severe) or 10% (mild) according to estimates by some organizations, including the British Dyslexia Association (Crisfield 1996). Such estimates are both theoretically and technically contentious. Establishing a resource allocation decision-making model that is explicit, open, fair and theoretically defensible, requires considerable professional knowledge. Inevitably, it involves subjectivities of professional judgement and the values and assumptions on which such judgements depend. Making the model accord to the law requires additional sensitivities. The management of provision for SDD requires considerable care (Pumfrey 1995c).

Measurement has many strengths; it also has considerable limitations. Figures can be used as a smokescreen, deliberately or unwittingly. On balance, Sutherland's comment concerning institutional decision-making that must be seen to be open and equitable in the interests of accountability, acknowledges the value of tests, despite their weaknesses.

In the *Division of Educational and Child Psychology Newsletter*, an article entitled 'Dyslexia, perplexia, mislexia' (Anon. 1994) spelled out some of the serious concerns that many professionals having responsibilities for all pupils and all disabilities will recognize. The issue of preferential help for particular groups of children with special educational needs, is a socio-political one (Cornwall 1995). Entirely legitimate pressure groups attempt to influence national policies, priorities and resource allocations.

## Q5 How might SDD be prevented?

Early identification, though fraught with the many dangers of false positive and false negative identifications, may help. So, too, would raising professional awareness of SDD and more clearly specifying constructive approaches to its identification and alleviation as a part of initial teacher training and INSET (Layton and Deeny 1995; Pumfrey 1995d). In relation to children with SpLDs, the Special Education Needs Training Consortium (SENTC) has presented a report which includes a specification of the professional competencies required by the teachers of such pupils

(SENTC 1996). More recently, the Teacher Training Agency (TTA) has issued a consultation paper concerning the standards of knowledge, understanding and skills required of Special Educational Needs Specialist Teachers (TTA 1998).

It is vital to distinguish between socio-political and scientific considerations in decision-making. In England and Wales, the government accepts that SDD exists and comprises a subset of SpLDs. SDD is acknowledged in law, in the Code of Practice on the Identification and Assessment of Special Educational Needs, in Circular 6/94, and in the beliefs of many citizens (Chastey and Friel 1993; DfE and Welsh Office 1994; DfE 1994a, 1994b; DfEE 1998a; Smythe 2000).

Despite this socio-political and legally enshrined confidence concerning the existence of SDD, some professionals disagree concerning the validity of the concept (Presland 1991; Young and Tyre 1983; McGuinness 1998). Those who accept the validity of the concept often differ when methods of identification are considered. It follows that professional opinions currently differ markedly concerning the nature of SDD, its identification, incidence and alleviation. Uncertainties exist and are likely to continue (Pumfrey and Reason 1992; Miles 1993; Nicholson and Fawcett 1995; Seymour 1994; Ellis et al. 1997a, 1997b; Frith 1995, 1997; Klein and McMullen 1999).

In connection with the case of a young person deemed to have SDD, the following comment was made by the Law Lords: 'The failure to treat his condition which would have improved had it been correctly diagnosed and treated, has disadvantaged the individual' (*The Times* 1995).

There is an interesting circularity in this argument based on the suspect assumption that a suitable treatment was available and would have been effective. It depends on what one means by effective. Does this imply that the individual's attainments in literacy skills should approximate some agreed index of intellectual ability?

Professionals should be aware of what can be regarded as the limits of their reasonable expertise. They should also be extremely careful in what they say, write or recommend in the service of their employers. Technical aspects of assessment and the interpretation of test results are important areas. The Association of Educational Psychologists (AEP) and the Division of Educational and Child Psychology of the British Psychological Society (DECP) have circulated a document providing guidance for educational psychologists concerning the statutory advice that they are required to provide to LEAs (AEP and DECP 1995). The Division of Educational and Child Psychology of the British Psychological Society Working Party's report entitled *Dyslexia, Literacy and Psychological Assessment* provides a current review of research (DECP, 1999).

In summary, socio-political considerations largely determine the official recognition of SDD. Only in part is such recognition a result of scientific knowledge. The prevention of SDD depends on capitalizing on the promise in existing imperfect knowledge and continuing to expand the existing multi-disciplinary professional knowledge base.

## Q6 How may SDD be alleviated?

Moving to the 1990s, promising educational practices are myriad (Pumfrey 1991; Pumfrey and Reason 1992; Reid 1993, 1994; Reason and Boote 1994; Reid 1996a, 1996b; Ott 1997; Reid 1998; Reitsma and Verhoeven 1998; Miles and Miles 1999; Robertson 1999). Some workers consider that it is possible theoretically to define, identify and remediate the core deficits of SDD. The situation may be summarized as 'Variety: neither consensus nor panacea'. We can learn from studies of the outcomes of interventions with pupils with SDD (Lovett 1999). When considering such studies, it is essential to consider the quality of the evidence on which the case for a particular intervention is based.

The potential of information technology in facilitating the identification and alleviation of SDD is immense and developing at a rapid rate (Singleton 1994; Boutskou 1995; Singleton et al. 1996; Blamires 1999). Special Educational Needs Information Technology (SENIT) is a computer-based network of individuals interested and involved in using and developing various applications of information technology in addressing obstacles to learning experienced by those with special educational needs in general. The SENIT list is supported by the government. Its address is <senit@ngfl.gov.uk> The British Dyslexia Association Computer Committee is a helpful source on Information Communications Technology (ICT) for dyslexic individuals (Cotgrove 2000).

Among the rapidly growing number of commercial suppliers of ICT for dyslexic students, Dyslectech from Iansyst Training Products merits consideration (its web page address is http://www.dyslexic.com). Multi-disciplinary interest is considerable as is the work of neuropsychologists such as Bakker (1990, 1994, 1997) and teachers (Robertson 1999) demonstrates. Research by vision scientists such as Wilkins, formerly of the Medical Research Council Applied Psychology Unit at Cambridge and now holder of a Chair in the Department of Psychology at the University of Essex (Wilkins et al. 1996), and Stein of the University Laboratory of Physiology at Oxford, testifies to activity in this field. In the USA the use of drug treatments, for example, ritalin, with dyslexic pupils is considerable, growing and controversial (Pumfrey and Reason 1992). The drug is also increasingly being prescribed for dyslexic pupils in the UK.

At a series of workshops with practising educational psychologists and specialist support teachers, the following information was elicited concerning psychomedical interventions available within their LEAs, albeit not necessarily through the LEA (Table 7.1). No claim for either comprehensiveness or representativeness of this 'convenience' sample of professionals is made. Despite this caveat, some interventions were more frequently reported than others. The table supports the proposition that SDD is not a unitary condition.

**Table 7.1** Pupils with SpLD (SDD): psychomedical interventions*

|  | Yes | Used in your LEA Rank order |
|---|---|---|
| **Neuropsychological interventions** |  |  |
| Perceptual development | 26 | 6 |
| Dominance training | 15 | =9 |
| Reprogramming | 0 | =20 |
| Neurological impress method | 1 | =18 |
| Hemispheric Specific Stimulation (HSS) | 1 | =18 |
| Hemispheric Alluding Stimulation (HAS) | 3 | =14 |
| ARROW (Aural, Read, Respond, Oral, Written) | 5 | 13 |
| Others | 0 | =20 |
| **Psycho-Ophthalmological interventions** |  |  |
| Occlusion | 74 | 2 |
| Cambridge optical lenses | 15 | =9 |
| Flicker distortions | 2 | =16 |
| Visual pattern distortions | 2 | =16 |
| Irlen coloured overlays | 96 | 1 |
| Irlen lenses | 45 | 3 |
| Binocular stability tracking | 18 | 8 |
| Prismatic lenses | 3 | =14 |
| Others | 0 | =20 |
| **Dietary and psychopharmaceutical interventions** |  |  |
| Vitamins | 43 | 4 |
| Trace elements | 19 | 7 |
| Antihistamines | 12 | 11 |
| Food additives | 40 | 5 |
| Psychostimulants (including ritalin) | 8 | 12 |
| Nootropics | 0 | =20 |
| Others | 0 | =20 |

*Replies from 81 educational psychologists and 291 specialist teachers (opportunity samples).

Based on earlier work by Stordy of the University of Surrey and published in the *Lancet* on 5 August 1995, a proposal to study the effects of docosahexaenoic acid in a randomized placebo-controlled study with children identified as dyslexic has been suggested. The aim is to test the effects on auditory information processing and phonological abilities in children identified as being dyslexic.

The simultaneous consideration of all children's literacy development must accompany the search for individuals and groups of pupils with SDD. Bakker's Balance Theory of the development of literacy addresses both normal development and the identification of groups of pupils showing important variations based on differential hemispheric development. Bakker is the former Head of the Research Department at the Paedological Institute and Professor of Child Neuropsychology at the Free University, Amsterdam. According to his Balance Theory of reading development, reading is initially mainly perceptual. If right-hemisphere strategies fail to shift to predominantly left-hemisphere strategies, children remain using right-hemisphere strategies. Such children remain particularly sensitive to the perceptual features of text and make characteristic mistakes when reading. These include a high frequency of fragmentation errors. Such pupils are called P- (Perceptual) type dyslexics. In contrast, other pupils generate mainly left-hemisphere strategies when starting to learn to read. They show a high frequency of substantive errors such as omissions and additions. These pupils are called L- (Linguistic) type dyslexics. Bakker argues for the stimulation of the underused hemispheric functions. He has developed two interventions. The first is called hemispheric-specific Stimulation (HSS); the second, hemispheric-alluding stimulation (HAS). The former is achieved by presenting reading materials in the left visual half-field of L-types and in the right visual half-field of P-types. This can be done by use of a specially devised computer program called HEMSTIM (Moerland and Bakker 1991) or by the use of a tactile training box. HAS for L-type dylsexics is based on the presentation of perceptually demanding text: for P- type dyslexics, a range of linguistically challenging materials is used (Licht and Spyer 1995).

Bakker's work in developing intervention programmes provides one of the better examples of a theoretically based identification of potentially important Aptitude Instruction interactions. What works for subjects of perceptual dyslexia (P-type) differs from interventions of value to subjects of linguistic dyslexia (L-type) (Bakker 1990, 1994; Bakker et al. 1994; Licht and Spyer 1995; Robertson 1999; Chapter 13; Robertson and Pumfrey, in press). The results from one of Bakker's major studies using a tactile training box are summarized below (Figure 7.2).

| 56 remedial teachers; 98 pupils; IQ >80 | |
|---|---|
| L-type<br>(N = 59)<br>Mean chronological age 10;06 years<br>Mean reading-age 7;05 years<br>HSS to right hemisphere<br>Use left hand to palpate letters<br>(out of sight) on board<br>Use words with concrete<br>meanings (e.g. bike) | P-type<br>(N = 49)<br>Mean chronological age 9;04 years<br>Mean reading age 7;02 years<br>HSS to left hemisphere<br>Use right hand to palpate letters<br>(out of sight) on board<br>Use more abstract words<br>(e.g. cold, love) |
| Single letters, words, sentences | |
| 20 sessions, 2 sessions per week | |
| Experimental group<br>(N = 28)<br><br>Predict decrease in<br>substantive errors<br><br>Control group<br>(N = 21) | Experimental group<br>(N = 26)<br><br>Predict increase in fluency<br><br><br>Control group<br>(N = 23) |
| RESULTS<br><br>L-type relative to control subjects: larger improvement in accuracy of reading<br>P-type relative to control subjects: larger improvement in fluency | |

**Figure 7.2** Effects of Hemispheric-specific stimulation (HSS)

The findings are promising. Work in this field is currently being carried out in Manchester (Robertson 1999; Robertson and Pumfrey, in press).

# Conclusion

SDD is a complex syndrome and its manifestations change as the child matures. There are no easy answers to understanding the complexities of SDD; no single agreed approach to its identification; no unequivocal method of estimating incidence, no unambiguous agreement on methods of either prevention or alleviation. On the positive side, there are many promising practices. Central to all of these, is the importance of making explicit and replicable whatever is done. Measurement matters.

The nature of research is Hydra-headed: one question answered raises others to be addressed. This suggests that pupils, parents, politicians and professionals would be well-advised to learn to live with legitimate doubts concerning the nature, identification, incidence, prognosis and alleviation of SDD. Acknowledging and accepting uncertainties is an essential prerequisite to addressing them. In this respect, the paradoxes identified and the tensions they represent, hold promise for the extension of knowledge in all the questions posed earlier. Parents say 'Neither we, nor our children, can afford to wait'. In my judgement, they are correct.

The socio-political dimensions of values, resources and priorities in a democratic society, including the involvement of the legal system in decisions concerning SDD, are ones in which individually and collectively citizens have a powerful voice. What type of society and educational system would we wish for our children and ourselves? How much are the citizens of our respective countries willing to pay in taxes to reduce the undoubted adverse effects on individuals of SDD?

Legitimate professional disagreements concerning the nature, identification, incidence and alleviation of SDD are viewed with great impatience by many parents. Simple solutions to complex learning difficulties are often, albeit unrealistically, expected. In England and Wales, an increasing number of cases of pupils with SDD are being taken by parents before the courts, to the Ombudsman and to SEN Tribunals in the quest for additional resources. If class sizes for pupils over seven years of age, increase, as advocated publicly by the current Chief HMI Woodhead in November 1995, this is unlikely to make it easier for teachers to provide the support that pupils with SDD require. Woodhead acknowledges that small classes do benefit pupils with special educational needs and also lower-attaining pupils in secondary schools. In 1995, reducing class size to a maximum of 30 for pupils under the age of seven was estimated to cost about £180 million per annum. In 2001 this class size reduction should be achieved. If, however, the resources required to reduce class size were used to improve teachers' skills in identifying and alleviating literacy difficulties in general, and SDD in particular, there could be benefits to many pupils. Raising public awareness concerning the antecedents, concomitants, consequences and costs of SDD inevitably increases parental expectations of the public services whose existence is to facilitate children's learning. Psychologists' and teachers' expertise, is central. So, too, is that of many other professions.

The answer to the question 'How much should the nation invest in improving the literacy of pupils deemed to have SDD?' lies in citizens' collective hands. It is a responsibility of all citizens, not solely that of experts.

In terms of professional knowledge, 'If a man begin with certainties, he shall end in doubts; but if he will be content to begin with doubts, he shall end in certainties'. Thus wrote Bacon 395 years ago in *The Advancement of Learning*. Forgiving the sexist anachronism, the maxim stands the test of time. Even though the horizon of 'certainties' in relation to SDD is unlikely to be reached in the near future, there is considerable evidence to show that progress is being made. There *are* professional basics to back.

# Chapter 8
# Adult dyslexia: research and practice

HANNA-SOFIA POUSSU-OLLI

---

Questions addressed in this chapter include:

- What kinds of literacy difficulties continue beyond school experience into adult life for dyslexic learners?
- Are there continuing disadvantages in education and vocational opportunities as a result of these difficulties?
- Are there any cases of successful literacy learning despite dyslexia?
- Do they completely overcome phonological processing problems?

---

## Introduction

Coping in today's society calls for good written communication and skilful use of both spoken and written language. It is not good enough that people are able to send messages by diverse technologies; they must also be capable of responding to messages with quick reciprocal communication. An error in literacy or language may turn out to be fatal. It is often thought that when compulsory schooldays are over the problem of dyslexia ends. This is not the case.

The study which is reported here investigated the literacy experiences of dyslexic and non-dyslexic adults. The literacy errors of both groups are analysed. The study took place in Finland, a country which is widely recognized for the value it places on literacy, and for its high standards of literacy. According to international assessments, 2% of the adult population suffers from severe dyslexia. One in ten Finnish adults suffers from a dyslexic disorder of some sort. In the present study the background of 20 dyslexic adults was studied along with their dyslexic difficulties, academic achievements, post-school studies and their ability to cope in Finnish society in the late-1990s. Their achievements are compared with those of adults with no symptoms of dyslexia.

# Realities of adult dyslexia

In Finland, considerable attention has been given to dyslexia only during the last five years. Acceptance of dyslexia in adults cannot be taken for granted. In fact, some dyslexic adults have had to bring their problems to the fore and have demanded remedial teaching to overcome their problems. Some dyslexia associations have been founded recently with the aim of addressing the concerns of dyslexic adults. Research and remedial methods focusing on adults are now being planned. Developments include various tests, rehabilitation programmes and network-models for diagnosis and 'rehabilitation'.

Even though dyslexia as a phenomenon in childhood has been studied for some time, studies of dyslexia in adults are extremely rare. Dyslexia has been thought only to concern the school population, and thus various supportive measures have been directed towards children and young people. The incidence of dyslexia in vocational institutions is approximately 10-15% and in upper secondary school (according to cautious estimates) 1-2%. The incidence of dyslexia among university students has not been studied. Adults have been given remedial teaching only at random and, for example, in upper secondary schools the probability of dyslexia is still rarely accepted or it is totally denied (Poussu-Olli 1996).

In the background of adult dyslexia, there is often a life-long problem relating to language processing, the difficulty being noticed in early childhood, but without any possibility of it being corrected during school years. The background of difficulties with words includes difficulties with sound differentiation, memory and verbal combinations. These factors cause reading errors (Schonhaul and Satz 1983) and thus also problems in writing performance.

It has been established in studies focused on dyslexic adults that, among other things, they make considerably more mistakes in reading aloud and in writing than non-dyslexic adults. Frequently, dyslexia has been noticed during their school years. Recurrent difficulties in reading performance have been emphasized in particular. Poor interpretation of text and difficulties in reading aloud were considered to be due to difficulties in pronunciation. Johnson (1987) states that these problems are caused by difficulties in auditory analysis, verbal consciousness and interpretation. An essential factor in the tests of reading comprehension is slow rate of reading, which (according to Johnson's studies) is due to a lack of verbal automaticity, interpretation problems, linguistic retardation and anxiety (Johnson 1987).

# Method and results of the study

The study was carried out in the Department for Special Education at the University of Turku between 1994 and 1996. The subjects were 20 dyslexic adults and a control group of 20 non-dyslexic adults. Their average age was 33 years. Forty per cent of subjects were female and 60% male. Subjects were tested in reading and writing comprehension. In addition, the subjects' auditory and visual memory was measured and their background information and current situations were noted. There were also two severely dyslexic adults who were investigated in the Neuro-Cognitive Institute of the University of Turku, using event-related potential (ERP), a technique which measures auditory perception. Measurements and analyses were based on tests developed by Korpilahti and Krause (1996).

# Results of literacy tests

### Reading

Reading aloud and reading comprehension were measured. The results show that the dyslexic subjects were statistically very significantly weaker in reading aloud. In reading comprehension they were statistically significantly weaker. In memory and rate of reading aloud the dyslexic subjects were very significantly weaker than the non-dyslexic group. In reading aloud they have been analysed both qualitatively and quantitatively (Figure 8.1).

When reading aloud, the dyslexic subjects made mistakes in word endings significantly more frequently than non-dyslexic subjects. After analysis of the errors it may be noticed that the errors made by both groups included wrong words, wrong endings and repetition of words. The dyslexic subjects were significantly weaker than the control group in reading comprehension.

### Writing

Tests included dictation and creative writing. In order to analyse the results the dyslexic group was divided into three subgroups, according to severity of difficulty (mild, moderate and severe). The male:female ratios of the subgroups were as follows:

- Mild: 2M:5F.
- Moderate: 5M:3F.
- Severe: 5M:3F.

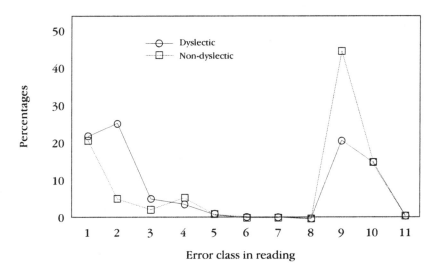

**Figure 8.1** Percentage distributions of error classes in reading, by research groups. Reading 1 = wrong word; Reading 2 = wrong word ending; Reading 3 = wrong letters; Reading 4 = missing words; Reading 5 = missing letters; Reading 6 = additional letters; Reading 7 = singular/plural; Reading 8 = breaks; Reading 9 = repetition; Reading 10 = corrections; Reading 11 = reversals.

There were more males than females in the most severely dyslexic groups. The errors made by the groups are represented in Figure 8.2.

In dictation the dyslexic group made statistically very significantly more mistakes than the control group. Dyslexic subjects made 89% of the total incidence of errors and non-dyslexic subjects, 11%. The errors of the dyslexic group included initial sounds and punctuation, omission of letters, mistakes with compound words as well as missing words, incorrect contractions of words and wrong word endings. The errors of the control group were mainly with initial sounds and compound words. In the 'severe' dyslexic subgroup, double consonants (geminates) and long vowel errors were evident as well as omissions of words, wrong word endings and incorrect contractions of words. These subjects showed word contraction, made non-word and compound word mistakes significantly more often than the other dyslexic subgroups (Figure 8.3).

In creative writing none of the dyslexic subjects fell into the 'excellent' group. In the 'severe' dyslexia subgroup 90% of cases belonged to the 'satisfactory' and 'weak' categories. In the 'moderate' dyslexia subgroup <60% of cases were in the 'good' category and in the 'mild' dyslexia subgroup 27% belonged to the same group. Statistically the differences were signficant.

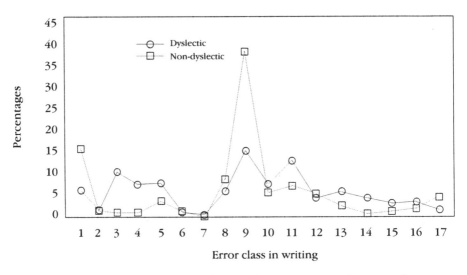

**Figure 8.2** Percentage distribution of error classes in writing, by research groups. Writing 1 = big or small initial; Writing 2 = reversal or rotation; Writing 3 = missing letter in a geminate; Writing 4 = missing letter in a long vowel; Writing 5 = other missing letter; Writing 6 = m/n mix up; Writing 7 = nk/ng mix up; Writing 8 = other wrong letter; Writing 9 = words together or apart; Writing 10 = missing punctuation; Writing 11 = missing word; Writing 12 = wrong meaning of word; Writing 13 = wrong word endings; Writing 14 = meaningless or non-word; Writing 15 = missing syllable; Writing 16 = additional letter; Writing 17 = other errors.

## Auditory and visual perception and memory

The results of the auditory and visual perception tests are shown in figures 8.4 and 8.5. Auditory perception comprises the following sub-areas: formation of a word from sounds; rhythm of words; syllable differentiation, and differentiation of the latency of a sound. The dyslexic group was statistically extremely significantly weaker than the control group in all items.

In visual perception, the perception of a sentence (compiling) and visual word differentiation were measured. There was no statistically significant difference between the groups (Figure 8.5)

In memory performance, short-term memory was measured both with numbers and syllables, and permanent memory with words. According to the results, the dyslexia group was statistically very significantly weaker than the control group ($p = .000$) (Figure 8.6).

## Event-related potential (ERP)

Auditory perception was examined in the two subjects diagnosed as suffering from reading and writing disorders, by measuring event-related

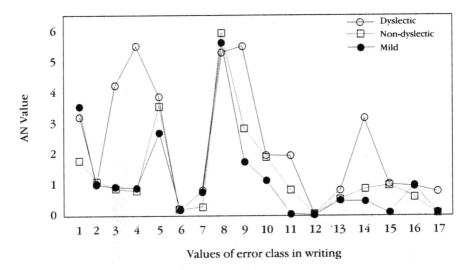

**Figure 8.3** Mean value distributions in writing, by dyslexic subgroups. Writing 1 = big or small initial; Writing 2 = reversal or rotation; Writing 3 = missing letter in a geminate; Writing 4 = missing letter in a long vowel; Writing 5 = other missing letter; Writing 6 = m/n mix up; Writing 7 = nk/ng mix up; Writing 8 = other wrong letter; Writing 9 = words together or apart; Writing 10 = missing punctuation; Writing 11 = missing word; Writing 12 = wrong meaning of word; Writing 13 = wrong word endings; Writing 14 = meaningless or non-word; Writing 15 = missing syllable; Writing 16 = additional letter; Writing 17 = other errors.

potentials (ERPs) in three passive oddball paradigms. The three experimental conditions were as follows:

- One with pure tones (standard 500 Hz) and deviant Hz).
- One with words (standard /tu:li/ 'wind' and deviant /tuli/ 'fire').
- One with pseudo-words (standard /tu:ni/ and deviant /tuni/) as stimuli (Korpilahti and Krause 1996).

The preliminary results indicate that the mismatch negativity (MMN) latencies for pure tones (eMMN) were longer (352 and 283 ms) in the two subjects, as compared with ten normal control subjects (190 ms). Further, the differences between the MMN latencies for words versus pseudo-words (lMMN) were smaller in the two dyslexic subjects than the normal control subjects. The MMN latencies are suggested to yield information about the mental speed of auditory encoding. Auditory information is time-related and mental speed is thus a very important factor for language processing. The results from this preliminary investigation suggest that the ERPs, especially the MMN, might provide valuable information about cortical dysfunctioning in reading and writing disorders.

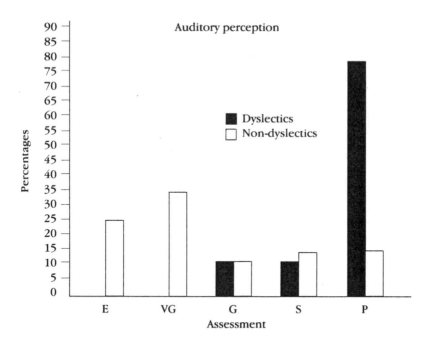

**Figure 8.4** Percentage distributions of auditory perception, by research groups. E = excellent; VG = very good; G = good; S = satisfactory; P = poor.

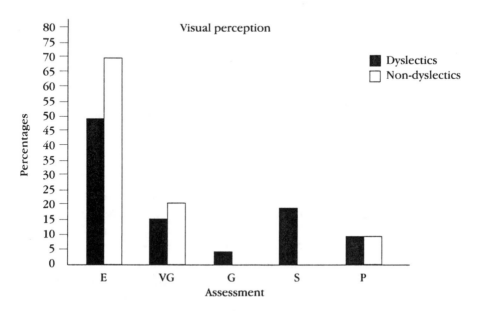

**Figure 8.5** Percentage distributions of visual perception, by research groups. E = excellent; VG = very good; G = good; S = satisfactory; P = poor.

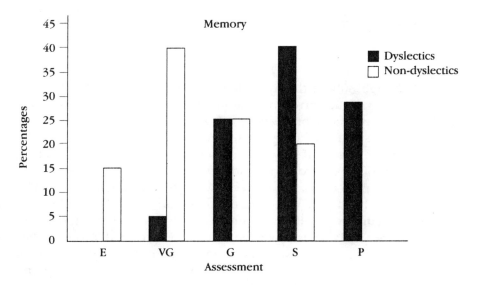

**Figure 8.6** Percentage distributions of memory, by research groups. E = excellent; VG = very good; G = good; S = satisfactory; P = poor.

## Laterality and cross-laterality

In the analysis of laterality of the whole sample, 83% of subjects were right-handed and 7% were left-handed; 63% were right-eyed and 37% left-eyed; 99% were right-legged and 1% left-legged. In the dyslexic group laterality was divided as follows: left-laterality and cross-laterality occurred statistically more frequently than in the non-dyslexic group (e.g. cross-laterality was found in 63% of the dyslexic group and 37% of non-dyslexic subjects).

## Background information

The existence of dyslexia in the rest of the family and close relatives was explored with the dyslexic adults. Eighty per cent of the dyslexic adults who answered had others with dyslexia among their families or close relatives. Twenty per cent of those who answered were not aware of dyslexia in their families. According to retrospective analysis, the dyslexic subjects (60%) had been ill more frequently in childhood than the non-dyslexic subjects (20%).

## Education and occupation

Figures 8.7 and 8.8 present the analysis of the education and socio-economic backgrounds of the sample. The results indicate that the adults with dyslexia were the most substantial group among those who were unemployed and those who had no vocational education. Eighteen per cent of the dyslexic subjects had no kind of vocational education, whereas everyone in the control group had further professional education at some level. Although 30% of the dyslexic subjects had attended vocational training colleges, the corresponding number for the control group was 12%. Twenty per cent of the control group passed examinations in colleges of institutes of higher education, compared with 6% of the dyslexic group. None of the dyslexic subjects studied in universities, whereas 12% of the control group did so (Figure 8.7).

Twenty-six per cent of the dyslexic subjects were unemployed, 37% were employed and 21% were in further education. In the control group, 7% were unemployed, 40% were employed and 40% were studying in various further and higher education colleges. However, the courses they were following involved basic education ('primary studying'). According to these results, dyslexic subjects had lower levels of education and achieved less than non-dyslexic subjects (Figure 8.8).

## Psychological and emotional factors

Eighty-two per cent of the dyslexic subjects stated that reading and writing difficulties had hindered their progress at school, recruitment in vocational education and their later placement in work. Many had not received remedial teaching during their compulsory school years. Often,

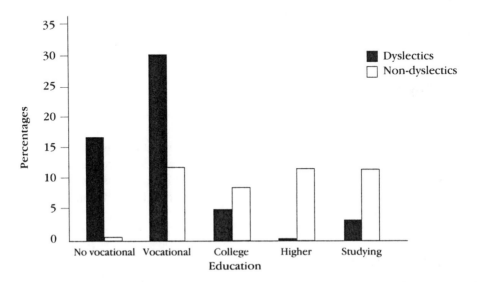

**Figure 8.7** Percentage distributions in education levels, by research groups.

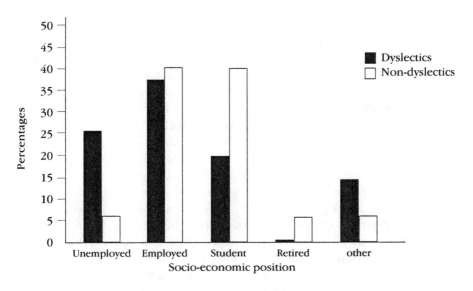

**Figure 8.8** Socio-economic position of research groups.

diagnosis of dyslexia had not been made, or if made, was deficient. Failures had a cumulative effect, so that if they got a job, subjects felt that they needed to try to hide their dyslexia in every way.

## Discussion

Changes are a part of everyday life today in Finland, even for adults. Getting employment or staying employed no longer holds the promise of a secure, life-long job. Unemployment, retraining and changes of workplace are facts of life for many adults. Today, working life demands creativity, knowledge of foreign languages, a wide general education, initiative, automatic data-processing skills and internationality. Efficiency requires continuing professional development and life-long study. The growing requirements of modern literacy (both reading and writing) call for continuous new efforts and these skills are expected to be developed on top of mastery of the basics. Literacy, language and communication skills are prerequisites for linguistic mobility and creativity. These skills are acquired as interactive processes in which reading and writing performance is dependent on both content and form and also on the experience and knowledge of the reader and writer.

The results of the study indicate that dyslexia may occur very severely – even in adult life – and affect the domains of both reading and writing. The mistakes that dyslexic adults make in their reading and writing are both qualitatively more serious and quantatively greater than those made by non-dyslexic adults. The performances of dyslexic subjects on various tests have been shown to be slower than those of non-dyslexic individuals.

The analysis of reading and writing errors reveals the fact that, for many dyslexic adults, the phonological processing problem continues and has caused a linguistic disorder, dyslexia. Background information has indicated that the disorder has its origins in early childhood. The findings endorse results of previous studies to the effect that linguistic disorders connected with development are causally related, both in learning language and in adopting a new language (second or other language learning). The subsystems for language learning include phonology, morphology, syntax and semantics. Pragmatics is connected with the use of a language (in different contexts and situations). The better the mastery of the various subsystems, the more skilful the use of words, phrases and sentences in various situations. A hierarchy exists between the subsystems of a language in which the phonological development is primary and the rest of the subsystems are formed on the basis of the previous systems. It is astonishing to discover that according to the results of the error analysis of reading and writing, certain mistakes can be identified as evidence of phonological processing difficulties and thus appear to be causally related to the prolongation of the primary phonological processes. In other words, the dyslexic adults' problems lie at the level of the basic subsystem of a language, on that of the mastery of phonological processes.

The results reveal that mistakes made by adults are similar to those made by beginner readers and writers (Poussu-Olli 1993, 1996). This phenomenon is especially evident in severe dyslexia. Support for the results gathered from error analysis is also given by diagnostic test results in which dyslexic adults' problems occur in the auditory and visual perception of a language and in short- and long-term memory performances. The weakest performances occur in the domain of auditory perception.

Reading comprehension and creative writing require the mastery of all linguistic domains. The results show that dyslexic adults' performances in these tests were weak. The results show clearly the hierarchy of linguistic development in that since the basic skills of dyslexic adults are deficient, they have also influenced the entire language subsystem.

According to the present results the central, critical problem of adult dyslexia can be found in the area of working memory. Baddeley (1990, 1992) suggests that working memory consists of three subsystems: the central executive and functioning under its control, the phonological loop, and the visuospatial sketch pad. Working memory can perform several functions simultaneously so that these functions do not disturb each other. But, if some sub-area of working memory is functioning deficiently, erroneous information in this part is transferred to the storage memory. According to the results of the study reported here, the deficient functioning of the phonological loop appears to be involved with dyslexic adults. Information which has been incorrectly stored in the long-term memory causes, amongst other things, prolongation of the phonological processes, defects and errors in the concept system and difficulties with text comprehension.

An interesting and encouraging finding among the research results is the fact that two subjects in the control group had reading and writing mistakes which suggest that their difficulties had been 'corrected' earlier. Their weaknesses in the auditory and visual items of the diagnostic tests were evident, yet their reading and writing performances were good. In other words, despite primary defects, they have been able to create, with the aid of corrective teaching, their own control system, especially for writing, through which they were able to write without mistakes.

The results of the laterality tests point to a phenomenon which has also been discovered in previous studies, namely that dyslexic subjects are more likely to be left-handed and have cross-laterality (Geschwind and Behan 1982; Poussu-Olli 1993). As a phenomenon, it refers to the possibility that the dyslexic subjects process language in a different way. In addition, the laterality result emphasizes the biological origins of dyslexia. Although ERP had been performed on only two dyslexic individuals, the results support the slowness of the dyslexic subjects' language processing. These kinds of studies will give more support to the diagnosis of dyslexia in the future.

In the present comprehensive school system in Finland, an efficiently functioning special teaching system helps dyslexic children by teaching through remedial methods. However, as noted earlier, all dyslexic subjects' problems cannot be correct during the compulsory education phase and it must be acknowledged that dyslexic children grow up into dyslexic adults. The results also indicate that this 'growth' is traumatic for many of them. There have been defects in school choices and in vocational education of dyslexic adults and problems also have to be faced in their working lives. The negative experiences reported by some adults have also been affected by the fact that there may not have been any part-time special teaching programmes in the schools they attended. Information from the research interviews suggests that almost every dyslexic adult seems to have undergone traumatic experiences in school. The following quotations provide some examples:

'The teacher just told me to read more to learn. I thought that I was somehow hard-headed or ungifted as I did not learn to read. I was ashamed and avoided

everything connected with schooling so much that I was relieved when I had
passed compulsory education age.'
'The other pupils teased me and the teachers did not understand. I did not get
support or encouragement, not even from home.'
'Well, Lena, what now? Not like that! Just try! Can't you see which letter comes
first? Not there.'

From the interview reports it would appear that dyslexic pupils have
often been used by teachers as a sort of warning to other children in
school. Neither the school nor home had the 'know-how' to guide them.
One of the interviewees made this statement about motivation to learn in
school:

'Difficulties in reading and writing lowered motivation before I ever got any.'

Many other dyslexic subjects agreed with this statement.

The results of the study indicate that dyslexia has crucially affected
subjects' possibilities for further studies and, therefore, also possible
career choices. The experiences of adult interviewees have been more
positive, however, compared with those reported by primary and
secondary school pupils, but on the other hand, further education has
involved a lot of extra work as students attempt to compensate:

'Dyslexia has certainly influenced my own studying, for I did not dream of
going to college.'
'Even in college when I was an 18-year-old, the training was focused on
practical subjects because of the "role" which I learnt in primary school.'
'I finished vocational school. I had accepted the fact that I could not write.'

Those dyslexic learners who had been successful in gaining employment had mostly had positive experiences. They appreciated the support
given at their workplace. However, problems related to dyslexia had
affected working life. When enquiring of dyslexic subjects about other
people's attitudes toward them, it looks as though some people did not
know about dyslexia, some think those with dyslexia are stupid or take
another kind of negative stance. The attitudes of close relatives were
reported to have been positive, but they had not been able to help with
the actual problems experienced.

One of the goals of the interviews was to map out dyslexic subjects'
own attitudes to their dyslexia. The results show that dyslexia has not
embittered them, although it has troubled them all their lives. Dyslexia has
been a fact which they have had to accept. One dyslexic adult crystallized
these thoughts as follows:

'Some thought I was stupid; others knew something. I, myself, take a humorous attitude towards it, although sometimes it annoys me.'

The instruction of a dyslexic adult involves 'rehabilitative teaching'. In addition to corrective teaching of dyslexic errors, it includes the development of compensatory abilities for linguistic shortcomings, the support of emotional life and the development of social skills. In order to realize this rehabilitative teaching more comprehensive information is required about the problem concerned and about its acceptance. Diagnostic tests for adults must be further developed and teaching methods directed and controlled by the adults themselves. Computer-based teaching will give wonderful opportunities for this in the future. In severe dyslexia, especially, the biological symptoms may be compared with those with dysphasic language disturbances. Compensatory rehabilitation services should be offered, particularly to individuals with severe dyslexia.

The hopes of the dyslexic adults themselves, regarding society at large, were as follows:

'I think the issue should be considered akin to blindness or deafness. Our difficulty is no worse. Considering that, support should be given to correct the circumstances.'
'People should learn to accept their diversity more readily. At school, in studying and in working life, we should try to take into consideration every person as an individual.'

# Chapter 9
# Partnerships with parents

Morag Hunter-Carsch

---

Questions addressed in this chapter include:

- What challenges and difficulties are faced by parents of children with literacy difficulties including dyslexia, in relationships between home and school?
- How can successful family literacy projects contribute to overcoming some of the difficulties?
- How can schools become 'dyslexia-friendly' places?

---

## Introduction

In September 1998, the *Times Education Supplement* publicized the findings of government-sponsored research under the title, 'Mums too afraid to ask' (Ghouri 1998). The article began with the statement that 'Mothers from low-income families are too intimidated by schools and teachers to ask for help with their children's learning'. This is the background against which the 'Family Learning Day/Weekend' was launched as part of the National Campaign for Learning. It is within the wider concerns for promoting effective learning, and in particular, literacy learning, that the above statement prompts the observation that it rings true not only for low-income mothers but also for mothers in prosperous home situations who also feel that their particular questions are not being heard. Some of these questions are explored in this chapter and the importance of the partnership between teachers and parents in promoting effective literacy learning is illustrated.

The first part of the chapter draws upon the author's experience of working closely with parents in a range of school and family literacy projects and in the context of local groups within the UK Reading Association and

The British Dyslexia Association over a number of years. The challenges, difficulties and questions faced by parents of dyslexic children are considered within the wider context of fostering family literacy, life-long learning and 'inclusive education'. In the second part, an attempt is made to suggest ways of overcoming some of the difficulties through establishing working partnerships with parents. The third part draws upon the findings of successful projects on family literacy and 'dyslexia-friendly schools' to illustrate issues being addressed through partnerships with parents.

The views expressed are those of the author, not of any single institution or LEA.

## Literacy context

As part of the government's five-year plan for 'building a literate nation' (McClelland 1997) through a strategic agenda designed 'to transform standards of literacy' (Barber 1997), there has been the National Year of Reading (1998-1999) and the follow-up campaign 'Read-on'. The strategy has brought together special contributions from a wide range of literacy agencies, including professional and voluntary associations. It has formally involved administrators, advisers and teachers in mainstream and special education at primary, secondary and in tertiary education and has sought to reach the public through diverse media projects involving also a range of library services.

Although there remains much to be done, there is also evidence of some success through small-scale, yet locally significant developments in communication, literacy and home–school relationships which have taken place in England (e.g. family reading groups: Beverton et al. 1993; Hunter-Carsch et al. 1996; Parents in Education Research Network (PERN), http://www.ioe. ac.uk/pern/; Wolfendale and Bastiani (2000)). This chapter is concerned with the extent to which the individual school is considered by parents of children with literacy difficulties to be 'welcoming'. The focus is thus on successful ways of improving the quality of communications between school, home and community with reference to literacy support so that there is widespread appreciation not only of the message of 'dyslexia-friendly schools' (Warwick 1999; Rule 1999) which is discussed later in the chapter, but even more fundamentally, that all parents should have the opportunity of experiencing visits to genuinely 'parent- friendly schools'.

## Policy and practices

Increasingly, schools are responding to the need for explicitly stated policy documents to be available for parents and the public in general. There have been dramatic changes in national policy regarding public access to information about academic achievement levels, schools' performance tables, OFSTED (Inspectors) Reports and school governors' reports. It is not only through locally printed materials that schools' results can be shared, but the internet can now be accessed for such information. Schools' websites are being developed along with training for their pupils in designing their own personal websites.

However, some parents still feel that matters of communication on an interpersonal basis with school staff are not satisfactory. There seem to be differences between policy statements and their translation into practice. Teachers may consider themselves to be friendly, not intimidating; accessible and not hard to reach, but the perceptions of teachers by some parents reflect a different picture. It is through listening to the messages from parents that the following points are shared with a view to shaping perceptions about what remains to be done if all parents are to have equal opportunities to feel not only that their views are heard but that they are able to regard their local school as welcoming to them and as 'dyslexia-friendly'.

## Challenges and difficulties for parents

The kinds of concerns that parents voice are exemplified in the following comments which have been selected as fairly representative, across a range of schools, over several years and arising repeatedly in the context of different literacy projects:

> 'If the school does not intervene soon, I can see that the situation will get worse and my daughter will slip further and further behind.'
> 'I don't understand why they are "keeping me on hold" – it has been ages since I asked about assessment for my son.'
> 'I know that there is something wrong. I've known it for a long time, and I can't deal with the idea that we have to wait to see – for the development to happen.'
> 'I can tell you my daughter is going to turn out like me. And they're not going to do anything in time to change that.'

These comments reflect concerns about early diagnosis of difficulties, understanding about the assessment procedures and both policy and practices regarding learning support. Some further examples illustrate concerns about the nature of dyslexia and exactly what can be done and who should help:

'I've asked the teacher but she doesn't seem to know much about dyslexia. She thinks that because my son can read and is about average in his class, that he can't be dyslexic.'

'I know my child is not very able, but I think he could do a lot better if he had more time from the teacher and really learnt his work. He is always having to finish work at home and it is not fair for him as his mates expect him to go out to play with them and he can't go out.'

'I've asked about how to help and I've tried at home, but it doesn't seem to work and I hate to keep asking. I don't know what to do. Maybe if they showed me, not just telling me.'

'Well, I don't find it easy to write and my spelling isn't good so I ask his sister first, then his father to help him, but he gets short-tempered with him, and it is not working out and I blame myself. Should I try to do something about my own spelling? How would I go about that?'

'Why can't they find a teacher to help? – Or even give him a chance not to have to write everything as it takes him so long and makes him so depressed.'

Parents are keen to help. They are interested in talking about the problems but apprehensive about the reception they may have if they try to talk with teachers. Some parents have themselves experienced problems in learning literacy and some may have negative thoughts about schools, based on their own unhappy schooldays. Some comment spontaneously in 'safe conversations' that as children, they were 'often in trouble in school' and may indicate that they do not wish to be reminded about that, and that every time they go near the school (often the very same building) they feel unable to say what they want to say.

In summary, the kinds of concerns illustrated by the above comments include:

- Early diagnosis of difficulties.
- Understanding of assessment procedures and policy about provision of support for learning as well as awareness about practices.
- Shared and sufficient understanding about the nature of dyslexia.
- Matters concerning special teaching methods and availability of specialist learning support.
- Help with homework.
- Help with parents' literacy skill development.
- Realistic and shared expectations.
- Reassurance about the quality of support and ready access to unthreatening, high-quality communication.

# Family literacy: life-long learning and 'inclusive education'

## Meeting the challenges and overcoming difficulties in communication

It might be suggested that there are two levels of concern expressed through examples of parents' comments and the summary of the issues. The first relates to the points of content in the above summary (e.g. putting in place the means by which early diagnosis can take place). The second relates to overriding concern about parents' feelings in relation to the extent to which the school is perceived to be a welcoming place and one in which people understand each others' interests. It is at this more holistic level, that the dynamics of human communication may need to be more fully considered. Individual sensitivity levels and interpersonal preferences and learning styles may also need to be taken into account. The following paragraphs provide some illustrations of ways in which parents suggest that communication between school and home can be improved.

### Making the meaning of printed communications more accessible

The most common form of communication with parents tends to be through sending printed materials, letters, notices and reports of various kinds. Teachers have recently been subjected to substantial amounts of documentation from the government. These include curriculum guide-lines and codes of practice. There are documents also from the LEA and the production of the school's policy documents about a wide range of matters, not only curriculum content. For example, most schools have readily available copies of school 'mission statements', governors' reports and policy statements, such as 'Coping with Bullying'. Some of these materials are shared with parents but not always presented in a manner which is accessible by all parents.

In particular, with reference to letters sent home with children, parents say that it would be helpful if there was less dense print on pages and presentation included well-spaced paragraphs with bold print labelled sections and bullet point style so that main points could be highlighted and would 'stand out'. Perhaps more importantly, however, parents' preference is often to talk to the teachers, not just to read about school matters. Many parents are happy to hear directly from teachers by telephone, if mutually suitable times can be found. Many prefer to talk than to read or write about matters which concern their child and the school.

## Talking and listening, not reading and writing

If parents receive and respond to written invitations to come to the school (e.g. for a scheduled meeting with their child's teacher, whether in primary or secondary school) it is often under less than ideal conditions in which time is very limited and other parents may also be waiting for fairly brief scheduled discussions at the end of the working day when teachers as well as parents may be tired and preoccupied with mundane matters such as practical planning for the next day.

What is wanted is time to be listened to in a manner that hears the real concerns and addresses them directly. This involves establishing a sense of mutual respect and trust. Such a relationship cannot be taken for granted. It may be easier for a parent to talk to a member of staff from the school in their own home, or in a parents' room in the school, or on the telephone rather than in the classroom. In some schools there are designated home-school liaison officers but they may not personally have the special information that may be in the province of the special educational needs co-ordinator (SENCO) or the curriculum subject specialist. In such cases the liaison officer may set up further contacts indirectly or directly with parents.

In some schools in the UK, in addition to open meetings in evenings, in order to inform parents about policy developments and matters such as how literacy is taught in the school, there is a policy of 'open visits' at any time and parents are encouraged to come in and assist informally. In others, special 'open days' are set up so that parents who are able to visit during the working day, can see the school in operation. Beyond the UK, in some schools in Germany, for example, special parent days are organized on a regular basis (every month) so that parents can make arrangements to spend some time in school during working hours, and talk with their child's teacher (with acknowledgement to Mrs Wohlfarth, a primary head teacher, for correspondence with the writer in 1999; see also Haase (2000) regarding parent–teacher partnerships in German schools).

More confident parents can pursue the information that they seek, but some may lack the confidence to be able to negotiate or to articulate their concerns sufficiently clearly for the liaison officer or teacher to grasp exactly what is required. In some instances, parents may also suffer from a combination of inhibitions stemming from the fact that they may also be dyslexic and possibly also from their past experiences of unsuccessful attempts to communicate their concerns to teachers. It can be the case that parents ask to speak to the headteacher assuming that since the headteacher is in authority that such contact would constitute the fastest route to resolution of their problems. The headteacher, however, may not be in possession of the kinds of detailed knowledge about special educational methods that parents may expect and for many reasons may not be as readily available as parents might wish. Delays or difficulties in arranging a meeting can add to a build-up of anxieties which can cumulatively result in a confrontational situation.

### Teacher training for partnership with parents

It may take a special kind of training to equip class teachers and specialist special educational needs (SEN) teachers as well as liaison officers to diffuse such anxieties and build the essential confidence levels in the course of acquiring a deeper understanding of how best to work together to overcome communication problems as well as SpLDs. It is encouraging that initial teacher-training courses are now introducing not only more information about the identification and support for dyslexic learners (e.g. TTA/BDA video package 1997) but also undertaking workshops on the topic of 'parents as partners' (e.g. Leicester University PGCE Primary course) and that continuing professional development courses are addressing some of these issues (for example, ensuring effective communication across the transition from primary to secondary; the implications for the student as negotiator in their own transition at secondary into tertiary education).

## Successful literacy initiatives

### Dyslexia-friendly schools

The 'partnership with parents' emphasis was echoed in the BDA's campaign towards 'dyslexia-friendly' schools (BDA and Swansea LEA 1999) Their message was effectively disseminated at teacher education courses such as the 'Sharing Good Practice' Conference at Leicester University, February 2000.

The message was mediated in a manner which revealed the harsh realities of the investment of time that LEAs and individual schools will need to make in the process of building effective communications with parents who are initially experiencing anger and frustration at delays in identifying the nature and severity of their children's literacy difficulties. Cliff Warwick and his team of SEN specialists pointed to the need 'to get beyond the will to blame when things go wrong and to find ways of working "from the top down" with the backing of the local authority' and, through a process of partnership, to agree a strategy, which in the Swansea situation, involved a series of steps over a period of about three years. It involved working through unpleasantness and times of feeling uncomfortable until through talking together (with children, parents, teachers and learning assistants), the policy of inclusion became shared practice at all levels.

The Swansea team was aware that 'it takes only one teacher with a negative attitude to seriously undermine the policy of the school', thus their focus was on 'getting everyone on board' (that is, all the school staff, learning assistants, social services and related services such as libraries, and working closely with the BDA at national, regional and local levels and with the Dyslexia Institute). The aim was to improve the quality of teaching at all levels. This was achieved through setting up specialist centres and providing inservice training in schools as well as specialist teacher training. At the time of writing they had reached about 70% of the target of working towards provision of a trained teacher in every school (see also the history of the Lancashire teacher training, Crossley 2001; and Lothian region's pioneering training with the support of the BDA, Chapter 15 in this volume).

The findings of the Swansea team are reflected also in other projects involving partnership with parents: as parents' confidence increased, relationships with teachers improved and collaboration became more effective between schools and the community. In Warwick's words 'there was a perception of a change from the sense of the school providing policing to its provision of "supportiveness"'. There were five main strands of this development. They included:

- Working towards improving management so that a coherent dyslexia policy was recognizable as including co-ordinated strategies for SEN, valuing the skills of all of the staff and maintaining school governors and pupils within the partnership.
- School development plans, including inservice training, perhaps through a series of seminars and courses.
- Improvements in identification and assessment through heightening awareness and putting in place a range of approaches for early assessing and for diagnostic assessment, including Fawcett and Nicholson's Dyslexia Early Screening Test (DEST).
- Engaging pupils and parents in partnerships which involved listening to their points of view and hearing what they said.
- Improving communication in the classroom by, for example, giving precise instructions in a manner which makes clear the purpose of the task ('Look so that you can recognize this sign' 'Look, and study it so you can draw it'), employing multi-sensory teaching and training in study skills.

In particular, partnerships between teachers and parents were illustrated as 'involving the development of a school and classroom climate in which pupils feel secure enough to confide concerns and have a chance to feel valued and of worth to society'. The words of the Swansea team have been employed in some detail in order to endorse the points that they have illuminated about the importance of the quality of communication and the time which is required to develop trust and true partnership. This process has been independently found to be vital to the success of family literacy projects, which, if they are to thrive, require comparable quality of partnership which takes investment of time, goodwill and participation of everyone in training. It is thus as a part of inclusive education, and with the purpose of relating the improvement of meeting the needs of dyslexic pupils as one part of the wider need to raise of the quality of literacy and communication in education, that some of the findings of the following five successful literacy projects are briefly mentioned. Each of the five projects reflected in varying degree the developmental stages of the process illustrated by the Swansea project.

## A family reading groups project

This project ran between 1994 and 1996 in order to set up family reading groups (FRGs) at Eyres Monsell Primary School, an urban fringe school serving a large council estate. FRGs are groups of children, parents and a leader (teacher/librarian or parent) who meet regularly to discuss, recommend and borrow books. Their aim is to promote the love of books and voluntary reading and to widen children's and adults' experience of children's books (Beverton et al. 1993). Although, normally, FRGs tended to be open and not to select a target group with particular achievement, some FRGs are designed particularly for 'able or gifted children', or for an age band (e.g. Key Stage 1, early years or Key Stage 3, secondary school). The Eyres Monsell FRGs were designed for nursery and beginners and to include, where possible, children likely to have literacy difficulties if not provided with early additional support.

The project was jointly supported by a small grant from ALBSU, the LEA (then Leicestershire) and the University of Leicester. Average attendance was ten parents with their ten children for a weekly meeting of one hour during school time. The meetings involved parents, teachers and librarians working together to promote the enjoyment of literature and to extend use of stories in school and at home. The project involved eight teachers at different times, five librarians, an adult basic education tutor and a university researcher in partnership with over 50 parents and their children in one year. From a target group of adults identified to have literacy difficulties, seven individuals completed a nationally accredited basic literacy course while also supporting their children's literacy development; 13 gained Open College accredited certificates for working with their children (that is, 265 of the adults participating in FRGs became involved in accredited continuing education). The FRGs continued to meet beyond the date of the project and to inspire other groups.

The findings of the project included the following developments for teachers:

> greater confidence and trust in parents' ability and enthusiasm, leading to higher expectations of their potential as partners in developing children's learning.

For parents and teachers together:

> more parents are taking opportunities to consult with staff informally before and after school, to visit school, use the parents' room for informal chats, work in classrooms alongside teachers, and seek opportunities to speak with their child's teacher. (Hunter-Carsch et al. 1996)

The research work associated with the project contributed towards the development of a screening test for rhyming (Rappaport and Hunter-Carsch 1999) and teaching materials for initial teacher training and special education training (e.g. a case study of one dyslexic and dyspraxic child who attended the FRGs).

## The Highfields literacy project

This project involving four inner-city multi-lingual schools was run during 1997-1999 with the support of Leicester City LEA, the Community and Schools Library Service, the University of Leicester and diverse small grants. Staff from all four schools were involved and over 200 parents contributed. A range of activities was undertaken. Among them were courses for parents, a series of separate meetings with parents on different topics (e.g. assisting their children with literacy learning at home and in school) and the production of a video in five languages as well as English, for home use in order to share with parents, information about the Literacy Hour, a part of the government's national literacy strategy. The video, produced in collaboration with Leicester University, is now available from Leicester City LEA.

## Four primary school projects

Typical of the successful local literacy initiatives, are four Midlands primary schools which were successful in obtaining government grants (standards funding) to support their literacy initiatives. Three strands of the combined projects involved:

- 'Keeping up with the Kids', a 12-week programme which involved providing adults with the Literacy Hour at an adult level which addressed their own literacy needs.
- The CEDC 'Share' initiative, a parental involvement project for parents of children at Key Stage 1 (beginning school and early years) with resource materials for home use.
- 'Parents as Partners in their Children's Learning' was designed to connect the school learning of the children with the curriculum which parents were working on at home. It sought to help parents to understand their children's own needs, curriculum and learning targets and direct home activity to supporting it.

Figure 9.1, an illustrative letter from Arsalam's parent, indicates the sense of shared value which was a typical response to all of the initiatives in all four schools and reflects similar responses resulting from effective teamwork in literacy initiatives.

### Developing literacy at 11

The Summer Literacy Schools evaluation of six summer schools in Leicester City, over two summers involved both quantitative assessment employing norm-referenced tests of reading and spelling and also tests of language and communication, individual interviews with parents, teachers, other adult staff and of pupils. The analysis of the qualitative data has generated a range of findings and recommendations amongst which are strong messages about the importance of self-esteem, listening skills and opportunities for informal yet structured discussion and the practice of handwriting to 'automatic level' as components in the development of basic literacy competences (Hunter-Carsch 1998; Chapter 1 in this volume).

In conclusion, to return to the questions posed at the beginning of the chapter, some of the major challenges and difficulties faced by parents of children with literacy difficulties including dyslexia, in relationships between home and school have been illustrated. They include the sense of frustration and anger which ensues if parents find that teachers do not appear to appreciate their concerns and to be able to answer their questions in ways that are readily understood and give a sense of working together in partnership.

Some examples have been provided of ways in which successful family literacy projects contribute to overcoming some of the difficulties. Discussion of parents' prompts the suggestion that parents of children

Describe what you and your children have gained from the Families Learning Together Course.
Write at least a page'.

Arsalaan has gained a lot from the Families Learning Together course. When we began Arsalaan didn't know his alphabet it took him a while, but can now say the alphabet correctly. He didn't know how to spell his name, he can now do this. He can also write the first letter of his name and surname in capitals, and the rest in lower case.

He didn't know any words before, he now knows a total of 28 new words and can also spell them all. He can count up to 20 and recognises the numbers 1-12. He can do sums (additions and subtractions). His handwriting has improved tremendously and he has a lot of confidence in himself.

There are a lot more things that Arsalaan has learnt.

I have gained from the course as well because I have more confidence in my role as an educator. My handwriting has improved a lot from before. And I now know how to help my child at home. Which is very comforting because I wanted to help him before but I didn't know how. I have learnt not to compare my child with other children because they all have different things that they are good at. So this course has been very educational to us both.

**Figure 9.1** Letter from Arsalam's parent.

with general as well as SpLDs, including dyslexia and dyspraxia, and parents of children with attention deficit disorder may, perhaps have more in common than may have been appreciated. All of them share a need for self-perception as a worthy contributor to supporting their child's learning, and in that sense are partners with teachers, in this process. Parents' appreciation of teachers' expertise depends to a large extent on teachers' manner of respecting parents' actual and potential contribution, and how effectively teachers communicate practically helpful advice about, for example, helping with homework, adapting circumstances at home and providing learning support which connects what is happening in the classroom and at home (Cortazzi and Hunter-Carsch 2000).

The work of Warwick and the Swansea team on promoting 'dyslexia-friendly' schools has been cited as providing inspiration and 'good practice'. It has been considered in relation to the wider need to provide an ethos which is welcoming to parents of children with the full range of literacy and learning difficulties, so that all have an equal opportunity of becoming partners in promoting children's successful learning.

## Acknowledgements

Thanks are due especially to Sue Barnes for inspiration and for collegial discussions over some years; also to Margaret Herrington for discussion and comments on an earlier draft of this chapter; Ted Hartshorn, formerly chair of Leicestershire primary head teachers' association and Clive Hawley, contributing tutors to the initial teacher training workshops at Leicester University School of Education on partnership with parents; Sam Fox, Chris Hossack and Sue Whiting, teachers and parent members of the Leicestershire Dyslexia Association for their discussion of the Swansea team's presentation at the conference on 'Dyslexia Friendly Schools'; Judy Dunning, Sue Barnes, Shanti Chanhan (Leicester City Education Authority) and John Shears (Leicester University A–V Department) for support in production of the video on Developing Literacy at Home and in School (in English, Bengali, Gujerati, Punjarbi and Urdu); and to all the teachers, parents, children, learning assistants and helpers participating in the range of family literacy projects with whom the author has had the privilege to work.

# Chapter 10
# Dyslexia and multi-lingual matters

LINDSAY PEER

Questions addressed in this chapter include:

- What is the incidence of bilingualism or multi-lingualism amongst the dyslexic population?
- What questions and issues affect the process of identification and diagnostic assessment of dyslexia in bilingual or multi-lingual learners?
- How might the teaching of dyslexic learners who are bilingual or multi-lingual be improved?

## Introduction

Although there is an already substantial and rapidly increasing body of research information about language, phonology and learning to read (Hulme and Snowling 1997; Snowling and Nation 1997) and about learning to read and spell in different orthographies (Leong 1987; Goswami 1997), until very recently there appears to have been relatively little research which focused directly on the complex issues associated with multi-lingualism and dyslexia (Landon et al 1999; Landon 2001).

The focus sharpened, however, with the event of the first international conference on multi-lingualism and dyslexia of the British Dyslexia Association, June 1999, in Manchester. It quickly became evident, from the exchanges between the 500 delegates from over 40 countries, that a new impetus had been given to make connections across the two areas of study: dyslexia and multi-lingualism, which have tended to remain separate in the past. In the words of Professor Tony Cline in his conference address, 'Some people in the field have been looking so hard for factors they expect to see, not learning to look from a different perspective'. The conference provided an opportunity to begin to appreciate the range of perspectives from which dyslexia and multi-lingual matters could be more fully appreciated and understood. For a brief report on the conference see Schwarz (http://ldonline.org/whats-new/multlingualism-conf699.html).

Research in progress on the development of an international test of dyslexia is perhaps one of the most exciting areas which was opened up to conference delegates. Delegates were invited to make their contribution to the ongoing process of refining and carrying out international trials with this instrument. For further information about this test readers may wish to contact Ian Smythe at the University of Surrey, Department of Psychology, or email: ian.smythe@ukonline.co.uk.

This chapter explores some of the issues which affect progress, not only in identifying and assessing multi-lingual and dyslexic learners, but also in providing appropriate learning support for them at different stages in their lives. It endorses the importance of collaborative research at all levels and extends an invitation to the reader to make a direct contribution to research by responding to a survey questionnaire designed to establish a baseline databank of an informal and reflective kind by taking into account dyslexic multi-lingual learners' views.

## Incidence of dyslexia and bi-/multi-lingualism

At present we have no clear picture of the incidence of bilingual or multi-lingual learners among the dyslexic population, nor detailed knowledge about the nature of the impact of dyslexia on their simultaneous language learning.

Although broad indications of the incidence of dyslexia across several countries is cited in the *International Book of Dyslexia* (Salter and Smythe 1997; see also Table 10.1 below), there is no detailed information provided there as to the range of languages spoken in the countries represented, nor those spoken by the dyslexic learners, whether indigenous, temporary residents or immigrants and whether they were in fact included in the relevant statistics.

The incidence of dyslexia is, of course, governed by the definition in use. We already know, for example, that in England and Wales dyslexic students' learning strengths are often regarded as characteristically greater in areas relating to speaking (oracy) but lower in areas relating to reading and writing (literacy). This tendency is noted in the DfEE Code of Practice definition of dyslexia as a specific learning difficulty:

> They may gain some skills in some subjects quickly and demonstrate a high level of ability orally, yet may encounter sustained difficulty in gaining literacy or numeracy skills. (DfEE 1994)

**Table 10.1** Incidence of dyslexia

| Belgium | 5% | Japan | 6% |
|---|---|---|---|
| Great Britain | 4% | Nigeria | 11% |
| Czech Republic | 2–3% | Norway | 3% |
| *Finland | 10% | Poland | 4% |
| Greece | 5% | Russia | 10% |
| Italy | 1.3–5% | Singapore | 3.3% |

*This figure refers to 'slow learners receiving special attention'.
(Adapted from Salter and Smythe 1997, p. 238, and reproduced with permission.)

It might be anticipated that this greater oral ability might be sustained over more than one language in those who are bilingual or multi-lingual. However, this is certainly not so.

## Dyslexia and language learning difficulty (monolingual and multi-lingual)

Further complications lie in the fact that the issue of dyslexia and bi-/multi-lingualism is not always clearly differentiated from the issue of difficulties with monolingual literacy learning. In the UK secondary school system, it is often assumed that monolingual students who already show difficulties in reading or writing in English would have significantly greater difficulty in coping with another (second) language. For some this is undoubtedly true, particularly with the written word. However, for others, given the appropriate teaching methodology, they would succeed. By automatically refusing them such access, they may be denied access to learning a second language which prompts concerns about equal opportunities and rights to education. We know, for example, that some dyslexic English-speaking students learning French in secondary school, experienced difficulties in processing English phonology which, Crombie (1997, 1999) suggests, affected their learning of French phonology and that the dyslexic students required more time to process phonological information. We will return later to the issue about phonological factors but meanwhile, to contextualize the question in the much wider concern that there is insufficient general awareness about the fact that, currently in the UK, in some areas students, including dyslexic students, are required to learn via other languages. Elaine Miles (1996) reminds us that:

> ... our dyslexics are required to learn some of them in school. Welsh, not English is the indigenous language of some of our British population, who need

to learn two working languages; some immigrant children start with assumptions about language which are very different from English ones. More recently the birth of the European Dyslexia Association has opened our eyes to the fact that other European languages may pose altogether different problems for dyslexics from the English language, and that some of the features we regard as the chief characteristics of dyslexics simply do not appear in a language of a different type. This is rather startling news if we had assumed that the methods that Americans and ourselves have refined over some 50 years for teaching dyslexics will be the ones that we will now teach to other Europeans. (Miles 1996)

The point Miles makes is an important one not only in the UK with its indigenous Welsh and Gaelic speakers and over 50 other languages represented in the families of children attending some inner-city schools, since a substantial increase in teachers' knowledge about language is required for their work with all their students, not only the dyslexic learners.

## Limitations of teachers' knowledge about language learning and dyslexia

The dyslexia and monolingual issue, however, must be differentiated from concern about the current limitations of non-specialist teachers' knowledge about the developmental patterns in relation to profiles of bilingual or multi-lingual dyslexic students.

It might be suggested that the introduction of the Literacy Strategy (DfEE 1998a) is making a strong contribution to increasing teachers' knowledge about basic linguistic terminology and structures (such as spelling 'rules') in English. However, it is the wider knowledge about differences in linguistic structures (e.g. grammatical sequences) in the other languages in use in the homes of their pupils, that may be required in order to understand and to differentiate between problems that relate to either language learning or dyslexia or both.

## Underfunctioning

Another area of concern which needs to be considered in a conceptually discrete manner is that of underfunctioning in terms of possibly associated causal factors, including deprivation and disadvantage. As long ago as the 1960s Hess and Shipman (1965) wrote that 'the meaning of deprivation is a deprivation of meaning'. They saw the deprivation which so limits learning and later achievement in school as arising from failure to understand and use language to facilitate a cognitive structure which enables parent and child, teacher and student, to represent and control the social and learning environment. Relatedly, in the 1970s Cashdan and Grugean (1972) wrote that:

A substantial minority of British schoolchildren underfunction in the educational system. After ten or more years of school attendence, their attainments are low. They are hostile to school, and remain in the system only as long as they are compelled to do so. They are the disadvantaged children in our culture. They, (or their parents) come from a wide variety of social and ethnic backgrounds, but most of them are still the indigenous British poor. Their accents, and their language also, differ in significant respects from those approved by the school and displayed 'naturally' by the children of the middle class. (p. 167)

The factors these authors highlight as being important may be classified as cognitive and related to the representation of ideas. In bi-/multi-lingual children, or children whose primary linguistic code differs significantly from the form of language used in school, the expression systems for delivering learners' thoughts and ideas through speech or writing are more complex and difficult to learn and to control (Sage 2000). Our concern here with secondary and adult dyslexic learners also requires that we take into account more recent work in the fields of phonology, language and literacy learning and dyslexia.

Phonological awareness might be defined as sensitivity to sound in spoken language (Gallagher 1995). Stanovich (1988) has gone as far as to suggest that a major key to the failure in the development of the reading process for some students is a weakness in the phonological processing system in the learning of grapheme–phoneme correspondences. Studies have been carried out highlighting the association of phonological processing and reading progress in primary schools (Stanovich et al. 1986a; Stanovich et al. 1986b), other studies of the longitudinal type have linked pre-readers' phonological skills with their later acquisition of reading (Bradley and Bryant 1983; Torgensen et al. 1994). Programmes have been developed which include the training of phonological skills and have proven that the progress made by students with difficulties in the acquisition of reading skills has been substantially enhanced (Hatcher et al. 1994).

## Questions still to be explored

There is a significant gap, however, in that none of these programmes have looked selectively at the specific difficulties experienced by dyslexic learners who speak two or more languages. Among the questions still to be more fully explored are:

- In what ways do their cognitive profiles differ?
- Do they differ in terms of processing spoken language, literacy and numeracy?
- What is the effect of stress on their learning?

Many countries demand that their students reach a high level of proficiency in a minimum of two languages before entering vocational or academic higher education. Failure to achieve the required competence in two languages at this level is not only a personal tragedy for the individual but also represents a substantial loss of skills to society, which neither developed or under-developed nations can afford. Furthermore, current studies among prison populations show that there is a high rate of offenders who have a poor level of literacy and numeracy. The question arises as to the linguistic contexts and experience of the population under consideration. A government-funded study in Sweden (Alm and Andersson 1996) highlighted the fact that 31% of such offenders were dyslexic. In countries in which bilingualism or multi-lingualism are the norm, it would be helpful at this point of our international research, to learn about the language characteristics of the relevant population, including those in prisons.

## Procedures for identification and diagnostic assessment

The above discussion raises some of the questions and issues which affect identification and diagnostic assessment of young dyslexic bi-/multi-lingual learners and are compounded for the older dyslexic students who may not have been diagnosed accurately. It draws attention, among other things, to the importance of distinguishing between levels of competence in basic interpersonal communicative skills (BICS) and cognitive/academic language proficiency (CALP). This point was made by Cummins (1984). BICS, although important, is not enough for educational success since learners must be able to use language for analysis, synthesis and evaluation of ideas if they are to succeed at the higher academic levels.

Thus any diagnostic assessment would need to include not only possibilities to observe characteristic 'dyslexic' difficulties but also opportunities to explore these dynamic aspects of language in use. Such an evaluation of the ability of learners to use language has been suggested by Cline and Fredrickson (1991) as needing to be considered from five different perspectives:

- competence in phonology and syntax;
- competence in semantics;
- pragmatic competence;
- conversational competence;
- socio-linguistic competence.

They consider that the proficiency of a bilingual speaker is best under-stood if all five of these factors are taken into account. Essential factors beyond listening and speaking include speakers' attitudes and feelings about situations in which each language is used. They firmly state that a proficient bilingual speaker requires not just competence but also confi-dence across a wider range of situations than faced by monolingual speakers. On the other hand, those learners who have a low verbal learning ability also need diagnostic approaches which take into account not only the linguistic processing and dyslexia characteristics but also the findings of recent work by Mellanby et al. (1996) on cognitive determi-nants of verbal underachievement at secondary school. Whilst not selec-tively working with dyslexic learners, their study may throw light on the range of factors involved in language-learning at secondary school level in relation to comparing reading and spelling abilities with learning 'pig-latin' in tests of phonological awareness in groups of students classified as 'discrepant'(non-verbal scores exceeding their verbal scores) and those classified as 'verbal' and 'non-verbal'. The results suggest that the discrepant group, which was not necessarily reading-retarded with respect to chronological age 'needs to be identified if they are to reach the poten-tial level of achievement predicted by their non-verbal CAT scores (cogni-tive abilities test)'. However, information about the research samples' home language(s) experience was not provided.

In summary, it might be suggested that the condition of being dyslexic and bi-/multi-lingual presents a substantial diagnostic challenge; one which is not solely the responsibility of any one linguistic group and which requires diagnostic assessment to include differential information about the following factors, any of which may contribute to reading, spelling and writing retardations:

- social, cultural and linguistic home and school experience;
- different or impoverished language skills, including imbalanced speech development or restriction of vocabulary in one or all languages;
- unusual learning profiles, including reference to memory competence.

## Successful teaching approaches

Recognizing the complexities of diagnostic assessment, nevertheless, points towards the importance and desirability of avoiding some of the difficulties and distress as well as costs of late intervention. This prompts the suggestion that funding go into early identification in the hope of prevention of later more complex problems.

Appropriate teaching approaches for younger and older dyslexic bi-/multi-lingual learners may in the future involve the increasing use of technology to bridge the speech-to-text and text-to-speech communication challenges and for prevention, via early intervention, of later literacy problems. However, the wider range of dyslexic symptoms will need to be addressed too, including areas such as speed of processing, visual/auditory perception and short-term memory weaknesses. Already there are some exciting developments in international communications about dyslexia and special teaching (for example, papers presented at the Fourth World Dyslexia Congress in 1997 and the BDA's first international conference on Dyslexia and Multi-lingualism in 1999, Peer and Reid 2000). New technology programmes for linguistic learning offer hope for increased effectiveness in language learning (and re-learning in the case of, for example, aphasia related to cerebral haemorrhage; see Haase 1999; Larsen 1999).

With or without the support of computer technology, there remains a need to share information about successful teaching and learning approaches for this particular group of dyslexic learners. One way in which an attempt has been made to identify a sample of such learners and to seek their reflections via self-reports is reported below. The question-naire which was employed in the 'first wave' of the study is included in full (see Appendix) and interested readers are invited to respond to the questions and, by doing so, contribute directly to one databank which is accruing and which may lead to further and more refined studies.

## Some preliminary findings of the 1999 survey on the nature of multi-lingualism and dyslexia

The questionnaire was designed by Morag Hunter-Carsch in collaboration with the writer and distributed to 500 delegates at the BDA's international conference on dyslexia and multi-lingualism in Manchester 1999. It comprises two parts, the first of which was for completion by conference delegates. The second part is for dyslexic multi-lingual speakers. Many of the conference delegates kindly completed the first section and then proceeded to find and 'interview' a friend or relative to complete the second part. A preliminary analysis (Hunter Carsch and Mailley 1999) of the returns from the first 74 delegates to complete the first part, and a sample of 12 dyslexic multi-lingual speakers, is reported below.

### The sample

The sample of respondents included 41 teachers of whom 21 were 'class teachers' (15 secondary or both secondary and primary level, one primary and five teachers of adults) and 20 were SpLD specialist teachers and/or SENCOs. There were also 14 teachers of English as another language

(EAL) and nine university-based respondents (seven tutors/researchers and two university students), as well as five educational therapists, two educational psychologists and one medical doctor.

The age range of the sample included respondents at every level, from age 20 years to over 60 years. There were 29 respondents of age 51–60 years; 19 who noted age 41–50 years; 12 indicated age 31–40 years and four at each end of the scale (20–30 years and 61+ years). This slightly skewed distribution curve indicates the weighting of the responses toward the 51–60-year age range, who might be anticipated to bring considerable experience to their shared views.

Respondents came from 22 countries. The largest number, 37, came from the UK (19 noted UK, nine from England, six from Scotland, two from Wales and one from Ireland). Respondents from other countries included eight from Sweden, five from the USA, three each from Denmark and Israel and two each from Belgium, Cyprus, Germany and Luxembourg. The remaining respondents were from the following 10 countries: China, Dubai (UAE), Greece, Hungary, Italy, Japan, Lebanon Norway, Poland and Spain.

In the case of 49 respondents, their first language was the same as that of the largest national group in their country of residence. For 25 respondents their first language was different from the main national language of their current country of residence. Eight of the 25 were bilingual and a further four had three 'first languages'. Sixty-six of the 74 respondents were bilingual; 42 were 'trilingual' and 23 had four languages; 10 had five languages and seven reported having a seventh language in which they considered themselves to be 'strugglers'.

Respondents' self-reports about their level of competence in the different languages were as follows: 35 considered that they were 'fluent' in their second language, 20 considered themselves 'competent' and nine 'strugglers'. Concerning the third language, eight respondents considered themselves to be 'fluent', 18 to be 'competent' and 13 to be 'strugglers'. For their fourth language, none of the respondents noted that they were 'fluent' but nine considered themselves 'competent' and 14 as 'strugglers'. Regarding their fifth language, again, no-one described themselves as 'fluent' but three respondents considered themselves to be 'competent' and seven to be 'strugglers'. For the sixth language, all seven respondents considered themselves to be at the 'struggler' level (Table 10.2).

Fifty-eight respondents noted that they knew someone who was dyslexic and multi-lingual and 56 of them were willing to contact that person and request that they complete the questionnaire (second part) or assist them, by 'interview' to complete the questionnaire. Thirty respondents indicated that they knew more than one person whom they could

**Table 10.2** Self-reported levels of competence in second or other languages (N=74)

|            | Second | Third | Fourth | Fifth | Sixth |
|------------|--------|-------|--------|-------|-------|
| Fluent     | 35     | 0     | 0      | 0     | 0     |
| Competent  | 20     | 18    | 9      | 3     | 0     |
| Struggler  | 9      | 13    | 14     | 7     | 7     |

invite to complete the questionnaire and some stated that they could find up to eight such people.

### Sample of responses from dyslexic multi-lingual learners

The second part of the questionnaire was designed for completion by (or with assistance) dyslexic multi-lingual learners. There were 12 returns arising from the efforts of the 74 respondents to the first part of the questionnaire within a few months of the conference in June 1999. Preliminary analysis of the first 12 returns is summarized below.

Four respondents who had completed the first part of the questionnaire went on to complete the second part as they themselves were dyslexic. A further eight respondents completed the second part in consultation with and on behalf of a multi-lingual dyslexic person.

### Current country of residence of the sample of 12

The 12 dyslexic multi-lingual learners included seven from the UK, two from Israel and one from each of Greece, Norway and Sweden. There were eight females and four males. Their ages ranged from under 20 to over 60 years. There were eight in the 12–20-year category, three aged between 21 and 30 years and one aged between 41 and 50 years. Six were students at school, two were adults, three were adult students and one was a secondary school teacher in England.

### Home languages

Only two of the sample of 12 were native English speakers living in England. For a further five living in the UK (four in England and one in Scotland), their home languages were French, Greek, Japanese, Swahili and Urdu respectively. The remaining five were bilingual at home. Their home languages and current residences were noted as follows:

- Two living in Israel, home languages Hebrew and English/English and Hebrew.
- One living in England, home languages English and Russian.

- One living in Norway, home languages English and Norwegian.
- One living in Sweden, home languages Swedish and German.

## School or work language

With reference to the question of home and work languages, there were only ten replies (two non-responses). The school or work languages for four of the dyslexic respondents were the same as their home language and for a further two (bilingual respondents) the school or work language was one of their two home languages. For four dyslexic learners, the school or work language was different from their home languages.

## Family history of dyslexia

Nine dyslexic respondents noted that there was a family history of dyslexia and three did not know if this was so.

The ages at which there was first awareness of dyslexia ranged between five and 15 years. Eight respondents became aware during the primary school phase, two at 12 years and two at 15 years. If the notional age of seven is taken as an 'earliest age for formal assessment' as has been the pattern in some countries, at least five of the 12 cases were aware before that point. Although for eight respondents the age at which awareness of dyslexia was noted and the age at which awareness of being dyslexic was 'confirmed' are regarded as the same, for four respondents there was a gap of two years in one instance (7–9 years of age) of five years in another (5–10 years of age), eight years for another (6–14 years old) and 10 years in another instance (15–25 years of age).

## Assessment of dyslexia

The age of assessment, whether informal or formal, was noted by ten respondents. Their responses ranged from one at age six years, to four at age 11 or 12, three at age 15 or 16 and two beyond this (one at 19 years and one at 25 years of age).

Of the ten respondents who completed the question about the language in which they were assessed, six were tested in their home language (two of the bilingual learners were tested in one of their home languages and one was tested in both home languages), four were tested in a language which was not their home language and in which, in at least two cases, was a language in which they did not consider themselves to be fluent. Formal testing took place in only seven of the 12 cases. Assessment was informal for five cases.

Nine respondents were able to comment on the occupational

background of their testers: seven assessments were made by educational psychologists and two by specialist trained teachers of students with specific learning difficulties.

## Strengths and difficulties

Taken collectively the multi-lingual dyslexic learners' strengths include the following (in the words noted): spatial, art (noted twice independently), creativity (noted twice independently), sports, (noted twice independently) photographic memory, verbal and spatial ability, oral work, vocabulary, analogies, logical reasoning and reading.

The noted areas of difficulty include: spelling (noted six times independently), writing (noted five times independently), reading (noted three times independently), auditory/visual sequencing (noted three times independently), memory (visual/auditory) noted twice independently and mathematics which was noted twice independently.

## Learning support

Learning support in primary school was noted by five respondents. Four respondents noted that they were given 'out of class, withdrawal learning support' during their primary schooling. Six noted learning support during secondary. Three noted 'in class' support. Three noted they were withdrawn for support (two noting both 'in class' and withdrawal support). One noted private tuition and another noted 'one-to-one support'. The language of mediation of the support was noted in six cases (English and Hebrew for one case and English only for the remaining five. For three of them, English was not their home language).

## Support found to be most helpful during school years

Five respondents did not answer this question and one mentioned only that the difficulties were attributed to bilingualism. Two considered that private tuition was most helpful. English teaching, targeted withdrawal in writing and mathematics and class support were noted by three and 'encouragement' specified by one. Having a reader in examinations was noted by one respondent as helpful.

## Most effective kind of support at home

Four respondents did not answer this question. Three of the remaining eight respondents mentioned the value of help with homework, especially with spelling, reading and written work. Other points mentioned as helpful were:

- Stopping the pressure; make the correct school choices.
- Having well-educated parents who paid attention to education.
- Private tuition.
- Elder sister (who helped with homework).
- Other read aloud school books.
- Specific multi-sensory spelling teaching.

### Advice about support for school-age students

No advice was offered by four respondents. The advice given by the remaining eight respondents regarding learning support for school-age students was:

- Ensure early recognition/pre-school screening; start as early as possible (two responses).
- Listen to the students; explain dyslexia; come to terms with it; don't bottle it up.
- Read worksheets to them and write for them when they are tired.
- Don't ask them to stay to work before or after school.
- It is important not to make them feel stupid; important to diagnose correctly.
- Teachers should be aware of the problems and give enough time and not care about spelling.

### Learning support as an adult student and learning support in adult working life

Only one respondent said they had learning support as an adult student. It was support with lectures and it was given in English. Five said that they had no support and six did not answer. Eight did not answer the question about support at work and four respondents indicated that they had no support.

### Dyslexia support for the family and advice to dyslexia support groups

Six respondents noted that they had been members of a local dyslexia support group. Four said they were not members and two did not answer. There were four comments about the ways in which the local group support was helpful. They were as follows:

- Can learn about dyslexia.
- It is helpful when making an appeal.
- They provided an excellent lecture series and support for parents.
- Mother works with dyslexic people and their families.

Five respondents gave points of advice for local dyslexia groups. They noted:

- Help to keep up the momentum.
- Inform dyslexic families and teach them.
- Speak to schools about dyslexia.
- Help children to believe in themselves and to use computers.
- Never give up fighting!

**Other comments**

The only other comment that was made was to emphasize the importance of raising dyslexia awareness and the value of early assessment. It should also be noted, however, that seven respondents were willing to be contacted with a view to assisting with further research.

## Comment about the findings of the survey

The willingness and generosity of all the 74 respondents and their dyslexic friends in making time to share their relevant views and to offer assistance with further research is encouraging. Their shared information provides endorsements for some of the feelings and hunches expressed in various ways at local dyslexia support gatherings and at national and international conferences by both professionals and laity. It is important that we listen to the multi-lingual dyslexic learners' own reflections. Their collective language experience is both diverse and substantial, as is their experience of dyslexia.

It is hoped that a follow-up 'wave' from this initial survey may generate further information about how best to proceed with this kind of investigative collaborative research, as well as to assist with illuminating directions for subsequent studies which may be able to explore selected issues and questions in greater depth.

## Conclusion

In order to answer the questions posed at the beginning of the chapter, there is a need for further research at many levels and for the effective dissemination of the research findings, for effective home–school and community projects and for parents as well as teachers to work together to bridge gaps in understanding both the language and cultural factors which affect dyslexic learners in particular contexts. Promising research and development projects are taking place at local, national and international levels within the wider literacy and communication framework (for example, Leicester's Highfields Project and its Literacy Hour Video in Asian languages for use at home (Barnes and Chauhan 2000); Edinburgh University's Scottish study of multi-lingual and dyslexia assessment procedures (Landon et al. 1999) and its research extensions beyond Scotland, concurrently with the development of the International (and multi-lingual) Test of Dyslexia (Smythe 1999).

In addition to the range of formal studies which is required to investigate diverse aspects of this challenging field (including identification, diagnostic assessment and teaching) readers may be interested in making their own direct contribution to the process of establishing a baseline and directions for future research. It is in the sharing of the experiences of learners, teachers, parents, researchers and others possibly from many professional and linguistic backgrounds that we can contribute to the more sensitive development of research procedures, not only the collation of information which may, in itself, lead to further understanding.

The dissemination of the questionnaire returns constitutes an attempt to contribute to increasing understanding about dyslexia and multi-lingualism within and beyond the UK, and in this way to assist with effecting what has been described as a much required 'sea change of attitude to language learning' on the part of some residents in the UK. This is needed since, even among the community of devoted and informed specialist teachers of dyslexic students, there remains a tendency to employ only methods suitable for teaching English to speakers of English as a first language. Along with the sharing of understanding about multi-lingual factors, and a welcoming of cultural diversity, we may be able to promote a recognition and celebration of the range of special skills and innovative ideas which also characterize many dyslexic learners.

## Acknowledgements

Thanks are due to Morag Hunter-Carsch for the inclusion of the preliminary report of the questionnaire findings and to Sue Mailley who assisted with the analysis of the data.

## Appendix

### Questionnaire on THE NATURE OF DYSLEXIA AND MULTI-LINGUALISM

If you are dyslexic and bi-/multi-lingual, or if you know such a person who is willing to assist with our survey, please copy this form, complete and return it to:

Lindsay Peer, Education Director,
British Dyslexia Association,
98 London Road,
Reading  RG1 5AU
UK

All contributions will be regarded as anonymous.
All contributors are warmly thanked for their contribution to the research.

I am completing this form relating to myself (please tick):          _____
I am completing it on behalf of someone else (please tick):          _____

## BACKGROUND

a)  Date of completing this form:          _____

b)  Name (optional):          _____

c)  Current Age (circle): 12–17 / 17–21 / 21–30 / 31–40 / 41–50 / 51–60 / Over 60

d)  Gender (tick):          Male:  _____  Female:  _____

e)  Current address (tick): UK: England/Ireland/Scotland/Wales/beyond UK

    If beyond UK please note country          _____

f)  Are you a school student?: (tick):          _____  an adult          _____

    If adult, please note occupation          _____

    Currently in a job  _____     not in work          _____

g)  What is/are your first language(s) [mother-tongue]?          _____

h)  What is your School/College/Work language?*:          _____

*For all languages please note whether fluent+++, competent++ or struggler+


i)  Other languages spoken?*:          _____

j)  Languages read?*:          _____

k)  Languages written?*:          _____

l)  Are there other dyslexic people in your family (whether or not they are formally

    identified)?:  Yes  _____  No  _____  Not Known  _____

## IDENTIFICATION/DIAGNOSIS

1.  At what age did you first become aware of dyslexia?:          _____

2.  At what age did you first become aware of being dyslexic?:          _____

3.  Was dyslexia identified informally  _____ or formally?  _____

4.  If assessed, how old were you at that time?:          _____

5.  By whom were you tested, e.g. a school psychologist/specialist teacher:  _____

6.  In what language(s) were you assessed:          _____

7. Where were you assessed? _____ school _____ college _____ clinic _____ home _____

8. What are your areas of special strength/ability: (give test results if you wish):

9. What are your areas of specific difficulty (give test results if you wish):

## LEARNING SUPPORT

10. Did you have any learning support in primary school (5-12) Yes _____ No _____
11. If yes, what kind of support? In class _____ withdrawn _____ other_____
12. If yes, in what language was support given? _____
13. Did you have any learning support in secondary school (12-17)? Yes _____ No _____
14. If yes, what kind of support? In class _____ withdrawn _____ other_____
15. If yes, in what language was support given? _____
16. What kind of support was most helpful during compulsory schooling years (Pr+Sec)?

17. What kind of help at home is/was most effective during school years?

18. What advice would you offer to teachers regarding support in school/community for school age students:

19. Do/did you have any learning support at college or university? Yes _____ No _____
20. If yes, what kind of support? In class _____ withdrawn _____ other (please specify) _____
21. If yes, in what language was the support given?
22. Do/did you have any kind of learning support at work? Yes _____ No _____
23. If yes, what kind of support? _____
24. Was the support appropriate? Please comment _____

## FAMILY DYSLEXIA SUPPORT

25. Are/were you/your family members of a local dyslexia support group? Yes _____ No _____
26. If yes, in what ways did you/they find this helpful? _____
27. What advice would you now offer to dyslexia support groups?

## OTHER

28. Please add/attach any further information/advice which you think may be helpful for others regarding policy decision-making or practical support.

_____

_____

_____

_____

_____

Thank you very much for making time to share your views and experience.

# Chapter 11
# Mathematically thinking

ANNE HENDERSON

---

Questions addressed in this chapter include:

- What learning styles are evident in learning mathematics?
- How do dyslexic students' styles of learning affect their learning of mathematics?
- What teaching strategies can be employed to assist dyslexic learners to overcome difficulties in learning mathematics?

---

## Introduction

In 1992, Miles and Miles stated that 'all or most dyslexics do, indeed, have difficulty with some aspects of mathematics'. Chinn and Ashcroft (1993) reinforced this with their statement 'we have become convinced that difficulties in mathematics go hand in hand with difficulties in language'. These difficulties include the language of mathematics, the immediate recall of simple number bonds, problems with learning multiplication facts and tables as well as sequencing and directional problems. This chapter will look at some aspects of these difficulties and will suggest possible ways of helping students to achieve success in mathematics. The methods recommended are based on both classroom and individual tutoring experience over the last 20 years.

Language is a splendid and powerful instrument and to be proficient with it, students must acquire automaticity in sequencing symbols as well as an awareness and understanding of the ordered structure of sentences. Dyslexic students who are experiencing some difficulties with reading, spelling and writing or, in fact any literacy skills, will probably have some problems with these skills as they occur in mathematics. In his video on 'The Teaching and Learning of Mathematics' Professor Sharma compares learning the language of mathematics to that of learning a second language which for many dyslexic students is an enormous, if not impossible, task. On the same video he highlights the importance of identifying the learning style of a student.

## Learning styles

Students are individuals who have differences in learning styles as well as preferences for particular teaching materials so these factors must be taken into account when trying to help them. Research into mathematical styles by Bath et al. (1986) and Sharma (1987) identifies two specific groups of mathematical learning styles. Bath et al. (1986) describe learners who are intuitive, seeking patterns, as 'Grasshoppers' and Sharma (1987) describes this type of learner as 'Qualitative'. In contrast to this group there are the ones named 'Inchworms' by Bath et al. or Sharma's 'Quantitative' group, who love to find a formula. Not all mathematicians fall into one particular group so there is a continuum that ranges from one end of the spectrum (where learners are holistic) to the other (where formula-seeking mathematicians may be found). Both styles may be observed among dyslexic students.

Identification of these categories leads to the realization that divergent mathematicians prefer different apparatus and their own distinct methods to record and problem-solve on paper. From observation, Inchworms are drawn to the use of concrete apparatus, such as multi-link and unifix cubes, as well as solving many calculations with a number line. Grasshoppers, on the other hand, use Cuisenaire rods, Dienes blocks and geoboards with equal ease. Bath et al. (1986) describe the student Inchworms as always looking for a formula and being prescriptive by nature. In practice it is these students who become 'bogged down' with the details given in mathematical questions, and in examinations, often find that they have spent so much time on the first few questions they are unable to complete the paper. In contrast, Grasshopper students, who are always looking for patterns and intuitive by nature, will quickly read questions, often misread important words, give a quick estimated answer, move on, complete the examination paper but be almost unable to write down a method they have used. Even when urged to write down something that an examiner can mark, Grasshopper students have considerable difficulty because they solve the problems by several different methods and cannot decide which is the easiest one to record.

To work successfully with both groups teachers need to begin early to help their Inchworm students to speed up by finding strategies to improve reading skills and to become more confident in their own ability and methods; Grasshoppers need to develop some way of choosing an appropriate method that they are both able to use and record with a certain amount of ease. If tutors are not aware of individual differences in learning styles and students' preferences for apparatus (e.g. selecting to work with two- rather than three-dimensional material) then tutors may inadvertently use methods incompatible with their students' preferred learning styles, thus creating more difficulties.

Identification of learning style is one that may be made by continual observation or by use of various tests that are on the market. Bath et al. (1986) and Sharma (1987) both reflect aspects of teaching which are of the utmost importance. These aspects involve the question of the current emotional, physical and intellectual state of students as they come into the lesson. There is little, if anything, that can be done immediately to alter these conditions except to be aware of them and offer empathy, sympathy and support. Teachers have to observe students carefully, as well as assessing their mathematical difficulties, so that their tutor's approach is holistic. Tutors who are aware of differences in learning styles will discuss these differences with students and this is an important part of successful tuition.

In relation to dyslexic students, Miles (1983) pointed out that the most successful pedagogical techniques are multi-sensory as well as being sequential, structured and cumulative. Hence, in developing effective methods, teachers must realize that students learn via different modalities: the main ones are kinaesthetic/tactile, auditory and visual. Feeling, touching and doing help the kinaesthetic group which remembers best concrete apparatus in two or three dimensions; listening, reading and talking give auditory learners a better opportunity of acquiring knowledge; whereas colour and imagery reinforced with experiences help visual learners. Audiotapes, calculators, computers plus appropriate, clearly typed and spaced worksheets all help with the learning process. The more knowledgeable and familiar teachers are about these, the more able they are to prepare material suited to their students' preferred method of working.

Assessing students' ability in mathematics is often rather a daunting task because published tests in mathematics often have a great deal of reading in them. Dyslexic students who have difficulty with both reading and speed of reading, for whatever reason, will find their ability in mathematics affected. Even if students have extra time, their concentration cannot be focused long enough for them to show their true ability. In college many tests have been tried, but even now, more than ten years later, the search continues to find the perfect assessment test that could be used with complete confidence. A test needs to be well-designed so that it is easy to read. Any illustrations used must add to the question, and the level of questions used must stretch students so that it will be clear just where they are experiencing difficulties. Designing a special marking table that allows not only a summative score for each student, but also one that enables test results to be used formatively is beneficial and can focus subsequent teaching on to specific problematic areas.

# Dyslexic difficulties and mathematical ability

As well as differences in learning styles students' mathematical abilities may be influenced by explicit features of their dyslexia. Specific language disabilities in reading, speaking, writing, spelling and understanding, as well as problems with direction, organization and poor short-term memory (all of which are on a continuum) may affect their mathematical ability. An individual working in mathematics may be affected in different ways by differing degrees of severity in each of the above areas. These are now discussed in detail below with key teaching points emphasized at the end of each section. For further information see also Henderson (1998) and Henderson and Miles (2001).

# Reading words in mathematics

Some dyslexic students develop their own strategies for reading whole words or phrases which give them a certain amount of fluency; others struggle with a few letters at a time, making words where possible, trying to make sense out of a seeming jumble of letters. Even if they use the same techniques that assist fluency in reading English textbooks, students appear to falter, mumble and generally make far more errors when reading problems in mathematics. It is difficult with mathematics textbooks to choose ones that are at the appropriate reading level for students.

Reading a story book often means that one reads from left to right along rows, allowing the eyes to move ahead in an orderly fashion. In fact, reading this type of material means that it is possible to scan, picking up contextual clues, using rapid reading techniques, almost reading in a superficial way, and still be able to follow the story reasonably well. What is different between reading a novel to reading a maths book? If a student has a particular reading problem then just reading the text in mathematics will cause difficulties, but in written mathematical problems every word has to be read (no scanning or speed reading allowed), for each word and symbol is crucial for the full, correct meaning of the question to be understood.

Often the text is interspersed with tables, graphs and/or diagrams; many are accompanied with separate instructions. It is easy to see why dyslexic students falter and eventually stop when they, who already have problems with direction, try to cope with information which may be written in a different direction (vertically or right to left). The tables are never placed in a regular fashion, so the eye has to become accustomed to 'jumping around' to find the relevant information.

Sometimes examples are worked out in the middle of the directions with instructions informing students about how to complete the calculations. If they are having difficulty reading the connecting text then there is every chance students will ignore the example, or not notice it. Students need practice to gain confidence in reading all types of word problems and even then, they will still come across some that they do not understand. The words used and the length of questions are important factors to consider; sometimes if a question is very long then students say that by the time they have read to the end they have forgotten the beginning. Often, reading is made harder because of the complex words or ones with multi-meanings that are used throughout mathematics. Here are three examples:

- Degree: degree from university/degree – temperature/degree – measure of an angle/third degree – intense questioning.
- Right: right – opposite to left/right – opposite to wrong/right – write/right – accurate/(right) size of an angle.
- Scale: scale – fish scale/scale – musical scale/scale – weighing scale/scale – to scale a mountain.

Dyslexic students who have difficulty with reading and yet are both anxious and eager to find a correct answer to a written mathematical problem, often decide quickly on the meaning of a word and, even if it is wrong, will not re-read to find a more correct one. This quick grasp of meaning is not limited to single words; whole questions may be misinterpreted or certain crucial parts ignored. For example, in a recent examination, students were asked to study two frequency diagrams. The first was a record of petrol purchased by 20 customers in the morning; the second showed the amount of petrol bought by 20 customers in the evening and students were asked to state with reference to the diagrams when most petrol was sold. One student listened to the question and then unhesitatingly wrote, 'The customers who bought petrol in the evening would buy most as they would be going out partying and would need more than morning customers who would only be parking their cars outside the office.' He never once glanced at the frequency diagrams which showed all the important information he needed to give him a correct answer.

Students need to be taught how to develop their own strategies for reading mathematical texts, such as covering up tables until they are ready to read them, using card to put under each line of writing and recognizing (rather than wasting time trying to pronounce) extra-hard first names which are used frequently in mathematics. In an examination situation things are worse and this point was emphasized by Feuerstein in Sharron (1987):

> The excitement, and the danger of failing, means that many children feel unable to spend those few vital but seemingly interminable minutes assessing the whole exam paper properly and then making sure they have read the questions correctly, before they start writing.  (p. 61)

Often, students become confused and full of despair when the problem does not make sense; old feelings of failure and lack of confidence in their ability to succeed take over, self-esteem falls to an all-time low and they give up.

### Key teaching points

- Explain how to read maths texts. Teach reading from text books.
- Build confidence to 'talk it through' to check understanding.
- Suggest ways of reading difficult first names perhaps by remembering the first three letters.

## Reading numbers in mathematics

Reading a number in mathematics is complex because to do it correctly means that students must understand place value, which seems to be particularly difficult for dyslexic students, i.e. 267 must be read as 'two-hundred and sixty-seven' (two lots of 100, six lots of 10 and seven lots of one's or units).

This number must also be read left to right. If there are noughts in the number they must be recognized and acknowledged, not ignored as many students do. If a number has a decimal point then that, too, needs to be read; and the tenths and hundredths after the point need to be understood.

When bigger numbers are to be read (e.g. 25689) students have to first look at it from right to left in order to identify the hundreds (thousands and millions) and to put in a space or a comma, for example; 25,689 or 25 689.

They then have to read the number from left to right as 25 thousand, six-hundred and eighty-nine.

**Key teaching point**

- Identify directional problems and provide cues (e.g. arrows).

# Speaking

Articulation is important with regard to understanding how students are thinking about a problem but often in a busy classroom there is neither the time nor the opportunity to do this. Students who have the privilege of one-to-one tuition have the chance to talk through difficulties, maximizing the value of their time with the tutor. Working with a peer group often produces good results as students can bounce ideas off each other. Of course, to interact well with a group requires students to be confident in their own ability and this takes some time, especially for dyslexic students, who may have failed so often that their self-esteem in the subject is nil.

It has become apparent that it is most important in mathematics for students and tutors to be able to discuss a problem together. To do this students must feel relaxed and free to say what they think; therefore, it is just as vital to build up good teacher/student relationships within mathematics as in literacy. In many ways it is more important because, frequently, students seem to have a great fear of mathematics. Henderson (1989) discovered that 'the very thought of maths puts fear into most adults, not just dyslexic students'. This fear needs to be allayed through the development of respect and trust by both tutors and tutees. Mathematics is a precise subject with definite and correct answers so that students with a history of failure in mathematics fear that they always produce the wrong answer and may be afraid to speak. Their need to share ideas and strategies with others in the process of developing confidence in the subject, is all the greater in order to overcome their lack of confidence.

**Key teaching points**

- Facilitate a relaxed discussion of maths problem.
- Allow enough time for students to voice their thoughts.

# Writing

Writing has become an important element of mathematics; students not only have to solve a set problem but also have to record it in a logical way which provides evidence for their readers of their method of reaching their conclusion. Many students find they can work out a solution to a problem but writing it down is another aspect altogether that they find almost impossible. They forget which bit they did first, lose important parts of their calculations and then do not remember how the solution relates to the question.

Once again, they find that language difficulties have encroached upon yet another subject. The loss of communication in mathematics coupled with the resultant feelings of rejection are compared with the loss of feelings of self worth, so not only is mathematical ability affected but confidence and self-esteem are seriously dented. Teachers would do well to remember the quote by Holmes (1996) 'Confidence is fragile'. However, if students are helped to record their work in small stages, to use a computer to make their work more presentable, and understand exactly what is being asked of them, then projects can be positively beneficial.

**Key teaching point**

- Provide help to record the steps towards reaching the answer.

# Spelling

Mathematical words are often difficult to read, spell and remember. Sometimes even if words are phonetically easy to spell, students still find them difficult and here are a few that always cause problems: *estimation, equidistant, perpendicular, horizontal, representation, polygon, hypotenuse* and *accuracy*. If students spell a word phonetically so that it is possible to read and understand it then, in maths, they should be assisted and counselled not to worry too much as the focus should be on the modes of reasoning. However, students should be encouraged to automatically check their own work for errors, but if reading is a particular problem this is difficult. In mathematics, teachers can help spelling in a positive way by giving a list of words that may occur in a particular topic before the topic is started. The student therefore has the correct words for easy reference which, in theory, means his spelling of technical words should improve.

**Key teaching point**

- Provide word list for mathematics topic work.

# Listening and understanding

Throughout their education, students have to acquire the art of listening. In mathematics, students say that if they stop understanding exactly what their teachers say then they stop listening because to continue would confuse them more. In fact, students often say the same thing in relation to almost all subjects across the curriculum. Even when dyslexic students listen carefully and store knowledge they tend to have poor ability to retrieve it quickly or to generalize the information once it has been remembered. Instructions put on to audiotape are able to be played back as often as is required by the student and sometimes help.

Students may have difficulty in transferring mathematical knowledge from one topic to another, so unless a particular teaching strategy (use of colour, audiotapes, concrete apparatus etc.) has been used to make that point particularly relevant, they will continue to struggle with skill transference. This disability causes great problems when students have to do mental tests which are on the syllabus for some present day examinations (WJEB). A variety of topics, such as measurement, time, speed, distance, fractions and percentages to name but a few, are tested within a single test and even students who do not have SpLDs become anxious. For many dyslexic students, these can constitute a nightmare. Help can be provided via good preparation incorporating strategic approaches to certain questions and with practice tests on an individual basis.

It is imperative to try to lay the bricks of new information on a good foundation of assimilated and understood knowledge, but with dyslexic students there are often many holes in the base which have to be filled before moving on. Assessment needs to be thorough so that these gaps can be identified – this procedure is often accelerated by encouraging students to talk and explain just where they are having trouble. As stated earlier, a good working relationship is vital as this enables students to relax, allowing them the privilege of discussion time. Orton (1992, p. 181) emphasizes this memory difficulty for many non-dyslexic students when he states that in the learning of mathematics 'for the memory to work efficiently, rehearsal and revision are important, but knowledge is retained better if it can be stored as part of a network of knowledge'. This is particularly true for dyslexic students who seem to understand new information more easily if it is related to concepts they have already grasped thoroughly.

### Key teaching points

- Understanding is essential for sustained listening.
- Make sure to fill in the gaps in prerequisite knowledge and skills before tackling new knowledge or skills.
- Provide plenty of preparation and practice for examinations.

## Direction

Directional problems in mathematics are compounded because words and numbers are read from left to right, as is the dividing computational method, but addition, subtraction and multiplication are all right to left. Dyslexic students often have difficulty learning a movement pattern, especially if it was one they supposedly learned long ago and never did. Equations cause severe problems for dyslexic students because there is often a great deal of left-to-right movement across the equals sign before correct solutions are found. To add to the confusion, negative and positive numbers are involved and many students with chronic difficulties with left and right cannot remember which symbol belongs to which digit. It is a good idea if students are having these difficulties to spend a little time actually writing out formulae with negative and positive numbers, using colours for the symbols and cutting up the letters with correct symbol attached. Students then begin to grasp the right connections.

**Key teaching points**

- Use movable materials (e.g. cut up concrete units in equations) in order to cue the mental movement.
- Teach sequencing of steps in reasoning to reach answers to maths problems.

# Organization

Students' difficulties in mathematics involve knowing where to start or how to set out work in a sensible way to make best use of the space. They continually cross out work and redo it, repeating this as many as ten times until the whole page is ruined. The frustration associated with this has to be seen to be believed. It is a good idea to start in the early lessons discussing with students the page size, use of rulers, straight columns and how work should be arranged generally. If instructions are given clearly so students know exactly what is required then eventually they become more logical in their approach and produce neat orderly work.

Time seems to present many problems that affect organization. Passage of time through the day, week, month and year all present special difficulties. Days and weeks affect timetables which affect remembering books and games kit for various lessons as well as punctuality for the same. Months and years affect future planning with regard to examination preparation and revision. Using clocks and doing much practice with telling the time helps, as does preparing individual daily, weekly and monthly timetables using different colours to highlight all important events.

**Key teaching point**

- Assist students to monitor the passage of time and to plan keeping track of time.

# Short-term memory

This shows itself in a failure to recall basic number facts, such as $5 + 7$, which in the middle of a long calculation quickly abolishes all thoughts of the main problem until the answer to this simple addition is found. Returning to the main problem causes confusion because students will have forgotten just what the problem was. Mostly, students will turn to their calculators which then creates other problems as they often cannot remember the names of the mathematical symbols. Students will say, 'multiply' but press the addition key, and a calculator needs to have the correct digits entered, correct symbol keys pressed plus correct reading of the display if a correct answer is to be had; all these are extremely hard for dyslexic students. Checking and re-checking answers slows down the process so that whilst students may know the procedure well, their progress begins to fall behind the rest of their group because of a lack of confidence.

Also, students cannot learn the verbal sequence of multiplication tables, mostly getting the answer wrong and often having to go right back to the beginning before being able to make any further progress. Many students have said that they think their failure with mathematics began with constantly being 'bottom of the class' in every table test they were given when they were in primary school. Several students have said, 'Once I knew all my tables, but now I cannot remember any of them!' Many students who have overcome their initial difficulties with mathematics and go on to study the subject at a higher level, say that they still cannot remember their tables, but find strategies which allow them to work out correct answers quickly.

A further difficulty with short-term memory in mathematics is that students forget what sort of calculation they are doing, perhaps subtraction, and may complete the calculation with addition. So even though they have read they question correctly and understood exactly which mathematical procedure to use and have applied it properly, all their work will be wasted because of a simple error part way through.

**Key points**

- Assist by gradually unravelling the 'connections' and re-building them along with confidence to go on working at finding ways of retrieving information.
- Create topic index cards alphabetically filed with notes about the topic plus an example to show a method the student understands.

## Further strategies

When students have their basic dyslexic difficulties identified, it is useful to assess and identify to see clearly their ability in mathematics and then identify their learning style. Working with each individual, building on strengths, a workbook is gradually built up. Games, wall charts, individual cards as well as any printed material appropriate for the age of the students are used. The important element is to allow self-esteem to develop as well as an enjoyment of the subject.

Students' books are usually begun by recording the symbols with the correct word but the actual number of words attached to each one depends entirely on their mathematical knowledge. As lessons progress it is easy to add to the words as they occur during normal teaching. It is very helpful to write down the symbol that is to be used in they same place each time, usually on the left of the calculation, and to highlight it with a strong colour to help students' memory. As students move on to progressively harder calculations the same method is possible by chunking sections of the calculation into manageable parts.

Topics that have assumed priority are:

- Estimation and approximation.
- Fractions.
- Decimals.
- Ratio and proportion.
- Percentages.
- Shape.
- Graphs.
- Algebraic and geometrical procedures.

Students struggle with Number and Algebra which is the first paper for GCSE because their greatest difficulties involving basic number (long multiplication and division), estimation, letters plus numbers, equations are a major part of the paper. Shape and Space, with Handling Data, both using more visual clues seem to present fewer problems. Pattern identification and appreciation are equally important for as West (1991) says:

From pattern recognition it is but a short step to 'problem solving', since, at least for its more common aspects, problem solving generally involves the recognition of a developing or repeating pattern and the carrying out of actions to obtain desired results based on one's understanding of this pattern (p. 22).

If teachers approach these topics in a methodical way, relating to understood strategies already used and understood in other subjects, then both teachers and students feel more confident about the topic.

Once the basic facts are understood, procedures sorted out and a strategic approach established, students are released from the overpowering fear of mathematics and are free to see and enjoy its patterns and capabilities. West (1991) reinforced this with a quote from a student, 'In mathematics, you didn't have to learn a lot of facts, you simply needed to learn the basic concepts. All the rest could be worked out from them'. If students have the confidence to apply a strategy to a problem because they have read, understood and know what action to take, they are able to find a successful solution. It may not be a method that is familiar to others but the answer will be correct. The vast subject of mathematics has been narrowed down to small simple steps both teachers and students can use in a positive way.

Vocational courses, which are popular with many dyslexic students, present mathematical difficulties of a practical nature, for very often they have to be confident in measuring capacity, finding exact lengths or quantities and at times converting from imperial to metric measures. The accuracy of their answers depends on their ability with this type of mathematics, so obviously they need to have been taught strategies which allow them to reach correct answers as well as to be familiar with the measuring instruments which they need to use. Encouraging the use of colour, prompt cards for certain measures or mnemonics that assist memory are all helpful.

The more advanced students are the further they are away from the 'basics' in mathematics, but it is often these fundamentals that cause problems when students ae studying more advanced mathematics or, indeed, any subject where mathematics is involved. Often, students will embark upon a course which contains a great deal of mathematics but this has not been clearly stated in the information they have received before beginning the course. They may find themselves having to do statistics which they have probably not studied to any depth before and will therefore need help to succeed. Specific Greek letters plus many important symbols will need to be written down with meanings, using colour where appropriate, so that students can become familiar with them and then begin to use them happily. Other areas of statistics, such as, for example, standard deviation, lend themselves to be presented in multi-sensory ways hence possibly alleviating fear.

# Conclusion

If multi-sensory techniques are used in a structured, systematic way applying visual, auditory and kinaesthetic methods where appropriate, there is more likelihood of students acquiring some mathematical knowledge that they can remember and use correctly. Students who have achieved skills and confidence in basic mathematics become motivated to study the subject to a higher level. Appropriate pedagogical techniques working closely with students' learning styles can give them the key to unlock their mathematical potential. Opening a door on such a vast store of knowledge for any student makes teaching mathematics a rewarding task, but to open it for dyslexic students, who previously only experienced failure in the subject, is immensely satisfying.

# Chapter 12
# ICT-based interactive learning

ALAN CROMBIE AND MARGARET CROMBIE

Questions addressed in this chapter include:

- As a result of the changing social and technical context of literacy, how must our response to dyslexia adapt?
- What are the technical skills needed to ensure that those with dyslexic difficulties can exploit new tools as they become available?
- What opportunities do emerging technologies present for teaching and learning?
- What are the implications for teacher training, and for classroom management and design?
- How will the demand for technician and auxiliary support change, and what skills will be required?
- What can research tell us about how to exploit the opportunities presented by the new technologies?

## Introduction

Around 100 years ago literacy was only just becoming important for the majority of the population. Dyslexia, until then unrecognized, had recently been acknowledged in the medical journals of the time (Hinshelwood 1895; Morgan 1896). Illiteracy then was not uncommon, but as work in manual jobs was relatively plentiful, those with literacy difficulties or inadequate schooling could find useful employment in a variety of practical jobs. In the last 100 years, however, literacy has reached such a level of importance that those without the skills feel themselves to lack one of the essentials of daily living which others take for granted. This is very much reinforced by an education system which assesses skills, including art, technology, design and even home economics, mostly in terms of ability to interpret by reading and to report by writing answers. In striving for objectivity in assessment, we may have sacrificed elements of creativity in those we seek to support. However, 'those who learn with great difficulty in one setting may learn with surprising ease in another' (West 1991, p. 11).

West has found, in many individuals, a link between difficulties in reading and writing and superior levels of creativity in fields such as art and design. Although the complex interactions of the two hemispheres of the brain are not fully understood, the idea that certain functions are specialized in the left, and others in the right hemisphere, is now widely accepted, with the left hemisphere being generally responsible for language and the sequential skills of arithmetic, logic, order and time, and the right hemisphere processing visual and three-dimensional images and pictures, spatial relationships and gesture. Although the notion of 'right-brained' and 'left-brained' people is a gross oversimplification, there is nonetheless strong evidence for the existence of different but complementary hemispheres of the brain (Springer and Deutsch, 1997)

Learning styles are inextricably linked to hemisphericity and the way in which we process information. Whilst we must be aware of the dangers of simplistic models of how the brain processes information, we can accept that certain students are better adapted to learning in particular ways, even though we accept that they, like all students, are also affected by social, cultural and developmental factors. Knowledge of students' best modes of learning, along with knowledge as to how to develop thinking and meta-cognitive skills should lead to advancing the learning of our students. Giving students control over their own learning therefore is of utmost importance.

All education is to some extent interactive, but Thomas C Reeves, writing in AACE (Association for the Advancement of Computing in Education) On-Line, the Web page for the *Journal of Interactive Learning Research* defines 'interactive learning' as referring to 'the presence of a "computer" with a significant role in the learning environment' (Reeves 1999). Within this concept of interactive learning the computer can be a microworld and a safe learning environment where information may be presented to students in a suitable form for them to use, or they may be directed into fruitful areas where their teachers know the students will find the information the teachers intend them to discover. The computer can offer a controlled and controllable environment where students can learn and develop in the manner which they find most suits their learning style. Among the questions we need to discuss are: 'How can the computer mediate?' and 'How can we define the learning objectives?'

As we progress into the twenty-first century, we are approaching a time when reading and writing of the printed word seems likely to become less important. Alternative means of transmitting knowledge and producing reading and writing will be available through the interactive world of computer technology. In such a context, what has the computer to offer to those for whom reading and writing does not progress as an integral part of the course of their development? How can the computer interact with the human being to alleviate learning problems and develop potential and creativity? And how can our own knowledge of how the human brain processes information affect provision and help us find the most suitable tools for those who find difficulty in learning by conventional methods?

## What is available to assist effective learning?

It is our belief that education should produce individuals who can take charge of their own learning and develop understanding of their own learning style. This process should be well-developed by the time the student reaches further or higher education and, ideally, this should produce life-long learners. However, writers such as Senge (1990) suggest that learning is a three-stage process: 'knowledge acquisition or information collection', 'skill acquisition' and 'mental model change'.

The computer or Information and Communications Technology (ICT) is conventionally seen as being mainly involved in the transfer or delivery of data and its processing into knowledge; in Senge's model of learning – 'knowledge acquisition or information collection'. Students can use ICT to learn by discovery: online searching, for example, will be less laborious than the use of conventional tools such as books in a library or a resource pack. However, interactive learning particularly supports the second of Senge's objectives – 'skill acquisition'. Through interactive learning, students' initiatives and reactions can determine the response which the computer makes, thus adapting to students' learning needs. It does not deliver the same material in the same sequence to students with differing starting points or current knowledge or targets. Students can work on material as often as they want until they are satisfied. They can choose to experiment or stick to tried and trusted methods; interactive learning is student-driven.

For some time, vital skills such as reading have been supported in many classrooms by interactive programs such Sherston's *Talking Stories*. The interactivity of the programs lies in the control which the child or young person has over what is produced in terms of pages, text and sound. Through simultaneous multi-sensory production of highlighted text on the screen (visual), words spoken (auditory), oral repetition and animated pictures (appealing to long-term memory), children's learning is aided through being able to control the number of presentations of the same page, same sentence or same word on the page, giving much of the repetitious practice necessary for words to become established. Although these 'books' have not become a substitute for the real thing, they give a support to learning for those who may require it. This may enable the children's journey through the real book to be a much more pleasant and successful one. In writing, too, the creativity of the human brain can be displayed by tools such as *Story Maker* which combine the graphical power of the computer with sound and print to produce animated stories with talking characters, not just pages of silent, static text.

In the area of written communication, interactive learning enables dyslexic students to develop and demonstrate their skills without having to expend significant amounts of energy on the mechanics of organization and presentation of the text. They can show that they have attained particular skills by producing clear printed evidence which may have otherwise remained hidden, buried, illegible and badly spelt under a layer of corrections and correction fluid. Those with dyslexic difficulties can demonstrate competence and exploit their strengths to compensate for their weaknesses.

A machine which has the 'patience' and ability to repeat instructions or points when necessary, which can present in a different way, facts which have been misunderstood, which can demonstrate and show and speak in the model of the most patient teacher, is indeed a challenge to the profession. Technology can produce a teaching machine which need never be sarcastic, never impatient, rewarding of small improvements, praising effort or nearly right answers, praising correct answers more so, and which never has an off-day, except perhaps a total power failure! This is indeed interactivity verging on the human, though without the inconsistencies. Can we teachers meet the challenge?

## Particular ways in which ICT can help dyslexic students

> One of the advantages of being disorderly is that one is constantly making exciting discoveries .
> AA Milne

### Visualizing

Dyslexic students often have good visual skills and prefer to think in pictures rather than words. They often use techniques such as mindmapping (Buzan and Buzan 1993) and build a visual map of the relationships between the concepts before starting writing. A structured approach to writing, working from a concept to a plan, from the first to a final draft through revisions, is possible. By use of programs such as *MindMan* to produce mindmaps, outlines can be created, stored and then copied into word processors for development and completion. Alternative versions can be created and compared at various stages in the developmental process.

## Organizing

Computers are good at routine, repetitive and detailed tasks, just the things which most humans find boring and many dyslexic students in particular find difficult, if not impossible. Searching, sorting, organizing, formatting, summarizing and generally formalizing are easily produced by computer systems – *Inspiration*, for example, can be used to create draft structures for essays from mindmap style charts. ICT allows students to demonstrate their strengths by co-ordinating both sides of the brain through the presentation of material visually without excessive demand for sequencing, structuring and formatting.

## Word processing

The benefits of conventional word processing packages for dyslexic students are well-documented (Crombie 1991, 1997; Scheib and Lillywhite 1994; Singleton 1994). The production of clean, legible, presentable material with all evidence of correction or editing removed is clearly attractive to both students and teachers. The use of spell-checking is conventionally described as 'highlighting' incorrect spellings. However, for those with dyslexic problems and the associated lack of confidence in their own spelling the converse is more important: spell-checkers 'lowlight' correct spelling! Thus, students with relatively mild difficulties, who can produce reasonably accurate phonic spelling, are freed of feelings of doubt as to whether spellings are right or wrong. The scenario where dyslexic students survey their own work and then change the correct spellings to wrong ones while leaving the incorrect ones, should now have gone. Dyslexic students will know which words to leave alone!

Interactive word processors can function as intelligent writing assistants which will take over some of the routine tasks and physical effort thus allowing dyslexic students to concentrate on higher-level processes. By predicting possible word choices or word endings on the screen, programs such as *Co:Writer*, reduce the number of keystrokes required by the typist. Following grammatical and syntactical rules such as subject-verb agreement, they allow students to recognize appropriate words. This is an easier process than the complete recall of these words. With the addition of speech, from a program such as *Write:Outloud*, all doubt about what a word actually says or spells will be gone. Recent speech recognition programs can also provide text-to-speech output from otherwise conventional word processors such as *Word*.

## Graphing and charting

Just as word processors carry out the physical conversion of words into shapes on paper and provide tools to aid construction and presentation of written material, spreadsheets allow for the automation and repeated application of numerical processes and automatic creation of graphs and charts. Graphics packages do the same for diagrams which can be melded into the final presentation or folio with a word processing or desktop publishing package. The use of special fonts, such as *Sassoon* which is similar to handwriting, allows for the consistent presentation of written material on screen or on paper in styles similar to those which have been taught to the students in handwriting. The consistency of presentation makes the content more easily assimilated and may also assist in the development of handwriting.

## Keyboarding

For many dyslexic students, a lack of keyboarding skills has until now prevented them from getting the best from the computer. They have not mastered the skills of touch-typing or at least 'finger picking' to a speed which matches or exceeds their handwriting. Although presentation may have improved beyond recognition, work has remained slow, and creativity has been stifled by concentration on finding the right keys. We have for many years been working with schools to ensure that keyboarding skills were taught to a level which would enable the greatest benefits to be gained from the technology. However, with the introduction of more interactive methods of processing words, such as speech recognition, the important question is whether time spent on teaching keyboarding or touch-typing skills is time which might be better spent on other areas. The answer may not be the same for all students.

## Speech

Speech output, where the computer talks to the user, can be a useful accompaniment for the above technique, helping dyslexic students recognize when they have inserted a wrong word, but for some it may become intrusive. However, it can be used simply for specific tasks on demand. Interactive word processors such as *Write:Outloud* will not only read out misspelt words or read back text, they will also help the student concentrate on content and style by alleviating the short-term memory load. With the talking spell-checker included, the program will highlight misspelled words and give audible feedback much as a human would didactically question a student. Speech feedback provides additional cues allowing more accurate choice by the student from lists of similar sounding or similarly spelt words.

A whole file may be read back which will help students to identify those errors where a correctly spelled but inappropriate word has been typed: *hat* in place of *that* or *hide* for *hid*. Hearing their own text read back, word by word or sentence by sentence, reaffirms word and sentence construction. The associated highlighting of individual words as they are spoken, provides reinforcement for associating words and sounds. These writing skills and the mental model change which would make them automatic would conventionally have been developed by encouraging students to read widely. This is not the most welcome advice to give to dyslexic students who are already struggling with course-related reading. However, paper-based text may be fed through a page scanner and into one of the many widely available optical character recognition (OCR) packages to produce a text file.

General purpose text-to-speech tools such as *textHELP!* or *ProVoice* or *Monologue* will read out these files or text from other applications such as Web pages, allowing students to concentrate on understanding the material rather than the mechanics of decoding graphemes.

## Speech recognition

Speech recognition systems convert spoken words into text. These are now relatively cheap and will run on most home computers. The systems require some training to enable them to recognize the voices of specific users. Users read some sample sentences from prompts on the screen and the computer builds a profile of the user's voice. This may take an hour or more but thereafter a word recognition rate of 60-100 words per minute can be attained. Dragon's *Naturally Speaking*, Kurzweil *Voice*, IBM's *Via Voice* and Philip's *Free Speech* all run on similar hardware and input into word processors and many other products, including spreadsheets and Web browsers. Voice control of the various menu functions is an added bonus with these applications.

Until recently, voice-based applications required the use of discrete speech – a rather artificial discontinuous form of speech – where users have to speak relatively slowly, clearly and with a gap between each word. New products such as IBM's *Via Voice* allow for continuous dictation where users speak normally without these staccato interruptions. However, this requires rather more training and this process relies on the reader accurately pronouncing the exact words on the screen. For children with dyslexic-type difficulties who may still have reading problems, this may prove particularly awkward. This is recognized as a problem and some companies have attempted to lower the reading age required. For example, IBM have produced an enrolment text with a reading age of 10. However, with help during the training phase, speech recognition allied with speech output from a computer will create a multi-modal and multi-sensory learning environment which can be used across the whole curriculum. Planning methods already familiar to pupils, together with computer-based planning tools, should accompany speech technology to facilitate efficient and effective production of written work.

Microphones are usually supplied with speech recognition systems but are often cheap and inadequate for classroom surroundings. Additional investment in good-quality noise-cancelling microphones, or headsets incorporating microphones, will enable computers to hear only their masters' voice over the background noise of a classroom. Headphones can allow students to hear only their own material. Unfortunately, there is no technology currently available which allows a teacher to retain the attention and control of their class under these circumstances! Classroom design and management skills will need to change and develop to accommodate the altered noise level. This must surely curtail the widespread use of such technology across the full range of subjects till such time as establishments can be adapted.

## Interactive video

Interactive video based on pre-recorded material is a tool which schools and colleges are already recognizing, but which should be more widely used in the future. The technology already exists for considerable increase in teaching by interactive video, not just reinforcing or creating material, but actually proceeding and progressing in the way the best teachers would – a potential threat to the future of the teaching profession?

## Video-conferencing

The pace of development of video conferencing has accelerated vastly over the last few years. The technology for real-time distance teaching by means of interactive video-conferencing tools is already in use in a number of educational establishments. These allow for two-way interaction between teachers and learners. Once every computer in a class has its own video camera, the use of computer-based video under the control of the classroom teacher could enable classroom management to take on a totally different perspective.

# Internet and intranets

The internet has been touted as the ultimate learning environment: its anarchy and richness cited as 'unparalleled stores of knowledge' (Gerstner, 1996), but its very anarchy and richness make it a daunting and dangerous world for the novice learner. Industry has faced these dangers and has domesticated the internet by taking its tools and concepts, house-training and harnessing them for internal use within organizations – developing intranets inside individual organizations, more directed or focused, more accountable to the aims of the organization. Where the internet is a store of knowledge which can be shared between organizations, an intranet is a shared knowledge system within one particular organization, tailored to the needs of that organization. Individual institutions need to develop their own educational intranets. An educational intranet harnessed and focused to the delivery of education is essential to interactive learning.

An intranet has four distinct but highly connected components, each with its own set of applications:

- World Wide Web and Web browsers.
- Electronic-mail (e-mail).
- File transfer.
- Newsgroups.

Each has developed rapidly over recent years and the full implications for education are not yet fully realized. However, it is clear that each of these has some very specific attractions for those with dyslexic difficulties and for the teachers working with them.

The fact that dyslexic individuals can interact with such high-profile devices, serves not only as an educational tool, but also improves their morale by providing an arena in which they can shine (Dougan and Turner 1996). The interactive nature of Internet-based applications suits the learning styles of many dyslexic students. They are non-sequential, holistic and multi-sensory, using text, graphics, sound and animation, appealing to many individuals with typically dyslexic characteristics.

The World Wide Web grew out of the needs of scientists to share their data with a wide audience. It is a vast and rapidly growing collection of data repositories, each owned and controlled individually but generally conforming to a few standard conventions as to how the data is stored and displayed.

Owners make their data available to anyone who is looking for it but deliver it on a 'take it or leave it' basis. The owner of the data sets it up with a default format but the presentation of the data on users' computers can be altered. The presentation of the data is handled by Web browsers which are programs that display Web pages and can access other programs or 'plug ins'. These handle specific types of data embedded in Web pages, such as video clips, music or even the human voice. This self-adaptation makes Web browsers highly customizable. Dyslexic students can utilize this to set up their own systems so that material is displayed in their preferred font, in their preferred size, with coloured backgrounds and foregrounds to suit their tastes or needs. Speech output is an obvious option.

Being able to display data is only the last part of the exercise, a far more important part is to find what you are looking for so it can be displayed. Web browsers have 'search engines' – programs which scan the Web and report back to users the addresses of sites which contain data on the subject users have specified. The Web browser can then display the contents. For dyslexic individuals who have difficulty with organization, sequential operations and presentation of information, these tools can prove invaluable. They can search reference materials without worrying about alphabetic sequence – the computer knows that! They can search using as much of the word as they can spell, then using their recognition skills rather than recall, they can cut out the word, words or part of a word they want and feed them back into the search – the computer does not get bored with repetition or get slipshod with exhaustion.

Newsgroups are like notice boards but on a global scale and just as each society in a school or college may have its own notice board, each interest group can have its own newsgroup which will distribute the notices to members of the group. Creating and submitting notices are done using word processing and e-mail and distribution uses file transfer. Dyslexic students do not identify themselves by displaying their erratic spelling or poor handwriting as all the notices are similarly presented and can be spellchecked and grammar-checked before being submitted.

Newsgroups can be made read-only or moderated so that the content can be centrally controlled. They can be publicly accessible on a world-wide basis or can be restricted to small groups either by subscription, when the data is pushed to specified users, or by password when the data is pulled as required by those authorized. These closed conferences are powerful pedagogic tools whose power we are only beginning to understand. Already they are being used for discussion of specific topics, for the delivery of teaching material, for example, to distance learners and for the production of group work.

As core elements of a computer-mediated self-help group for students with disabilities they have proved useful educationally. They allow shared insights and discussions on appropriate techniques, but have also been useful socially, allowing mutually supportive peer groups to develop a 'virtual campus' (Debenham 1996) where true peer support can be given on the basis of shared common characteristics, mirroring the social structure of a conventional campus.

The benefits of being able to produce and obtain materials for the internet or intranets by the use of tools such as speech-text and text-speech processing and spellchecking facilities have innumerable advantages, not only for dyslexic people, but for all those whose typing skills do not match or outweigh their speech abilities. Through the use of scanners, which will replicate pictures to be further individualized for the task in hand, graphic images can be added to inform and enhance the quality of the presentation, releasing the creative potential of the individual however great their literacy difficulties.

## The implications

There are major implications for ICT-based interactive learning in terms of resourcing, teacher training, computer support roles and classroom organization. The potential of technology at present seems unlimited. Just where technology will end is the preserve of science fiction. The realities of the situations students find themselves in are quite the reverse. Education itself has not been slow to acknowledge the potential of technology, but the realities of accessing this technology has involved frustration for a sizable proportion of the present generation of students at all stages through the system. Few current classrooms are designed with ICT potential in mind and yet the technology presents us with implications for major change in thinking about classroom and school layout and management. How far will existing arrangements suffice? There are major budgetary implications at all levels from government down.

Technology is often touted as eliminating people, but in reality it changes the demand for people and their specific skills. New skills are required. The range of auxiliary and technician support in schools will be extended. Legal implications such as Disability Discrimination Data Protection and Health and Safety are being addressed in step with the adoption of interactive learning into mainstream education. The skills and procedures of network management need to become commonplace.

As investment in technology grows, so must the ICT skills of all teachers. This, of course, has major implications for teacher-training, in that all teachers will need to learn skills of technology in order to be able to transfer their knowledge in the most effective and efficient ways. Knowledge of the many uses of technology may be as important as knowledge of specific subject areas. Interactive learning will also extend the range of skills required by teachers. All teachers will become facilitators of others' learning, promoting discovery and skill acquisition.

Recent years have seen changes in attitudes towards class organization. Moves away from whole-class teaching have been stemmed and the pendulum seems to be swinging back. In terms of classroom management, technology challenges us once more to look at our practice from the nursery stage on, right through to college. If we are to develop the potential of our young people we require not only appropriate teaching but also auxiliary and technician support. We also need those with the ability to research and evaluate practice in a systematic and scientific way and to produce valid and reliable findings. Most important of all, we need to look at how our young people react to the technology. Technology can be found in the playground in the form of computer game machines, in the home in various forms and even in furry toys such as 'Furbies'. How will all this technology affect children's development and social skills? How will it affect their thinking and meta-cognitive ability? We can be sure of one thing: not all students will adapt in the same way as others. How can we be sure we are tapping the potential of all?

Healy (1990) presents the challenge:

> Computers offer extraordinary potential as brain accessories, coaches for certain types of skills, and motivators. Their greatest asset may ultimately lie in their limitations – which force the human brain to stand back and reflect on the issues beyond the data – if it has developed that ability. (p. 329)

Healy's challenge is that of developing our children's thinking skills to the level that can see beyond the obvious. We have reached a time when dependence on literacy by conventional means seems likely to decline, even for those who have no specific difficulties. The development and advancement of computer technology to compensate will be limited only by the creativity of the human mind.

# Appendix

### UK suppliers for software referred to in this chapter

| | |
|---|---|
| CO:WRITER | Warrington: Don Johnston Special Needs Ltd. |
| DRAGON DICTATE | Cambridge: iANSYST Ltd. |
| IBM VIA VOICE | Portsmouth: IBM Customer Response Centre. |

| | |
|---|---|
| INSPIRATION | Cambridge: iANSYST Ltd. |
| KURZWEIL VOICE | Cambridge: iANSYST Ltd. |
| MINDMAN | Sausalito, CA: Mindjet LLC. |
| MONOLOGUE | Cambridge: iANSYST Ltd. |
| PROVOICE | Cambridge: iANSYST Ltd. |
| SASSOON FONT | Redhill: Adrian Williams Design Ltd. |
| SCHOOL FONT COLLECTION | Warrington: Don Johnston Special Needs Ltd. |
| STORY MAKER | Tewkesbury: SPA. |
| TALKING SOFTWARE | Malmesbury: Sherston Software. |
| TEXTHELP! | Cambridge: iANSYST Ltd. |
| WRITE:OUTLOUD | Warrington: Don Johnston Special Needs Ltd. |

**Useful Web pages for software, and suppliers referred to in this chapter:**

| | |
|---|---|
| Don Johnston Special Needs Ltd | http://www.donjohnston.com/uk/ |
| Dragon Systems, Inc. | http://www.dragonsys.com/ |
| iANSYST Ltd | http://www.dyslexic.com/iansyst.htm |
| IBM ViaVoice | http://www.ibm.com/software/ speech/uk/ |
| Inspiration | http://www.dyslexic.com/inspir.htm |
| L&H Kurzweil Educational Systems | http://www.lhsl.com/education/ |
| Mindjet | http://www.mindman.com/ |
| Philips - Freespeech 2000 | http://www.speech.be.philips.com/ |
| SPA Education Software | http://www.spasoft.co.uk/ |
| *Sassoon* font | http://www.clubtype.co.uk/ |
| Sherston Online | http://www.sherston.com/ |
| TextHelp! | http://discovertechnology.com/Text Help.htm |

# Chapter 13
# Neuropsychological approaches to intervention

JEAN ROBERTSON AND GILLY CZERWONKA

Questions addressed in this chapter include:

- Is there merit in short-term intervention for dyslexic pupils by withdrawing them from the classroom for one-to-one teaching?
- How will nine- or ten-year-old primary school pupils with severe reading difficulty respond to teaching based on Bakker's Balance Model of Reading?
- How will 12-year-old secondary school pupils who are two years behind their chronological age in reading and spelling respond to teaching based on an amalgam of Bakker's methods?
- What are the implications of the research findings for teachers?

## Introduction

This chapter is organized in two parts. Both parts report research with school pupils. The first part, written by Jean Robertson, a university tutor and researcher, is based on a paper presented at the Fourth World Congress on Dyslexia in 1997. The second part is written by Gilly Czerwonka, a secondary school co-ordinating teacher specializing in teaching pupils with SpLDs. Both researchers were inspired by Bakker's work and have engaged in practical investigations of neuropsychological approaches to teaching based on Bakker's Balance Model of Reading (1990).

## Short-term withdrawal intervention for dyslexic pupils may be justified by wider curriculum access in the long-term

Jean Robertson

## Background to the studies

The background to this research was the need to investigate alternative methods of increasing the reading skills of dyslexic pupils in mainstream primary and secondary schools. Within the compulsory education sector, debate on the disadvantages and advantages of withdrawal or in-class support for pupils with dyslexia is ongoing. The debate is important and should also include research funding regarding the potential of each support model for long-term literacy. Provision will vary between LEAs and, in certain LEAs, may include different guidelines for primary- or secondary-aged pupils. One goal of support for all pupils will ultimately be to increase access to printed texts and competence with written work but whether this can be achieved by an in-class support model can be argued. Some would argue that provision of intensive individual teaching in the short-term can have a greater impact on the acquisition of reading skills. This research constituted an attempt to investigate intervention from one theoretical background on pupils, statemented as having SpLDs (dyslexia).

## Theoretical background

The theoretical background involves the Balance Theory of Reading proposed by Professor Dirk Bakker in the Netherlands. In this theory, the demands of initial and advanced reading are perceived as being qualitatively different. In initial reading the child needs to pay close attention to the orientation of the letters within words. There can be confusion between similarly shaped letters (e.g. p/q, b/d, n/u, m/w). Attention also needs to be paid to letter order (e.g. saw/was, no/on) and to the order of words within sentences (e.g. questions contain the same components as statements but require a different response). Furthermore the concept of 'perceptual constancy' needs to be appreciated as a vital part of children's acquisition of grapheme-phoneme correspondence (the relationship of the written form of a letter to the sound it represents).

Familiarity with these 'basic bonds' is prerequisite for the development of 'automatic' speedy and fluent reading without attention to the minute details of letter or word order. Skilled readers can fill in gaps on the basis of experience and do not need to process every letter or every word as they can go straight to the meaning of the text. These skills relating, on the one hand, to differentiating detailed aspects of visual perceptual features and, on the other, to tackling meaning, are considered to be mediated primarily by the different hemispheres of the brain. Generally speaking the right hemisphere is responsible for attention to the visuo-spatial aspects of form and direction and the left hemisphere for linguistic aspects.

Bakker's Theory involves the notion of balance between both functions and the engagement of both hemispheres in the process of developing skilled 'automatic' reading. Bakker considers that there are two distinct subtypes amongst those who do not develop reading skills at the usual rate, and who might be described as dyslexic. He describes these subtypes as 'P-type' (perceptual) and 'L-type' (linguistic).

### P-type subjects

P-type subjects demonstrate fragmented, almost letter-by-letter, reading. Their performance appears to be 'fixed' in right hemisphere functioning (with attention to visual perceptual detail). For example, subjects might decode separately each letter of the word 'had', repeating the procedure each time the same word is encountered, even on the same page. This is not because the word is 'unknown' but because of the signal to approach the text in this particular way.

### L-type subjects

In contrast, L-type subjects appear to have 'matured' through an observed stage of characteristic 'switching' to the use of the left hemisphere (linguistic strategies), but this maturation is illusory (i.e. the switch is being made prematurely). Subjects attempt to engage speedy and fluent reading before they have mastered the perceptual challenges of the text. Characteristically these readers read quickly and fluently but 'superficially' and with many errors.

These two subtypes are readily recognized by teachers and in that sense demonstrate a kind of face-validity for teachers. They also seem to reflect two common reading behaviours of readers described as 'dyslexic'. Experimentally these subtypes are revealed by electro-encephalography (EEG) and event-related potential (ERP) studies, as differential activity can be seen in the right and left cerebral hemispheres respectively.

### Allocation to subtype

This is carried out by error analysis similar to 'miscue analysis' procedure (Slingerland 1970, Goodman and Burke 1972, Arnold 1992, Campbell 1993) but with somewhat extended categories. This allows the type of error to be categorized and analysis of the neuropsychological processes to be assessed. The error analysis concerns the number of substantive and fragmentation errors. Substantive errors are substitutions, omissions, additions, reversals and mispronunciations: in other words, all real 'mistakes'. In contrast, fragmentation errors are time-consuming and comprise spelling-like-reading, repetitions (both words and sentences), self-corrections and hesitations.

Subjects making above-average substantive errors and below-average fragmentation errors are classified as L-types. Subjects making below-average substantive errors and above-average fragmentation errors are classified as P-types. Differentiated intervention can then be designed and provided. Intervention is designed to work directly on deficient or under-used brain regions and stimulate them.

## Intervention methods

There are two major methods. These are delivered thorough Hemisphere Specific Stimulation (HSS) or Hemisphere Alluding Stimulation (HAS).

HSS can be delivered by the tactile medium using a tactile training box or haptically via computer program. One study in this research focused on intervention by the tactile medium. This is differentiated according to the subtype of pupils. P-type pupils use the right hand (theoretically to stimulate the left hemisphere directly). Words and sentences are read and exercises to facilitate access to the linguistic content of the words are carried out. L-types (using the left-hand) read words and sentences through the fingers of the left hand. Exercises are designed to emphasize the perceptual aspects of the text.

HAS uses adapted text and is again differentiated for the different subtypes. For L-type subjects the text is made perceptually challenging, whereas for P-type subjects the linguistic aspects of the text are emphasized.

## The studies

The studies were carried out between 1993 and 1995 on pupils 'statemented' according to the DfEE (1994) *Code of Practice for Identification and Assessment of Pupils with Special Educational Needs* as having SpLDs, e.g. dyslexia.

They took place in three LEAs and involved 15 teachers. Intervention was over a period of 12 weeks and involved 37 pupils for the HAS study (one P-type, 21 L-types and 14 M(ixed)-types). This research posited the existence of a mixed subtype following reading error analysis and aimed to increase the reliability and coverage of the classification procedure.

The HSS study involved six pupils (two P-types, three L-types and one M-type) and intervention was carried out according to the theory. The measurement instrument for both studies was the *Neale Analysis of Reading Ability*. The testing schedule involved pre-test, then post-test 14 weeks after the intervention commenced. Follow-up testing was carried out 16 weeks after the post-test.

### Research design for the HAS study

The research design for the HAS study was a 'challenge design' as pupils were randomly allocated to groups using L- or P-type materials. In all cases materials were at an interest level appropriate for the pupils' age. The challenge design was considered appropriate as opinion is divided as to whether it is better to teach to pupil strengths or to aim to improve pupils' weaknesses. As evidence is lacking, an experimental approach was devised to investigate this central issue.

The main hypotheses were that pupils could be reliably classified and differential responses to intervention found. This allowed Aptitude Instruction Interactions to be explored.

### Results of the HAS study

In the study using HAS, significant results were found for L-type pupils using L-type materials. For reading accuracy, improvements between pre-test and follow up test were in a range from one year four months to two years 11 months. Reading comprehension increases were in a range from one year six months to three years five months. The theory does not address the use of comprehension but it can be suggested that if access to text improves, comprehension may increase accordingly.

### Research design for the HSS study

In this study, an additional criterion was of severe reading difficulty as all six pupils had reading age deficits of more than four years compared with their chronological ages. They were thus judged to have extreme difficulty with any text access (three of the six pupils did not score on a standardized test of reading). Their extreme difficulty and the intensive individual teaching they were to receive, rendered the challenge model inappropriate. Instead non-readers were treated according to either the developmental model and the right hemisphere stimulated or according to the subtype group to which they belonged.

### Results of the HSS study

In the HSS study differential results were found.

Results for two of the L-type pupils were educationally significant. Both of the pupils (aged nine and ten years respectively) had initially not scored at pre-testing but had begun to score on the Neale Analysis by post-testing. This increase improved between post-test and follow-up testing, despite the cessation of intervention and a long summer holiday. This kind of improvement has also been found by other workers. In both cases independent spelling ability had also improved markedly, although this had not been targeted for intervention.

## Conclusions

The following conclusions can be tentatively proposed:

- Pupils can be reliably classified according to the theoretical framework of the Balance Model of Dyslexia.
- When given suitable intervention, results can show that an Aptitude Instruction Interaction of utility had been found.
- With certain pupils these methods hold promise.
- Results were maintained over a period of no intervention, so could indicate that pupils had maintained a more effective system of accessing text.
- Follow-up studies showed that many of the pupils involved in the original research had ceased needing support from an outside agency and were no longer holders of a Statement of Special Educational Needs.

# Effect of simultaneous hemisphere stimulation on learning-disabled pupils' reading ability

Gilly Czerwonka

## Introduction

Many children moving from primary to secondary education were found to be without the reading ability required to cope with the extended curriculum. Specialist reading schemes and programmes were not always available due to additional costs of specialist trained staff, equipment and materials. Other factors include timetabling constraints due to the requirements of the National Curriculum.

The objective of this study was to find a 'classroom-friendly' method of improving literacy skills using materials that were easily accessible and in line with the National Curriculum framework and content.

Bakker's (1990) theory, described above by Robertson, seemed to present just such a possible approach. In summary, Bakker found that a group he described as 'L-type' readers read hurriedly and made many substantive (real) errors, such as omissions and additions. This group differed from 'P-type' readers who read very slowly and accurately. Their errors were mainly hesitations, word repetitions and fragmentations.

To initiate a change in the balance of the use of the cerebral hemispheres in the process of reading, Bakker postulated that an approach to stimulating the underused right hemisphere activity would need to be introduced to L-type readers who tended to rely heavily on activity of the left hemisphere of the brain. He designed an approach to

stimulate the right hemisphere in order to increase attention to visuo-
spatial factors and thus to slow down their pace of reading while emphasizing details within the printed words (Figure 13.1). This he found to
have a successfully positive effect in increasing the accuracy of pupils'
reading.

Bakker developed successful intervention for P-type readers by
activating their left hemisphere through use of cloze procedure. Pupils
had to use semantic and syntactic cues to make sense of the text (Figure
13.2). The text is printed in black ink on white paper and in a common
typeface to keep perceptual complexity to a minimum.

Every night Fred went to bed

With his cuddly little Ted

His dog, his cat, his little red hen

Altogether his bed held ten

**Figure 13.1** Perceptually complex text used to stimulate the right hemisphere.

Every night Fred went to bed

With his cuddly little _____

His dogs, his cat, his little red hen

Altogether his bed held _____

**Figure 13.2** Cloze procedure used to stimulate the left hemisphere.

Licht (1989) recognized further traits consistent with Bakker's L- and P-
types. He found that L-types relied on a direct visual word recognition
(lexical) strategy. They are 'whole-word' readers. P-types were found to
use an indirect phonological (non-lexical) strategy. They are recoders.
These types are in line with the 'top-down' and 'bottom-up' reading
models identified at least two decades ago (Kamil and Pearson 1979).

A combination of the 'top-down' and the 'bottom-up' processes, called
the 'interactive-compensatory' process is thought to be the most efficient
method of reading (Jorm 1981, 1983). Vellutino (1987) stressed that

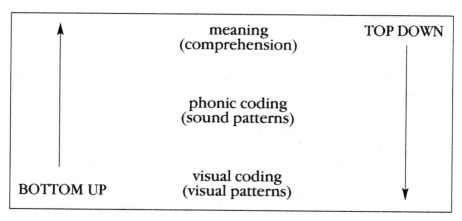

meaning
(comprehension)                    TOP DOWN

phonic coding
(sound patterns)

visual coding
BOTTOM UP          (visual patterns)

**Figure 13.3** Representation of 'top-down' and 'bottom-up' reading models.

success in reading may depend upon the combination of 'top-down' and 'bottom-up' approaches (Figure 13.3).

For the study, it was thus surmised that by combining Bakker's two methods (cloze procedure along with perceptually complex texts), both hemispheres would be involved simultaneously as well as having the added benefit of increasing interhemisphere exchange. This combined method for the purpose of this study was therefore called 'simultaneous hemisphere stimulation' (SHS). Both visual-spatial awareness and semantic and syntactic cues would be activated which should move the reader towards an interactive–compensatory model of reading (Figure 13.4).

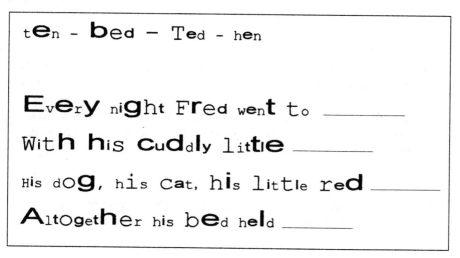

ten - bed – Ted - hen

Every night Fred went to _____

With his cuddly little _____

His dog, his cat, his little red _____

Altogether his bed held _____

**Figure 13.4** Perceptually complex text including cloze procedure.

### Research method

The sample involved all pupils beginning their first year in a comprehensive school in Lancashire who had a raw score of below 35 on the *London Primary Reading Test* which had been administered in their primary schools.

These pupils were given individual reading tests using the *New Macmillan Reading Analysis (A)* (Vincent and De la Mare 1992). Each test was recorded and timed to enable the researcher to scrutinize subjects' reading miscues and behaviour. These miscues were recorded following Bakker's criteria. All pupils were also given a spelling test using Young's Spelling (A) (first tier) (Young 1983).

Nineteen pupils were identified as learning-disabled (two years below chronological age in both reading and spelling) and subtyped according to Bakker's (1990) subtypes. There were 10 pupils who were linguistically able L-types, and nine pupils with visuo-spatial abilities, P-types.

The post-test reading test results were used to place the subjects into three groups whose reading accuracy levels were similar. Each group contained both L- and P-types. Pupils were chosen, at random, from each group to become the experimental subjects. The remaining subjects made up the control group.

The environment of the experimental group of five L- and five P-type subjects, was enriched by their engaging simultaneous hemisphere stimulation (SHS). Perceptually complex texts, including cloze procedure and rhyme, were given to these subjects to stimulate the right and left hemispheres of the brain simultaneously and so activate both visual-spatial and linguistic strategies enhancing interhemispheric exchange. The control subjects were given the same texts to read in Arial font, 14 pt without cloze procedure.

Individual educational programmes were devised for both experimental and control subjects. The programmes ran for 12 weeks. Pupils were taught in 'their groups' for one 50-minute session every week. After this time all subjects were retested using the *New Macmillan Reading Analysis (B)* (Vincent and De la Mare 1992) and Young's Spelling (A) (second tier) (Young 1983).

### Discussion of results

The findings of the study are represented in the tables and discussed in the following paragraphs. Table 13.1 represents the results for P-type subjects.

**Table 13.1** Overall average change in P-type subjects

|  | Experimental P | Control P |
|---|---|---|
| Reading accuracy | 21 months' increase | 11 months' increase |
| Reading comprehension | 17 months' increase | 9 months' increase |
| Spelling | 3 months' increase | 6 months' increase |
| Fragmented errors | 18% decrease | 18% increase |
| Reading speed | 43% increase | 20% increase |

Compared to control subjects, experimental subjects:

- Increased reading accuracy (by 10 months).
- Increased reading comprehension (eight months).
- Increased reading speed (by 23%).
- Decreased spelling accuracy (three months).

From these results it can be deduced that SHS had a positive effect upon reading comprehension and reading speed which may indicate there was improvement in the use of left hemisphere strategies.

As other researchers (Jorm 1981, Stanovich 1980) have also found, the more proficient use of sound analysis schema allows the subjects to consolidate sound/symbol correspondence more readily and so allows more attention to be devoted to understanding and so comprehension improves. Improvement in reading accuracy indicates a move towards an interactive–compensatory model of reading.

### L-type subjects

Table 13.2 represents the results for the L-type subjects.

Table 13.2 Overall average change in L-type subjects

|  | Experimental L | Control L |
|---|---|---|
| Reading accuracy | 16 months' increase | 7 months' increase |
| Reading comprehension | 14 months' increase | 5 months' increase |
| Spelling | 2 months' decrease | 7 months' increase |
| Fragmented errors | 65% increase | 27% decrease |
| Reading speed | 5% decrease | 9% increase |

Compared to control subjects, experimental subjects:

- Increased reading accuracy (by nine months).
- Increased reading comprehension (by nine months).
- Increased fragmented errors (by 92%).
- Decreased reading speed (by 14%).
- Decreased spelling accuracy (by nine months).

The increase in reading accuracy and fragmented errors and the decrease in reading speed were expected outcomes indicating stimulation of the right hemisphere. The increase in comprehension shows increased left hemisphere involvement. Again, the results indicate a move towards an interactive–compensatory reading model.

SHS has shown to have an adverse effect upon spelling. One explanation for this could be the increased use of phonic cues when spelling. Spelling involves identifying phonemes which involves speech/sound analysis and ordering of sounds which are skills mainly attributed to left hemisphere schema. These sounds have to be related to graphic structures which requires the use of right hemisphere skills. Using both skills simultaneously will be difficult for L-type subjects as they ideally work in one mode. It may be that further SHS is needed to balance the working of each hemisphere and allow intermodal enhancement. The experimental L-type subjects showed an increase in good phonic equivalents in their post-test spelling analysis. Table 13.3 represents the results of the control subjects.

**Table 13.3** Comparison of overall average results for P- and L-type control subjects

|                       | Control P            | Control L            |
|-----------------------|----------------------|----------------------|
| Reading accuracy      | 11 months' increase  | 7 months' increase   |
| Reading comprehension | 9 months' increase   | 5 months' increase   |
| Spelling              | 6 months' increase   | 7 months' increase   |
| Fragmented errors     | 18% increase         | 27% decrease         |
| Reading speed         | 20% increase         | 9% increase          |

The improvement shown in the control groups can be accounted for by the individual educational programme each subject was following as well as the continued curriculum teaching.

As P-type control subjects have shown a four-month increase in both reading accuracy and reading comprehension compared to L-type control subjects this gives credence to the maturational lag prognosis suggested by Pirozzolo (1979). The extra reading practice has allowed P-type subjects to consolidate sound/symbol correspondence whilst L-type subjects improved their grapheme/phoneme schema, allowing both types to show an increase in reading speed.

The increase in the fragmented error score of P-type subjects indicate that they are primarily using phonic cueing systems when reading. The decrease in fragmented errors in L-type subjects indicates a direct lexical, whole-word approach. These results would be expected by the definition of subtyping into L- and P-types. This gives face validity to the groupings. Table 13.4 presents a comparison of the results of the experimental subjects.

Table 13.4 Comparison of overall average results for P- and L-type experimental subjects

|  | Experimental P | Experimental L |
|---|---|---|
| Reading accuracy | 21 months' increase | 16 months' increase |
| Reading comprehension | 7 months' increase | 14 months' increase |
| Spelling | 3 months' increase | 2 months' decrease |
| Fragmented errors | 18% decrease | 65% increase |
| Reading speed | 43% increase | 5% decrease |

Compared to L-type subjects, P-types:

- Improved reading accuracy (by five months).
- Increased reading comprehension (by three months).
- Increased spelling (by five months).
- Decreased fragmented errors (by 83%).
- Increased reading speed (by 48%).

These findings confirm results obtained by Bakker (1990) that activating the right or left hemisphere, in this case simultaneously (SHS) has a positive effect on literacy levels, especially for P-type subjects. This improvement in reading accuracy, reading comprehension and spelling may imply that P-types may indeed have a maturational lag (Pirozzola 1979) and that addressing their literacy problems allows them to make significant maturational strides. Maybe the stimulation of the left hemisphere has allowed the P-type subjects an added mode in which to decode and recode text which will allow the simultaneous use of visual–spatial strategies with sound analysis (Goldberg and Costa 1981).

L-type subjects, however, use a direct lexical system of reading and spelling, therefore accessing the indirect phonological route will be new, and so by terms of novelty, will allude to the right hemisphere. As L-type subjects also work best in single mode then improvements will undoubtedly take more time.

## Conclusions

Several tentative conclusions emerge from the data:

- Simultaneous Hemisphere Stimulation has had a positive effect upon reading accuracy and reading comprehension for all pupils.
- Simultaneous Hemisphere Stimulation has had a detrimental effect upon spelling, especially for L-type subjects with a reading accuracy of above eight years.
- A reading accuracy of above approximately eight years four months allows a pupil to improve reading accuracy and reading comprehension substantially using Simultaneous Hemisphere Stimulation.
- Devising individual educational programmes for pupils on their miscues in reading and spelling seems to be a futile practice compared to SHS for those pupils with a reading accuracy of approximately eight years four months and beyond.

It appears from the evidence that large improvements can be made by learning-disabled subjects if they undergo SHS. It would seem feasible that National Curriculum materials can be written in fonts that are perceptually complex, including cloze procedure, to be used in the classroom and these would benefit literacy levels. Pupils using the materials would not have to be subtyped into L- or P-types as both types made similar and significant improvements in their literacy skills.

The question arises as to what results might be achieved if 'ordinary' readers underwent SHS?

Ongoing research is addressing this question. An accelerated literacy programme is being trialled in two forms, one for summer schools and one for Key Stage 3 intervention. A reading and spelling programme has been written by the researcher on the basis of research findings to date. SHS is included in this programme in the form of poems which are written in perceptually complex texts along with cloze procedure and rhyme. The programme is being delivered successfully by 'ordinary' teachers in a Blackburn school to pupils in years 7, 8 and 9. The Accelerated Literacy Programme is due for publication in 2001.

# Chapter 14
# The role of counselling in supporting adults with dyslexia

CHARMAINE MCKISSOCK

Questions raised in this chapter include:

- What might be the position, nature and value of counselling in the support of adult dyslexic learners?
- Whose responsibility is it to provide counselling?
- How can counselling theory inform teaching practice?
- How can dyslexia be reframed as a positive experience?

## Introduction

This chapter is derived from the experiences and reflections of one practitioner, involved for over a decade in the support of adults with dyslexia. It starts by describing the emotional difficulties often associated with dyslexia, and then explores in some detail the position, nature and value of counselling in helping adult learners with dyslexia to fulfil their educational goals. It thus raises questions about three of the major factors which affect individuals' learning outcomes:

- the emotional experience of learning;
- the teacher-learner relationship;
- the individual's dyslexic identity.

The very process of asking and exploring these questions contributes to reflective practitioners' ongoing professional development. It should be noted, however, that the chapter does not attempt a comprehensive evaluation of traditional counselling practices and belief systems. Instead, some of the most promising insights will be selected from a range of sources, including psychoanalytic, humanistic and cognitive approaches to counselling.

# Rationale for counselling

SpLDs may seep over a lifetime throughout individuals' thoughts, emotions, behaviour and relationships. Their effects may be as subtle and changeful as watermarks on silk or as overpowering as a river bursting its banks. Adult students – with either acknowledged or unidentified dyslexia – often only seek professional help when their emotions have become impossible to bear, hide, deny or explain away. Edwards (1994) cites a number of authorities who:

> ... from their different disciplines and perspectives, converge in projecting an image of dyslexic students as being seriously affected at home and school by academic failure. (pp 145-50)

Through structured interviews with eight young male survivors of disabling educational experiences, Edwards details the childhood sources, manifestations, consequences and scars of the painful feelings often associated with dyslexia. These feelings can include all shades of fear, shame, anger, frustration, sadness or confusion. A desolate picture of personal alienation, violence, ritual humiliation, unfair treatment and inappropriate help is built up. The bewildered narrators struggle to reconcile old labels of stupidity, laziness and disruptiveness with intuitive feelings about their own potential. Ironically, they convey with considerable eloquence how it feels to be unable to communicate the abilities which they know to be locked within the private self.

Other extreme reactions to dyslexia, such as nervous breakdowns, suicide attempts, delinquency, aggression and psychosomatic illness, which indicate the need for specialist help, are described by Hampshire (1990):

> 'After I had been diagnosed as being dyslexic I couldn't be helped to overcome my dyslexia, because by that time I had got myself into such a state that I had a nervous breakdown. ... I went catatonic and I was totally agoraphobic . I literally sat at home next to a radiator rocking back and forwards, for months and months. ... When I tried to kill myself they put a care order on me and put me away in a special unit. ... I was given all sorts of drugs . (pp 33-9)

These encounters with the sharper end of dyslexia have supported the impression from a number of studies by educationalists, psychologists, support groups and some dyslexics themselves – that many adults with dyslexia would benefit from counselling (Miles 1988; Ryden 1989). Undeniably, when anxiety about learning:

... ceases to rouse us to a special effort ... when it becomes a source of disorganisation, as when we panic at everyday tasks ... when it paralyses a person like a deer before an oncoming headlight ... it is time to seek help. (Kovel 1991).

However, the notion that all those with dyslexia would benefit from the formal counselling of the consulting room is difficult to defend.

## Some limitations

Though 'attracted by the use of counselling with children with reading difficulties', Pumfrey (1977) feels that results of:

research evaluating self-esteem enhancement or stress reduction procedures have generally been equivocal.

Lawrence (1985) demonstrates that extra reading tuition is far more effective when accompanied by an approach aimed at developing self-esteem. However Pumfrey (1991) wonders if this conclusion is not somewhat obvious to practitioners, and argues that:

the assistance might not require additional drama or counselling sessions but plenty of opportunity for discussion with a sympathetic adult who supports the learner in reading and writing. (p. 72)

This argument is strengthened by the fact that there does not appear to be a single shared definition of counselling or any consensus about the most appropriate form in this context. Nor is it clear whose responsibility it is to deliver it, how it should be paid for, where and when it should take place and what specialist training is necessary.

Moreover, many adult students are averse to the mention of formal counselling, which can often become a taboo word, unfortunately associated with moral weakness or mental illness. Many consider it condescending to assume that any person with dyslexia 'needs' counselling on any other basis than the fact that they are human beings first and foremost, and may wish for help to feel and live better. They may not have the desire, commitment, opportunity, or belief needed to benefit from the formal counselling procedure of the consulting room.

## Counselling skills within teaching roles: aptitudes and boundaries

This inaccessibility to formal counselling crystallizes the need to explore how counselling skills can be successfully embedded into tutor/lecturers' approaches to dyslexia support. Though counselling is notoriously difficult to define (British Association of Counselling 1996), there appears to be some agreement about the following principles and processes between the different perspectives:

- Counselling largely takes place through the verbal communication between the counsellor and the counselled.
- In times of crisis, anxiety, unhappiness or confusion, a 'good counsellor is one who provides emotional support, intellectual clarification and some attention to environmental problems'.
- The ideal therapeutic relationship is 'intense but dispassionate', which allows the troubled person to safely let go of bottled up feelings without fear of consequences or value judgments (Kovel 1991).

Edwards (1994) places the responsibility of unlocking the dyslexic student's hidden potential squarely with support teachers who have received, 'a basic training in counselling'. She recommends that teaching methods should take account of the 'dyslexic's need for individual attention, to have their say and to be listened to' (p. 164). Thus, teachers retain their right to give instructions, information, advice, feedback, alongside counsellors' roles of non-judgmental support, clarification and guidance.

However, Kovel (1991) reminds us that all principles need to be applied by human beings, who must have certain skills and personal attributes:

> He or she should be able to sense what is going on psychologically within another person; be attuned to communications both as a receiver and sender; form balanced rational judgments while keeping himself open to feelings; be able to flexibly adapt to changing circumstances without losing identity or purpose; and most essential of all, maturely care for the well being of the patient.

If the word 'patient' is changed to 'student', the person specification could well fit learning support tutors, trained in non-judgemental and empathetic communication skills which are always required for:

- negotiation of a clear learning contract;
- helping students identify their needs;
- setting realistic aims;
- supportive yet honest analysis of strengths and weaknesses;
- exploration of learning blocks and negative self-concepts;
- discussing progress;
- developing advocacy roles;

- identification of discriminatory practices;
- respect for individuals' culture, language history and learning styles.

It is, however, difficult to estimate how many tutors and lecturers are able or willing to adopt this approach to their work. Further, it is possible to speculate that if and when Edwards' (1994) scarred teenagers enter higher education, they will encounter an environment where the cathartic effect of 'talking therapies' is considered less important than the acquisition of functional skills and intellectual excellence; and in which some lecturers are unaware of the force and complexity of their students' personal and learning difficulties.

Such lecturers may decide to distance themselves from their students or from the very notion of dyslexia. Weighed down by their own worries about managing large numbers of students, modules, assignments and conflicting demands, they may, in the words of Salzberger-Wittenberg et al. (1990), 'find quick and forceful ways of managing [their burden]'. They may be inclined to dismiss students' problems as a natural reaction to the higher-powered challenges of a new learning situation. They may also feel that their role is only to pass on the flame of knowledge and that, therefore, the emotional problems of their students are either the responsibility of the students themselves or else of a counsellor/clinician. They may feel totally ill-equipped to 'deliver counselling', especially if they view it with a medical perspective or that of 'the more ambitious psychotherapy which attempts to go beyond the limits of counselling into the incursions made by the unconscious' (Kovel 1991).

## Specialist staff: insights from counselling

Other staff, however, (ranging from personal tutors, learning support coordinators or disability officers) may have more opportunity and inclination to concern themselves with students in a more holistic way. Students with dyslexia may at some point need these individuals in order to communicate their bottled up distress in the hope that it might be understood and they might be helped to bear it. However, Salzberger-Wittenberg et al. (1990) warn 'some people will dump their problems into another person, wishing simply to get rid of them' (pp 58–60), presumably in the childlike hope that the all-powerful parent figure will take them away. Without having some counselling techniques to hand, would-be helpers are soon overwhelmed by students' personal and academic problems.

Salzberger-Wittenberg et al. go on to stress that receptiveness to anxiety, together with an intolerance of such a state, may leave members of staff overwhelmed by the feelings projected into them. There is a risk that sensitivity to students' painful memories, as they resurface, without the inner resources to respond in a helpful manner, may leave both individuals feeling exhausted, empty and powerless. She therefore suggests how a psychoanalytic approach to counselling could be usefully embedded into the teaching/learning situation. If tutor–counsellors can tolerate 'the pain put in her [them] without becoming overwhelmed, she [they] acts as a container for the feared emotion. The individual finding his anxiety, aggression and despair accepted and contained, is enabled at a feeling level to realise that someone who is capable of living with a feared or rejected aspect of himself does in fact exist' and therefore these parts become less frightening, powerful or painful. The aim of this approach is for students to invest less psychic energy on hidden feelings and fantasies – which have become confusing and unmanageable – and more on the process of learning.

Saltzberger-Wittenberg et al. also stress the importance of recognizing the nature of interaction between students and teachers as having a powerful influence on learning outcomes: this may be achieved by the building of self-esteem and confidence as well as 'the hopefulness required to remain curious and open to new experiences, the capacity to perceive connections and to discover meaning' (p. ix). Indeed, many personal accounts of dyslexia attest to the saving grace of a special learner/teacher relationship (Edwards 1994).

Humanistic counselling practice also stresses the importance of the counsellor–client relationship. With its emphasis on problems of self-esteem, it is especially well-suited for counselling dyslexic students 'in times of stress when the environmental situation is not in itself overwhelming, but it brings out self-defeating feelings of inferiority or insecurity' (Kovel 1991). Thus, tutor-counsellors' main aim is to get students to feel better about themselves: this is achieved by tutor-counsellors setting their own positive regard for students against students' internalized negative self-image. Tutor-counsellors have to 'engage in a good deal of positive yet realistic reinforcement' (Kovel 1991, p. 157-64).

Research into the field of 'Explanatory Style' could also offer new insight for the support of dyslexic students. In *Learned Optimism*, psychologist Martin Seligman (1990) acts like a kind of linguistic detective, offering a new perspective on the way not only our thoughts, but the very words we use, explain our negative experiences in life (our 'Explanatory Style') and the way we construct our individual worlds. By use of content analysis of verbatim explanations (CAVE), a subtle and exciting technique of linguistic analysis, Seligman is able to estimate the powerful effect of preferred cognitive style on life experiences.

Finally, Gerber et al. (1992) suggest that 'the patterns of successful functioning that promote high levels of vocational success' among adults with learning disabilities are as follows:

> ...the quest to gain control of their lives; goal orientation; reinterpreting the disability experience; adaptability; persistence; learned creativity and social support. (pp 475-87)

It is suggested that through training, individuals can learn to copy and interiorize these predictors of success. Many learning support tutors have been successfully practising these strategies with dyslexic students for many years. Seligman, however, holds out the possibility of taking these ideas into a different realm. With his techniques it becomes possible to detect barriers to achievement or seeds of success even amongst the deceased or absent, providing that a piece of recorded or written autobiographical material is available. It would be fascinating to apply the CAVE technique to the writings of an Albert Einstein or Thomas Edison (who are reputed retrospectively to have been dyslexic) in an attempt to understand how some people with dyslexia succeed – on their own terms – against all odds, and how others may best be helped to do so.

## Solution Focused Brief Therapy (SFBT)

Recent developments in counselling with adults include adaptations of solution-focused brief therapy. This originated from family therapy practice in the USA in the 1980s and is a form of therapy in which therapists attempt to make maximum impact in minimum time; some even argue the case for a single session.

Its main focus is on clients' resources rather than their deficits. John Parke, a dyslexia-centred counsellor and the exponent of SFBT, finds that exploring 'Exceptions to Problems' and use of the 'Miracle Question' are two particularly effective ways of empowering adults with dyslexia. With the former, tutor–counsellors help students to recall – and repeat if appropriate – situations in which the problem was not happening or was being managed better: for example when students successfully use self-talk and breathing techniques to curtail a panic attack at the start of an exam. By use of the 'Miracle Question', tutor–counsellors prompt students to imagine and describe (in as much detail as possible) what life will be like once the problem is solved or is being managed better. Individuals may be helped to believe in their own ability to find solutions and change their lives. This is particularly useful when contact time is limited and study outcomes are a priority.

# Reframing and rethinking

Being dyslexic can be lucky. If I could read, I could have been driving the No. 47
bus for the rest of my life. (Ron, business magnate)
(Hampshire 1990, p. 54)

The cognitive approach to reframing the dyslexic experience is a
precursor to a current and alternative view of dyslexia as a multi-faceted
phenomenon, involving strengths as well as weaknesses. Researchers,
such as Susan Parkinson from the Arts Dyslexia Trust, have highlighted the
paradoxes of the dyslexic condition. From her own teaching experience,
she has observed that the same intellectual make-up which can undermine
achievements in specific areas and result in loss of self esteem, has turned
out to be an advantage in many other situations and occupations;
especially those requiring visual–spatial skills, determination, problem
solving, survival humour, intuition, creativity and holistic thought.

West (1991) adventures further in his belief that the basic literacy skills
of 'the mediaeval clerk', such as handwriting and orthographic accuracy,
will become obsolete in the twenty-first century and the 'special' skills that
can accompany dyslexia will become indispensable and therefore highly
prized. Much of the pain of dyslexia which comes from not being able to
automatize those socially prized literacy and communication skills that
others seem to acquire with ease, will be relieved. These are important
ideas for staff who are involved in counselling adults with dyslexia; it is
clearly essential to assess and re-assess one's own conscious or unconscious belief/value system in relation to this dis-ability.

Currently, the term 'dyslexia' is often used to imply disability; and this
term itself often carries negative connotations. In *An Anthropologist on
Mars* (Sacks 1995) it is stated that this need not happen. Sacks describes,
with all the beauty and art of the poet–scientist, 'the narratives of nature
and the human spirit, as these have collided in unexpected ways amongst
people visited by neurological conditions'. His exploration of the inner
landscapes of people who are travellers to unimaginable lands leads him
to conclude that 'all my patients, so it seems to me, whatever their
problems, reach out to life – and not only despite their conditions, but
often because of them, and even with their aid'. Sacks' approach to
collecting case histories has much to inform tutors' interviewing practice
when noting autobiographical clues leading to diagnosis and, indeed, to
the deeper and respectful understanding of the rich personal variations in
dyslexia. We also learn that whether individuals' private and public selves
are tarnished or burnished by their difficult experiences depends on many
diverse considerations such as their personal response to education,
culture, fortune, faith, self-knowledge and the receipt of respectful love
and informed help.

# Conclusion and implications

Despite the apparent value of some counselling perspectives for providing support for dyslexic learners, no study has yet been conducted which evaluates the items on Sacks' list. It is difficult to find evidence about the relative outcomes from counselling alone, tuition alone, cognitive programmes, or from a mixture of these approaches. Nor is there any conclusion available about the type of personality or problem best matched with a specific approach. The issue of who should ultimately deliver the appropriate counselling within an educational setting and how, where and when it should be delivered is still unresolved. More investigation is clearly needed into the nature of effective student–tutor interactions.

Wherever counselling perspectives are identified as being of value, there are training implications. Any course which purports to train specialist staff should perhaps recognize this at the outset. It also seems, that however sketchy our understanding of the human heart and mind, the exploration of these questions appears to have a positive effect on both the giver and receiver of counselling within the tutor/student relationship.

# Chapter 15
# Specialist teacher-training in the UK: issues, considerations and future directions

GAVIN REID

Questions addressed in this chapter include:

- What are the trends in specialist teacher training?
- What issues affect the development of courses?
- How are these issues taken into account?
- What directions might future teacher training take?

## Introduction

This final chapter examines some of the factors involved in the development of specialist training courses in SpLDs, e.g. dyslexia in the UK. These factors include course content and structure, accreditation and dissemination of courses and issues of on-going controversy within the field of dyslexia (such as definitions of dyslexia and the roles of different groups of professionals, e.g. educational psychologists, clinical medical officers, school management and class and learning support teachers). Additionally, some future directions in relation to teacher-training will be highlighted.

The principal thrust for this chapter emerged from the experience of the author in developing specialist courses for experienced teachers and for students undergoing initial teacher-training at Moray House, Faculty of Education in Edinburgh. Reference will be made to these developments throughout this chapter and, in particular, to the importance of the different phases of development, from initial consultation to validation and accreditation.

# The trend for training

One of the interesting factors to emerge in this field is the increase in availability of specialist training in dyslexia. At present, the British Dyslexia Association has accredited 16 UK university courses in dyslexia. These courses have been validated by the universities concerned and are offered by them at a range of levels, from Certificate to Masters. Additionally, five independent dyslexia centres also run accredited courses at Associate Member of the British Dyslexia Association (AMBDA) level and five Local Education Authorities (LEAs) also run courses accredited by the British Dyslexia Association. This is consistent with growing awareness of the need to train not only specialist teachers in teaching dyslexic children but also classroom teachers. It also coincides with greater government commitment to dyslexia awareness and teacher-training. The Department for Education and Employment (DfEE) funded the development and dissemination of 'dyslexia-friendly schools packs' to every school in England and Wales.

In 1996 in Scotland, the Scottish Education and Industry Department (SOEID) funded a programme of early literacy initiatives, including dyslexia, called the Early Intervention Programme; initially for a three-year period, the programme has been extended to 2002. This programme provides funding for a range of early intervention initiatives, including research programmes, staff development and purchase of resources. In its first year, 700 schools and 44,000 children benefited from the initiatives and, during 1997–1998, 5,600 staff undertook early intervention training and 3,300 staff undertook training specifically in special educational needs (SEN) issues. Dyslexia is clearly considered within the SEN training programmes, but additionally, a programme of dyslexia training was funded by the SOEID in conjunction with the Scottish Dyslexia Trust in 11 locations in Scotland where 165 primary 1 and 2 class teachers all undertook the first module of the Moray House Dyslexia course.

With this increasing trend to run courses in dyslexia there is a greater need to ensure that courses are of an appropriate standard and that the tutors writing and running them have up-to-date knowledge of dyslexia. Tutors also need to possess the necessary tutoring skills to run and evaluate the performances of course participants; in some cases this is acquired through experience.

In a pioneering initiative, the British Dyslexia Association sought to deal with this issue by developing a three-year programme of tutor-training for those who run accredited courses in dyslexia. As well as focusing on current initiatives in dyslexia, recent research and other aspects which can be associated with dyslexia (such as dyspraxia), this programme also included discussion groups on running tutorials, marking assignments and providing feedback to students. Evaluation of this initiative from participants has been very promising, with those attending appreciating the opportunity to discuss issues relating to running courses and sharing experiences with others.

## Issues for consideration

There are a number of issues which can affect the development of courses, participation of teachers and support of education authorities in courses in dyslexia.

Some of the fundamental issues which continue to be debated strongly by researchers and practitioners include definitions of dyslexia, appropriate methods of assessment, the nature of the teaching approaches, access to the curriculum and the role of parents, external agencies and what constitutes appropriate provision. In this context, it is interesting to note how Lancashire LEA and its local university (Central Lancashire) worked collaboratively to develop courses which recognized and accredited teachers' competences as well as developing further their relevant professional knowledge, teaching and research skills (Crossley 2000).

The area of assessment was the focus of a working party by the British Psychological Society and the resulting report (BPS 1999) provided ten different hypotheses each seeking to provide a theoretical explanation of dyslexia. These factors and the working definition of dyslexia indicated in the report will have an influence on education authority perceptions and practices and therefore will influence the development and content of courses. This does raise some concern as the definition used in the report is hotly disputed by the British Dyslexia Association. The BPS (1999) definition that 'dyslexia is evident when accurate and fluent word reading and/or spelling develops very incompletely or with great difficulty' (p. 18) appears extremely open-ended and is disputed by the British Dyslexia Association (BDA press release, 29 October 1999) on two counts; first, it makes early identification less likely because authorities will wait until there is evidence of reading failure before intervening and, second, the definition focuses only on literacy yet dyslexia can be evident in other areas apart from reading and spelling (Nicolson 1996).

Much of this debate is encapsulated in an earlier study conducted by Stirling University on policy, practice and provision for children with SpLDs (Duffield et al. 1995). The research questions addressed three main aspects:

- To what extent are pupils with SpLDs recognized as a group with distinctive needs and how is the nature of their difficulties perceived?

- Where SpLDs are recognized, how are they identified?
- How are the needs of these pupils met and their identified difficulties remedied?

In attempting to answer these questions, the research drew on perspectives from local policymakers which included principal educational psychologists, education officers and SEN advisers, parents and voluntary associations, learning support teachers, teacher educators and pre-service teachers and Scottish Examination Board officers and medical personnel.

A measure of the controversy and disagreement which existed at the time can be seen in Table 15.1, which shows the differences in the conceptual understanding of specific learning difficulties between those occupying key policymaking powers in education authorities.

**Table 15.1** Definition of specific learning difficulties: local authority views*

|  | Discrete | Continuum | Anti-categorization | Total |
|---|---|---|---|---|
| Psychologists | 3 | 12 | 2 | 17 |
| Education Officers | 4 | 5 | 2 | 11 |
| Advisers | 6 | 4 | 6 | 16 |
| Total | 13 | 21 | 10 | 44 |

*Reproduced with permission (Duffield et al. 1995).

For the purposes of teacher-training courses in SpLDs the views of learning support teachers, the principal recipients of the course, are interesting to note.

There was clear disagreement within this group regarding the use of labels in particular, and also in other issues, such as assessment, and in teaching strategies. These differences are perhaps encapsulated in the following statement from one learning support teacher:

'I dislike the term specific learning difficulties: it is unwieldy, vague and nobody understands what it means. Having used it, you have to launch into further explanations. I actually prefer 'dyslexia' but only use it with qualification because of people's varying reactions. Learning support colleagues are aware of the ambiguities and controversy surrounding the word.'

With regard to identification, the responses indicated that the majority of learning support teachers were apprehensive about their abilities to identify SpLDs, e.g. dyslexia. From a sample of 206 learning support teachers, around 75% were able to make at least one means of diagnosis of

SpLDs in their school, but a total of 50 different tests were named! In the BPS report (BPS 1999) 12 tests were described which draw on theoretical rationales of dyslexia.

In view of the issues and controversies which arose from the Stirling University Research in Scotland, it was felt that the Moray House course (because it was located in Scotland) had an important role to play in clarifying the debate among policymakers and learning support teachers in particular, and clarifying the issues in relation to definitions, assessment and teaching approaches. This, it was felt, could pave the way for greater confidence and greater awareness among teachers, learning support teachers and other professionals who would participate in the course. Similarly, course leaders of all courses in dyslexia within the UK need to incorporate the latest thinking, debates and controversies, and clarify and contextualize these for course participants and, indeed, for Education Authority policymakers. It was interesting to note that in the Moray House course some of the first recruits to the course were Education Authority advisers.

## Course aims and rationale

Although education authorities may differ on the desired focus of the course there appear to be some common elements (source: BDA Teacher Training Accreditation Board). The expectation is that course participants, on completion of courses, will have competence in the following:

- A sound framework of the theoretical issues relating to SpLDs, e.g. dyslexia.
- Critical awareness of assessment, teaching and curriculum issues.
- Heightened awareness of the existence of relevant research and an understanding that knowledge in this area is continually developing.
- An ability to link ongoing research with practice.
- An appreciation of the location of SpLDs, e.g. dyslexia within the framework of SEN and mainstream provision.
- Experience and competence in practical aspects relating to the assessment and teaching of learners with SpLDs, e.g. dyslexia.
- Awareness of the holistic dimensions associated with SpLDs, e.g. dyslexia, including social and emotional factors, parental involvement, multi-disciplinary approaches (including the role of other professionals) and whole-school issues.

The emphasis, therefore, throughout many courses is on a broader conceptual definition of SpLDs, e.g. dyslexia and how such difficulties can be addressed by professionals within the context of the curriculum and the school.

## Course content

Course content is clearly an important area. This is particularly the case in relation to dyslexia where course participants can come from different teaching backgrounds but normally expect the course to have a direct impact on their working practice. Practical elements of the course must be balanced with sufficient theoretical knowledge and these aspects must then be applied to different educational contexts.

It is usually wise to begin a specialist course of training with a theoretical overview since the field of SpLDs is a complex one with different views and perspectives. Such an overview may include the following:

- definitions of dyslexia;
- assessment and early identification;
- teaching and curriculum access;
- study skills and learning styles;
- the importance of counselling and self-esteem;
- the role of parents and external agencies.

The remainder of the course can investigate these and other elements associated with SpLDs, e.g. dyslexia in greater detail: assessment, teaching approaches, curriculum aspects, whole-school approaches, motor factors, emotional considerations and factors relating to policy and provision. It is also useful to introduce some flexibility to provide course participants with some choices, since there is a considerable number of areas which can be associated with dyslexia and a number of different support approaches can be investigated and evaluated. For example in assessment the range of tests which can be used for different purposes include the role of discrepancies, qualitative tests of phonological awareness, qualitative error analysis (such as miscue analysis), behaviourist approaches and observation assessment from a child and a whole-school perspective. This can influence teachers in consultation and utilizing a team approach within the school. It can also influence education authorities in the development of policy therefore providing management with a formula or framework consistent with authorities' guidelines and the Code of Practice (DfEE 1994).

Different practices in assessment occur in different areas of the country. For example, one education authority with a sound policy on dyslexia only uses psychometric assessment reluctantly, whereas another may lean heavily on this form of assessment – to the extent that only the educational psychologist can diagnose dyslexia. Many, of course, fall somewhere between these two extremes. This example, however, highlights one of the issues in relation to assessment. Course textbooks for teacher-training in dyslexia (Reid 1996, 1998) highlight this and other issues within the framework shown below:

- What? What aspects of the child's cognitive abilities or curriculum performance are to be assessed?
- Why? Why should an assessment be carried out and what purpose does this serve?
- How? The issue of how an assessment should be conducted is an important one.
- Effect? A consideration throughout the assessment process of the effect of the assessment – the assessment outcome. It is important to ensure that the assessment provides information which can be readily linked to a teaching programme, or which can be used to help the child cope more effectively with the curriculum.

The controversies related to assessment for SpLDs, e.g. dyslexia highlight the benefits of developing a contextualized course which can accommodate different perspectives in different areas of the country.

## Education authority: policy and provision

It is important that courses recognize Education Authority policies on SpLDs and the range of provision which can help to meet the needs of both children and teachers. The range of provision possibilities, such as mainstream, team teaching, withdrawal, on- and off-site unit provision and separate school provision, need to be discussed. One specific focus of a course may be directed towards education authorities' particular preferences on provision and much of this depends on the availability of resources and trained teachers. Issues relating to each of these, however, should be addressed.

## Consultation and development

Since it is important to be aware of the particular needs of education authorities and the teachers whom the course will serve, consultation during the development and review of courses is of paramount importance. With regard to Scotland, before reorganization in 1996, this included authorities with densely populated areas (such as Strathclyde) and others with a rural, widely-dispersed school population (such as the Highland Region which also incorporated Island populations). This consultation was effected by convening task groups which comprised professionals representing the perspectives of teachers, policymakers, psychologists and other professionals such as speech therapists. Task group meetings were held regularly during the development stages and were convened by the course leader. Mode of delivery was also considered then.

Since the course was to be delivered in different locations it was decided to offer a range of delivery options. These included taught course, open learning and distance learning. It was also felt that the course should be within the award-bearing system. This meant in relation to Moray House, that the course should be within the Masters' framework validated by the University. Placing the course within the University Masters framework allowed the development of a higher award in dyslexia, such as the Masters in Education (M.Ed). The M.Ed award (which was validated in 1994) became a discrete named Award in Specific Learning Difficulties (Dyslexia). It was felt this was a major achievement in the field of dyslexia. This offers an example of a desirable and accept-able product resulting from consultation and co-operation between course developers and recipients. Other such examples have been noted elsewhere in the country with most course providers now linking very closely with LEAs.

## Interface between policy and practice

It is now clear that a specialist course on teacher-training in SpLDs, e.g. dyslexia should not be developed in isolation, and that those whom the course will serve need to be consulted throughout development of the course. There is now some evidence that educational authorities and schools are developing guidelines and policies in SpLDs, e.g. dyslexia (Fife Council 1996; Durham LEA 1999; East Renfrewshire 1999). It is important that there is liaison between training and policy, and there should be two-way dialogue as training can influence policy and vice versa.

## Whole-school needs

Teacher-training in dyslexia should move beyond specialist teacher-training of individual staff and address the needs of the whole school. School management systems and personnel should be included in training programmes as policy issues relating to identification, assessment and teaching can be greatly influenced by them.

Class teachers clearly have a role to play in relation to whole-school requirements necessary to deal with the needs of dyslexic students. Too often the in-service training needs of class teachers are overlooked, yet they are in a prime position to identify and deal with dyslexic difficulties at an early stage.

## Monitoring and maintaining standards

As indicated earlier, there is an increasing trend in the UK for universities and colleges to develop specialist courses in dyslexia. Although this is welcome, it is important that standards, in particular in relation to course balance and the training and expertise of those running it, are consistent. In order to ensure this consistency, the British Dyslexia Association recommends that courses should be accredited by them. The BDA Accreditation Board includes experienced professionals from different areas in the UK, drawn from universities and other bodies who run courses in dyslexia. The Accreditation Board appoints two of its members who take principle responsibility for examining particular courses in terms of construction, content, assessment tasks, balance between theory and practice, length and general standard. The Accreditation Board undertakes to monitor and review procedures to ensure course quality remains consistent with accredited status. Although universities have internal and external validation procedures which contribute to the maintaining and monitoring of standards it may well be desirable for all such courses to gain accreditation from the BDA Accreditation Board.

## Initial teacher education

Initial teacher education should be recognized as a priority area since awareness of classroom teachers is important for the early identification and recognition of the needs of dyslexic children. At present, such teachers often lack confidence in dealing with dyslexia because of their lack of knowledge and training. Courses in initial teacher education are characterized by competing priorities – curriculum development, child development, teaching principles and practice and, as a result, competition for specific input in initial teacher-training programmes is fierce. Despite this, it is desirable that new teachers have at least an awareness of dyslexia and it is possible for this to be achieved within the constraints of an already full teacher-training programme.

To provide continuing professional development and resource materials for initial teacher-trainers from all over the UK, the Teacher Training Agency (TTA) and the BDA have run a series of half-day courses in

London and Manchester during 1998–2000. A potentially far-reaching initiative has also been implemented by Manchester Metropolitan University, a discrete module within its B.Ed course specifically on dyslexia. Other universities may have some dyslexia input located within courses dealing with special education needs or reading and literacy.

## Responses from teachers

Feedback on course content, delivery and potential impact on practice is important. A summary of some comments from teachers on various courses they have undertaken is shown below:

- Teachers were heartened by the fact that the course helped them become familiar with a range of materials and strategies.
- They acknowledged that no one single resource or programme is suitable for all dyslexic children.
- They understood as well as considering the child, one needs to consider the school and teaching context.
- A specialist course in dyslexia needs to acknowledge the curriculum demands which confront dyslexic students.
- Teachers need to discuss and gain some insight into how they can help to differentiate and access the curriculum for dyslexic students.

## Future directions

Teacher-training in dyslexia has made considerable progress over the last five years. There are several reasons for this, ranging from convincing research evidence which provides a sounder theoretical basis for dyslexia, an increase in public awareness, increased awareness among professionals and potential course developers and the quality of the courses developed. This latter point has helped educational authorities realize the potential benefits of teacher-training in dyslexia and there now appears a considerable will among them to ensure that the training needs of teachers in this area are met (Peer 1999).

It appears that many course leaders are embarking on the task in a similar way, that is, ensuring that courses are not only available to specialists but also to classroom teachers and school management. Additionally, there is now a trend to offer courses for those engaged in supporting people with dyslexia undergoing further and higher education (Singleton 1999). This is commendable since many more dyslexic young people are now able to access higher education and therefore the opportunity of fulfilling their potential is greater. It has been noted that many dyslexic young people have low academic self-esteem and this can be addressed with adequate support at college and university (Reid and Kirk 2000). It is important that course tutors and advisers have some awareness competence in recognizing the needs of students with dyslexia and supporting them in an appropriate manner. There are also some developments in providing courses for employers and dyslexic adults themselves, for example the Armed Forces (Myers 1999). This is desirable as there are indications that awareness of dyslexia among employers is low (Kirk and Reid 1999).

In view of these developments it appears that awareness of dyslexia and the needs of teachers, trainers, college and university staff and employers in providing support for those with dyslexia is increasing and there is every indication that this momentum will be maintained (Peer 1999).

## Conclusion

The controversies related to dyslexia are unlikely to disappear. Despite them, however, there is a clearer and more credible view of the concept of dyslexia witnessed by the considerable research activity in this area and the increase in appropriate teaching programmes related to the outcomes of research. It is important that teacher-training incorporates the two elements of research and practice and paves the way for a new generation of trained teachers confident in the recognition and teaching of dyslexic children.

# References

Adams MJ (1990) Beginning to Read: Thinking and Learning about Print. Cambridge, MA: MIT Press.

Adey P, Shayer M (1994) Cognitive intervention and academic achievement. London: Routledge.

Aldridge TM (1995) Special Educational Needs Tribunal Annual Report. London: SEN Tribunal.

Alm J, Anderson J (1996) Reading and Writing Difficulties at Prisons in the County of Uppsala. Uppsala: The Dyslexia Project for the National Labour Market Board of Sweden at the Employability Institute of Uppsala.

Alston J, Taylor J (1990) Handwriting: Theory, Research and Practice. London: Routledge.

Anon (1994) Dyslexia, perplexia, mislexia. Division of Educational & Child Psychology Newsletter 62: 37–8.

Archer M (1995) Editorial: When the writs hit the fan. Special Children September: 2.

Arnold H (1992) UKRA Diagnostic Reading Record. London: Hodder and Stoughton.

Ashton AF, Conway NF (1997) An Introduction to Cognitive Education. London: Routledge.

Association of Educational Psychologists and the Division of Educational and Child Psychology of the British Psychological Society (1995) Statutory Advice to the LEA: Guidance for Educational Psychologists. Leicester: British Psychological Society.

Augur J (1990) Is three too young to know? Dyslexia Contact 9: 10–11.

Augur J, Briggs S (1993) The Hickey Multisensory Language Course (Second edition). London: Whurr.

Banaji MR, Dasgupta N (1998) The consciousness of social beliefs: a programme of research on stereotyping and prejudice. In: VY Yzerbyt, G Lories, B Dardenne. Metacognition: Cognitive and Social Dimensions. London: Sage; 157–70.

Baddeley AD (1990) Human Memory: Theory and Practice. London: Lawrence Erlbaum Association.

Baddeley AD (1992) Working Memory. Science 255: 556–59.

Bakker DJ (1990) Neuropsychological Treatment of Dyslexia. New York: Oxford University Press.

Bakker DJ, Licht R, Kappers EJ (1994) Techniques in children with dyslexia. In: MG Tramontana, SR Hooper (eds). Advances in Child Neuropsychology. Vol 3. New York: Springer Verlag; 144–47.

Bakker DJ (1994) Dyslexia and the ecological brain. Journal of Clinical and Experimental Neuropsychology 16: 734–43.

Bakker DJ (1997) Dyslexia in terms of space and time. Abstracts. Fourth World Congress on Dyslexia, Halkidiki, Macedonia, Greece, 23–26 September; 7.

Barber M (1997) Transforming standards of literacy. In: N McClelland (ed). Building a Literate Nation. Stoke on Trent: Methuan Books; 3–8.

Barnes S, Chauhan S (2000) Highfields Literacy Project Video. Leicester: Leicester City Education Department.

Barrs M, Ellis S, Hester H, Thomas A (1988) The Primary Language Record. London: Centre for Language Information.

Barsch R (1965) The Movigenic Curriculum. USA.

Bath J, Chinn S, Knox D (1986) The Test of Cognitive Style in Mathematics. East Aurora, NY: Slosson.

Bentley T (1998) Learning beyond the Classroom, Education for a Changing World. London: Routledge.

Bettleheim B (1960) The Informed Heart. Glencoe, IL: The Free Press.

Beverton S, Hunter-Carsch M, Obrist C, Stuart A (1993) Running Family Reading Groups. Widnes: UK Reading Association (UKRA).

Bielby N (1994) Making Sense of Reading: The New Phonics and Its Practical Implications. Leamington Spa: Scholastic.

Biesta G (1998) Where are You? Where am I? Education, Identity and the Question of Location. Paper presented at the Annual Conference of the British Educational Research Association, Queen's University, Belfast: contact at the Department of Educational Science, Philosophy and History of Education, Utrecht University, Netherlands.

Bindra D, Stewart J (1968) Motivation (second edition). Harmondsworth: Penguin.

Binns R (1978) From Speech to Writing. Occasional Paper. Edinburgh: Centre for English, Moray House College of Education.

Binns R (1989) Re-creation through writing. In: M Hunter-Carsch. The Art of Reading. Oxford: Basil Blackwell; 100–110.

Blamires M (Ed.) (1999) Enabling Technology for Inclusion. London: Paul Chapman Publishing.

Bless H, Strack H (1998) Social influences on memory. In: VY Yzerbyt, G Lories, B Dardenne. Metacognition: Cognitive and Social Dimensions. London: Sage; 90–106.

Blyth C, Faulkner J (1994) To test or not to test, that is the question. Division of Educational and Child Psychology Newsletter 62: 27–35.

Boutskou E (1995) Computers and Specific Learning Difficulties (Literacy) in the Primary School. Unpublished MEd dissertation, Centre for Special Needs, School of Education, The University of Manchester.

Boyle J, Dinham H, Rust JN, Williams T, Bland S (1995) Checklist of Competences in Educational Testing: Foundation Level. Consultation document. Leicester: British Psychological Society Steering Committee on Test Standards, September.

BPS/DECP (1999) Dyslexia, Literacy and Psychological Assessment. Report by a working party of the Division of Educational and Child Psychologists of the British Psychological Society. Leicester: British Psychological Society.

Bradley L, Bryant P (1983) Categorizing sounds and learning to read: a causal connexion. Nature 301: 419–21.

British Dyslexia Association (1999) Dyslexia Handbook. Reading: BDA.

British Association of Counselling (1996) The BAC Counselling Reader. London: Sage.

British Psychological Society Standing Committee on Test Standards (1992) Psychological Testing: A Guide. Leicester: British Psychological Society.

British Psychological Society (1999) Dyslexia, Literacy and Psychological Assessment. Report by a working party of the Division of Educational and Child Psychology of the British Psychological Society (DECP) (see also DECP p. 269). Leicester: British Psychological Society.

Brook A (1997) Approaches to abstraction; a commentary. International Journal of Educational Research 27: 77–88.

Brooks G, Harman J, Hutchinson D, Kendall S and Wilkin A (1999) Family Literacy for NewGroups: The NFER Evaluation of Family Literacy with Linguistic Minorities, Year 4 and Year 7. London: Basic Skills Agency (website: www.basic-skills.co.uk/).

Brown R (1980) Metacognitive development and reading. In: R Spiro, B Bruce and W Brewer (eds) Theoretical Issues in Reading Comprehention. Hillsdale NJ: Lawrence Erlbaum.

Burton A, Radford J (1978) Thinking in Perspective: Critical Essays in the Study of Thought Processes. London: Methuen.

Buzan T, Buzan B (1993) The Mindmap Book. London: BBC Books.

Campbell R (1993) UKRA Minibook No. 3 Miscue Analysis in the Classroom. Widness: UKRA.

Cashdan A, Grugeon E (1972) Language in Education. Buckingham: Open University Press.

Cassidy J (1997) Multiple Intelligences: An Update on the Model and Implications for Literacy Instruction. Paper presented at the Tenth European Conference on Reading, Reading Choices: Bringing Cultures Closer Together, Brussels, August.

Cassidy S (1998) 'Tests are unreliable' says chief inspector. Times Educational Supplement 18 December.

Catts HW (1989) Phonological processing deficits and reading disabilities. In: AG Kamhi, HW Catts (eds). Reading Disabilities: A Developmental Language Perspective. Boston, MA: Little Brown; 101–32.

Chapman JW, Tunmer WE (1993) The Reading Self-Concept Scale. Unpublished scale. New Zealand: Palmerstone North, New Zealand Educational Research and Development Centre, Massey University.

Chapman V (1998) Praxis makes perfect too: an essential guide for parents and teachers. In: P Hunt (ed) The Voice of Experience: Parental Perceptions of Dyspraxia. Hitchin: Dyspraxia Foundation. 55–67.

Chappell D, Walker M (2000) Effective support for adult learners. In: M Hunter-Carsch, M Herrington (eds). Dyslexia and Effective Learning in Secondary and Tertiary Education. London: Whurr Publishers.

Chase CH, Rosen GD, Sherman GF (1996) Developmental Dyslexia: Neural, Cognitive and Genetic Mechanisms. Parkland, MD: York Press.

Chastey H, Friel J (1993) Children with Special Needs. Assessment, Law and Practice – Caught in the Act (second edition). London: Kingsley.

Chinn ST, Ashcroft JR (1993) Mathematics for Dyslexics: A Teaching Handbook. London: Whurr Publishers.

Chrisfield J (1996) The Dyslexia Handbook 1996. Reading: British Dyslexia Association.

Clark MM (1976) Young Fluent Readers: What Can They Teach Us? London: Heinemann Educational Books.

Clark MM (1994) Young Literacy Learners: How We Can Help Them. Leamington Spa: Scholastic.

Claxton G (1998a) Investigating human intuition: knowing without knowing why. Psychologist 11: 217–20.

Claxton G (1998b) Hare Brain, Tortoise Mind. London: Fourth Estate.

Clay M (1979) The Patterning of Complex Behaviour (2nd edition). Auckland, NZ: Heinemann.

Clay M (1991) Becoming Literate: The Construction of Inner Control. Auckland, NZ: Heinemann.

Clay M (1993) An Observation Survey of Early Literacy Achievement. London: Heineman.

Cline T, Fredrickson N (1991) Bilingual Pupils and the National Curriculum: Overcoming Difficulties in Teaching and Learning. London: University College.

Cockcroft Report (1982) Mathematics Counts. DfES. London: HMSO.

Coles G (2000) Misreading Reading. The Bad Science that Hurts Children. Portsmouth, NH: Heinemann.

Collins J (1996) The Quiet Child, and discussion of papers presented at the British Educational Research Conference, Belfast, August 1998.

Committee of Enquiry into the Education of Handicapped Children and Young People (1978). Special Educational Needs. (Warnock Report) Cmnd. 7212. London: HMSO.

Connor MJ (1994) Dyslexia (SpLD): assessing assessment. Educational Psychology in Practice 10: 131–9.

Coon KB, Waguespack MM, Polk MJ (1994) Dyslexia Screening Instrument. San Antonio, CA: The Psychological Corporation.

Cornelissen PL, Richardson A, Mason A, Fowler S, Stein J (1995) Contrast sensitivity and coherent motion detection measured at photopic luminance levels in dyslexics and controls. Vision Research 35: 1483–94.

Cornwall J (Ed.) (1995) Psychology, disability and equal opportunity. The Psychologist (Special Issue) 8: 396–418.

Cortazzi M, Hunter-Carsch M (2000) Multilingualism and Literacy Difficulties: Bridging home and school. Reading, Vol 34, No 1: 43–49.

Cotgrove A (2000) Voice activated systems. In: I Smythe (ed). The Dyslexia Handbook 2000. Reading: British Dyslexia Association; 189–96.

Cratty BJ (1975) Remedial Motor Activity for Children. Philadelphia, PA: Lea & Febiger

Cratty BJ, Goldman RL (1996) Learning Disabilities: Contemporary Viewpoints. Amsterdam: Harwood Academic Publications.

Crisfield J (1996) The Dyslexia Handbook 1996. Reading, British Dyslexic Association.

Crombie A (1991) Use of portable word processors by dyslexic students. In: C Singleton (ed). Computers and Literacy Skills. University of Hull: Computer Resource Centre; 137–48.

Crombie M (1997) Specific Learning Difficulties (Dyslexia): A Teachers' Guide (second edition). Belford: Ann Arbor.

Crombie M (1997) The effects of dyslexia on the learning of a modern foreign language in school. Dyslexia 3: 27–47.

Crombie M (1999) The Effects of Dyslexia on Learning a Modern Foreign Language. Paper presented at the BDA's first International Conference on Multilingualism and Dyslexia, Manchester, June.

Crossley S (2001) Shaping policy and practices in secondary schools: support for learning. In: M Hunter-Carsch, M Herrington (eds). Dyslexia and Effective Learning in Secondary and Tertiary Education. London: Whurr Publishers.

Crozier WR (1997) Individual Learners: Personality Differences in Education. London: Routledge.

Cruickshank W, Bentzen FA, Ratzeburg FG, Tannhauser MT (1961) A Teaching Method for the Hyperactive Brain-injured Child. Syracuse: Syracuse University Press.

Cummins J (1984) Construct of Learning Disability – Bilingualism and Special Education: Issues in Assessment and Pedagogy. Clevedon: Multilingual Matters.

Dadds M (1999) Teachers' Values and the Literacy Hour. Cambridge Journal of Education 29(1): 7–19.

Davies J, Brember I (1998) Boys Outperforming Girls: An eight-year cross-sectional study of attainment and self esteem in Year 6. Paper presented at the British Educational Research Conference in Belfast, August.

Debenham M (1996) Barriers to Study for Open University Students with Long Term Health Problems: A Survey. (Report 105). Milton Keynes: Open University Student Research Centre.

DeFries JC (1991) Genetics and dyslexia: an overview. In: M Snowling, M Thomson (eds). Dyslexia: Integrating Theory and Practice. London: Whurr Publishers. 3–20.

DeFries JC, Alarcon M, Olson RK (1997) Genetic aetiologies of reading and spelling deficits: developmental differences. In: C Hulme, M Snowling (eds). Dyslexia: Biology, Cognition and Intervention. London: Whurr Publishers; 20–37.

Dewsbury A and the Education Department of Western Australia (1995) First Steps: Parents as Partners: Helping your child's literacy and language development. Melbourne, Australia: Longman.

DfE (1994a) The Organisation of Special Educational Provision. Circular No 6/94. London: DfE.

DfE (1994b) Special Educational Needs Tribunal: How to Appeal. London: DfE.

DfEE and the Welsh Office (1994) Code of Practice on the Identification and Assessment of Special Educational Needs. London: Central Office of Information.

DfEE (1998a) The National Literacy Strategy Framework for Teaching, including additional guidance for Children with English as an additional language (EAL) and Children with Special Educational Needs (SEN). London: DfEE.

DfEE (1998b) Pamphlet: How can I tell if a child may be dyslexic? Handy Hints for Primary School Teachers. London: DfEE.

DfEE (2000) Draft Revision of the Code of Practice on the Identification and Assessment of Special Educational Needs. London: Central Office of Information.

Division of Educational and Child Psychology of the British Psychological Society (DECP)(1999) Dyslexia, Literacy and Psychological Assessment. Report by a Working Party Chaired by Dr R Reason. Leicester: British Psychological Society.

Dobbins A (1994) Expected reading scores of pupils in Years 3 to 6. British Journal of Educational Psychology 64: 491–6.

Donaldson M (1992) Human Minds: An Exploration. London: Penguin.

Dougan M, Turner G (1996) Information technology and specific learning difficulties. In: G Reid (ed). Dimensions of Dyslexia, Volume 1. Edinburgh: Moray House Publications. 397–414.

Downing J, Schaefer B, Ayres D (1993) LARR Test of Emergent Literacy (The Linguistic Awareness in Reading Readiness Tests (LARR)). Slough: NFER.

Drever (1952) A Dictionary of Psychology. Harmondsworth: Penguin.

Drew PY, Watkins D (1998) Affective variables, learning approaches and academic achievement: a causal modelling investigation with Hong Kong tertiary students. British Journal of Educational Psychology 68: 173–88.

Duane DD (1991) Neurobiological issues in dyslexia. In: M Snowling, M Thomson (eds). Dyslexia: Integrating Theory and Practice. London: Whurr Publishers; 21–30.

Duffield J (1998) Learning experiences, effective schools and social context. Support for Learning 13: 3–8.

Duffield J, Riddell S, Brown S (1995) Policy, Practice and Provision for Children with Specific Learning Difficulties. New York: Avebury Publishing.

Dunn K, Dunn R, Price GE (1989) Learning Styles Inventory. Lawrence: KS Price Systems.

Durham Education Authority (1999) Course Documentation on Dyslexia. Durham.

East Renfrewshire Council (1999) Policy on Dyslexia. East Renfrewshire.

Edgar B (2000) Effective learning in the secondary school: teaching students with dyslexia to develop thinking skills. In: M Hunter-Carsch, M Herrington (eds). Dyslexia and Effective Learning in Secondary and Tertiary Education. London: Whurr Publishers.

Edwards J (1994) The Scars of Dyslexia: Eight Case Studies in Emotional Reactions. London: Cassell.

Elbrow C (1998) Reading – listening discrepancy definitions of dyslexia. In: P Reitsma, L Verhoeven (eds). Problems and Interventions in Literacy Development. London: Kluwer. 129–46.

Elliott CD (1990) The definition and identification of specific learning difficulties. In: PD Pumfrey, CD Elliott (eds). Children's Difficulties in Reading, Spelling and Writing (third edition). Basingstoke: Falmer Press; 14–28.

Elliott CD (1994) British Ability Scales: A 'G-enhanced' Short-form IQ. Windsor: NFER-Nelson.

Elliott J, Figg J (1993) Assessment issues. Educational and Child Psychology 10: 80 (whole edition).

Elliott CD, Daniel MH (in preparation) Evaluation of ability–achievement discrepancies: some problems with the WIAT/WISC-III Tables. Circle Pines, MN: Guidance Service Inc.

Ellis AW, McDougall SJP, Monk AF (1997a) Are dyslexics different? III. Of course they are! Dyslexia: An International Journal of Research and Practice 3: 2–8.

Ellis AW, McDougall SJP, Monk AF (1997b) Are dyslexics different? IV. In defence of uncertainty. Dyslexia: An International Journal of Research and Practice 3: 12–14.

Ellis NC, Miles TR (1977) Dyslexia as a limitation in the ability to process information. Bulletin of the Orton Society 27: 72–81.

Erikson E (1968) Identity, Youth and Crisis. Toronto: WW Norton.

Evans BJW, Wilkins AJ, Brown J, Busby A, Wingfield A, Jeanes R, Bald J. (1996) A preliminary investigation into the aetiology of Meares-Irlen syndrome. Ophthalmic and Physiological Optics, Physiolology Opt 16; 286–96.

Ewing J (1982) Attitude to Reading Scales ATR1 and ATR2. Department of Educational Studies, Northern College, Dundee Campus, Dundee DD5 1NY.

Faupel A, Herrick E, Sharp P (1998) Anger Management, A Practical Guide. London: David Fulton.

Fawcett A (1996) Case Studies and some recent research. In: TR Miles, VP Varma (eds). Dylexia and Stress. London: Whurr Publishers. 5–32.

Fawcett A, Nicolson R (eds) (1994) Dyslexia in Children: Multidisciplinary Perspectives. Hemel Hempstead: Prentice-Hall.

Fernald G (1943) Remedial Techniques in Basic School Subjects. New York: McGraw-Hill.

Feuerstein R, Rand Y, Hoffiman MB, Muller R (1980) Instrumental Enrichment. Baltimore, MD: University Park Press.

Fife Council (1996) Guidelines and Policies in Specific Learning Difficulties (Dyslexia). Fife, Scotland.

Forness S (1996) Social and emotional dimensions of learning disabilities. In BJ Cratty, RL Goldman (eds). Learning Disabilities: Contemporary Viewpoints. Amsterdam: Harwood Academic Publications. 61–86.

Fox R (1996) The struggling writer: strategies for teaching. Reading 30: 13–19.

Francis H (1997) Teaching beginning reading: a case for monitoring feelings and attitudes. Reading 31: 5–8.

Frankenberger W, Fronzaglio K (1991) 'A review of states' criteria and procedures for identifying children with learning disabilities. Journal of Learning Disabilities 24: 495–500.

Frederickson N, Reason R (1995a) Discrepancy definitions of specific learning difficulties. Educational Psychology in Practice 10: 195–205.

Frederickson N, Reason R (1995b) Phonological assessment of specific learning Difficulties. Educational and Child Psychology 12: whole edition; 88 pp.

Frederickson N, Frith U, Reason R (1997) Phonological Assessment Battery (PhAB). Windsor: NFER-Nelson.

Frith U (1995) Dyslexia: Can we have a shared theoretical framework? Education and Child Psychology 12: 6–17.

Frith U (1997) Brain, mind and behaviour in dyslexia. In: C Hulme, M Snowling. Dyslexia: Biology, Cognition and Intervention. London: Whurr Publishers; 1-19.

Frost R (1955) The Road Not Taken. Penguin Poets Series. London: Penguin. 78.

Frostig M, Horne D (1970) Education for Dignity. New York: Grune and Stratton.

Funnell E, Stuart M (1995) Learning to Read: Psychology in the Classroom. Oxford: Blackwell.

Gains C, Wray D (1995) Reading: Issues and Directions. Stafford: National Association for Special Educational Needs (NASEN).

Galaburda AM (1999) Developmental dyslexia: a multilevel syndrome. Dyslexia: An International Journal of Research and Practice 5: 183–91.

Galaburda AM, Corsiglia J, Rosen GD, Sherman GF (1987) Planum temporale asymmetry: reappraisal since Geschwind and Levitsky. Neuropsychologia 25: 853–68.

Galaburda AM, Livingstone MS (1993) Evidence for a magnocellular defect in developmental dyslexia. In: P Tallal. Annals of the New York Academy of Sciences: 70–81.

Gallagher A (1995) The development of a phonological assessment battery: research background. Educational and Child Psychology 12: 18-24.

Gallagher A, Fredrickson N (1995) The Phonological Assessment Battery (PhAB): An Initial Assessment of Its Theoretical and Practical Utility. Educational and Child Psychology 12.

Gardner H (1985) Frames of Mind: The Theory of Multiple Intelligences (tenth edition). Arizona: Zephyr.

Garner RS, Alexander PA (1994) Beliefs about Text and Instruction with Text. Hillsdale, NJ: Lawrence Erlbaum Associates.

Gardner H (1995) Reflections on multiple intelligences: myths and messages. Phi Delta Kappa (November): 200–9.

Gathercole SE, Baddeley AD (1996) The Children's Test of Nonword Recognition. New York: The Psychological Corporation (Harcourt Brace).

Gerber P, Ginsberg R, Reiff H (1992) Identifying alterable patterns in employment success for highly successful adults with learning disabilities. Journal of Learning Disability 25: 475–87.

Gerstner L (1996) Speech at the AGM of IBM Corporation. Atlanta, USA.

Geschwind N, Behan P(1982) Left-handedness: association with immune disease, migraine and developmental learning disorders. Proceedings of the National Academy of Sciences of USA 79: 5097–5100.

Getman GN, Kane ER, Halgren RM McKee (1964) The Physiology of Readiness. Minneapolis, MN: PASS Inc.

Ghouri S (1998) Mum's too afraid to ask. Times Educational Supplement 4th September p. 4.

Gillingham A, Stillman B (1940) Remedial Training for Children with Specific Disability in Reading, Spelling and Penmanship. New York: Sackett & Wilhelms.

Gilroy DE, Miles TR (1996) Dyslexia at College. London: Routledge.

Given B, Reid G (1999) Learning Styles: A Guide for Teachers and Parents. St Anne's on Sea: Red Rose Publications.

Gjessing HJ, Karlson B (1989) A Longitudinal Study of Dyslexia. New York: Springer-Verlag.

Gleitman H, Fridlund AJ, Reisberg D (1999) Psychology (fifth edition). London: WW Norton.

Goldberg E, Costa LD (1981) Hemisphere differences in the acquisition and use of descriptive systems. Brain and Language 14: 144–73.

Goodman YM, Burke CL (1972) Reading Miscue Inventory: Procedure for Diagnosis and Evaluation. New York: Macmillan.

Gordon N, McKinley I (1980) Helping the Clumsy Child. Edinburgh: Churchill Livingstone.

Goswami U (1997) Learning to read in different orthographies. In: C Hulme, M Snowling (eds). Dyslexia: Biology, Cognition and Intervention. London: Whurr Publishers; 131–52.

Goswami U (1991) Causal connections in beginning reading: the importance of rhyme. Research in Reading 22: 217–40.

Goswami U (1999) Causal connections in beginning reading: the importance of rhyme. Journal of Research in Reading 22(3): 217–40.

Gough PB (1995) The New Literacy: caveat emptor. Journal of Research in Reading 18: 79–86.

Goulandris N, Snowling M, Walker I (2001) Dyslexia in adolescents: a five-year follow-up study. In: M Hunter-Carsch, M Herrington (eds). Dyslexia and Effective Learning in Secondary and Tertiary Education. London: Whurr Publishers.

Greaney J, Reason R (1999) Phonological processing in Braille. Dyslexia: An International Journal of Research and Practice 5(4): 8–20.

Guilford JP (1952) Psychometric Methods. New York: McGraw-Hill.

Haase P (1999) Linguae Mundi: A Multilingual System for Early Intervention in Dyslexia and Aphasia. Workshop session with Morag Hunter-Carsch at the BDA's first International Conference on Multilingualism and Dyslexia, Manchester, June.

Haase P (ed.) (2000) Schreiben und lesen sicher lehren und lernen. Dortmund: Borgmann.

Hall K (1997) Metacognition, Reading and Nine-year-olds in Ireland and England. Paper presented at the Tenth European Conference on Reading: Literacy a Human Right: Bringing Cultures Closer, Brussels.

Hall K (1998) Discussion at the seminar on metacognition at the British Educational Research Conference, Belfast, August.

Hall K, Myers J (1997) 'That's just the way I am': metacognition, personal intelligence and reading. Reading 32: 8-13.

Hammersley M (1995) Opening up the quantitative-qualitative divide. Education Section Review 19: 2-9.

Hampshire S (1990) Every Letter Counts. London: Corgi.

Hargreaves L, Comber C (1998) Leicestershire Literacy Projects (January-March 1998). Final Evaluation Report. School of Education, University of Leicester, 21 University Road, Leicester LE1 7RF.

Hart S (1997) Beyond Special Needs. London: Paul Chapman.

Hartland S, Harcourt K (1995) Discovering readers. Reading 29: 38-46.

Hatcher P, Hulme C, Ellis AW (1994) Ameliorating early reading failure by integrating the teaching of reading and phonological skills. Child Development vol 65 No. 1: 41–7.

Hayes N (1991) Introduction to the Cognitive Processes. Leicester: British Psychological Society Open Learning Units.

Hayes AE, Hegarty P (1999) The Apple Project Report 8/22/99. Action on Principal Pedogogy and Learning Evaluation, Department of Educational Research, University of Lancaster.

Healy JM (1990) Endangered Minds: Why Children don't Think and What we can Do About It. New York: Touchstone.

Henderson A (1989) Maths and Dyslexics. Llandudno: St David's College.

Henderson A (1998) Maths for the Dyslexic: A Practical Guide. London: David Fulton.

Henderson A, Miles, E. (2001) Basic Topics in Mathematics. London: Whurr Publishers.

Henderson S, Markee A, Sheib B, Taylor J (1999) Tools of the Trade. From the Handwriting Interest Group, c/o A Markee, Blackthorn Farm, Snows Lane, Keyham, Leices LE7 9JJ, UK.

Henry M, Ganschew L, Miles, TR (2000) The issue of definition: some problems. In: Perspectives in Dyslexia. Baltimore, MD: International Dyslexia Association 26(1) 28–43.

Herrington M (2001a) Adult dyslexia: partners in learning. In: M Hunter-Carsch, M Herrington (eds). Dyslexia and Effective Learning in Secondary and Tertiary Education, London: Whurr Publishers.

Herrington M (2001b) An approach to Learning Support in higher education. In M Hunter-Carsch, M Herrington (eds.) Dyslexia and Effective Learning in Secondary and Tertiary Education. London: Whurr.

Herrington M (2001c) Conversation about spelling in higher education. In M Hunter-Carsch, M Herrington (eds.) Dyslexia and Effective Learning in Secondary and Tertiary Education. London: Whurr.

Hess RD, Shipman VC (1965) Early experience and the socialization of cognitive modes in children. Child Development 36.

Hewstone M, Stroebe W, Stephenson GM (1996) Introduction to Social Psychology. Oxford: Blackwell.

Hickey K (1977) Dyslexia: A Language Training Course for Teachers and Learners. Private publisher: 3 Montague Road, London SW19.

Hinshelwood J (1895) Word-blindness and visual memory. Lancet 2: 1564–70.

Holland KC (1986) The detection and remediation of learning difficulties. Optician, 31 October: 21–2, 27–8.

Holland KC (1988) Reading with Vision. Eleventh Turvill Memorial Lecture. Optometry Today 2 January: 8–10.

Holmes P (1996) Specific Learning Difficulties and Mathematics: Supporting Teachers, Parents and Children in the Primary Years. UWB: MEd.

Horkheimer M (1947) The Eclipse of Reason. New York: Oxford University Press, pp. 54–7; 112–5; 133.

Hornsby B (1992) Overcoming Dyslexia, London: McDonald Option.

Hornsby B, Miles TR (1980) The effects of a dyslexic centred teachers program Br. J. Ed Psychgol, 50(3), 236–42.

Hornsby B, Shear F (1976) Alpha to Omega (second edition). London: Heinemann.

Howe CJ (1998) Conceptual Structure in Childhood and Adolescence: The Case of Everyday Physics. London: Routledge.

Hughes M, Hunter-Carsch M (2001) Spelling support in secondary education. In: M Hunter-Carsh, M Herrington (eds) Dyslexia and Effective Learning in Secondary and Tertiary Education. London: Whurr.

Hulme C, Snowling M (eds)(1994) Reading Development and Dyslexia. London: Whurr Publishers.

Hulme C, Snowling M (1997) Dyslexia: Biology, Cognition and Intervention. London: Whurr Publishers.

Hulme C, Joshi RM (1998) Reading and Spelling: Development and Disorders. London: Lawrence Erlbaum.

Hunter CM (1969) A Handbook for Teachers of Children with Learning Difficulties. Unpublished report for the Ontario Government Special Education Department.

Hunter CM (1970) Learning Difficulties: Collected papers by teachers on Option 209 Course. Unpublished report for the Ontario Government Special Education Department.

Hunter CM (1972) Remedial Exercises for Children with Learning Difficulties. Unpublished compendium of papers by MSc Educational Psychology students at Strathclyde University as part of their work for the course on 'Prescriptive Teaching'.

Hunter CM (1973) Screening for Specific Learning Difficulties. Unpublished MEd thesis, Glasgow University.

Hunter CM (1981) A Maxtrix for Diagnosing Inappropriate Learning Strategies. Paper presented at the British Psychological Society Cognitive Section Conference on Dyslexia, The University of Manchester.

Hunter CM (1982) Reading and learning difficulties: relationships and responsibilities. In: A Hendry (ed). Reading: The Key Issues. London: Heinemann.

Hunter-Carsch M (1984) The Talking-with-Books Project Report. Occasional Paper, School of Education, University of Leicester.

Hunter CM (1985) Exploring Reading Problems. Unit 17. In: R Dawson (ed). Teacher Information Pack (Special Educational Needs). London: Macmillan Educational.

Hunter-Carsch CM (ed) (1989) The Art of Reading. Oxford: Blackwell.

Hunter-Carsch CM (1990) Learning strategies for pupils with literacy difficulties: motivation, meaning and imagery. In: PD Pumfrey, CD Elliott. Children's Difficulties in Reading, Spelling and Writing, London: Falmer Press; 222–36.

Hunter-Carsch M (1993a) Stance, meaning and voluntary reading. In: P Owen, P Pumfrey (eds). Emergent and Developing Reading: International Concerns. London: Falmer Press; 137–60.

Hunter-Carsch CM (1993b) Pre-requisites for teaching reading to dyslexic children in mainstream classes. In: B Hornsby. Literacy 2000 International Dyslexia Conference Proceedings. London: The Hornsby International Centre; 52–62.

Hunter-Carsch M, Barnes S, Millward S, Ranson P (1996) The Eyres Monsell Family Reading Groups Project Report. Occasional Paper School of Education, University of Leicester.

Hunter-Carsch M. (1997a) Seeing the wood *and* the trees, specific learning difficulties and dyslexia, papers presented at the World Congresion Dyslexia, Halkidiki, Greece.

Hunter-Carsch CM (1997b) What's in a name? Literacy and linguistic awareness; knowledge, understanding and the teaching of reading. In: Paper presented at: Literacy: A Human Right: Bringing Cultures Closer, Tenth European Conference on Reading, Brussels.

Hunter-Carsch M, (1998) Developing Literacy at 11: Evaluations of the Leicester Summer Literacy Schools: Unpublished report to Leicester City LEA. Copy available from the author at: Leicester University School of Education.

Hunter-Carsch M, Mailley S (1999) A Preliminary Analysis of Responses to the Multilingualisim and Dyslexia Questionnaire, unpublished papers. Leicester University School of Education.

Hunter-Carsch M, Herrington M (eds) (2001) Dyslexia and Effective Learning in Secondary and Tertiary Education. London: Whurr.

Irlen H (1991) Reading by the Colors. New York: Avery Press.

Irlen H, Lass MJ (1989) Improving Reading Problems due to symptoms of Scotopic Sensitivity Syndrome using Irlen Lenses and overlaps, Education, Vol. 109 no 4 pp 413–417.

Jackson W, Michael W (1985) The Foundations of Writing Reports. Glasgow: Jordanhill College of Education.

Jeanes R, Martin J, Lewis E, Stevenson N, Pointon D, Wilkins AJ (1997) Prolonged use of coloured overlays for classroom reading. British Journal of Psychology 88: 531–48.

Johnson M, Phillips S, Peers L (1999) A Multisensory Teaching System for Reading (MSTSR). Manchester: Manchester Metropolitan University.

Johnston D (1987) Reading disabilities. In: D Johnson, J Blalock (eds). Young Adults with Learning Disabilities. Orlando, FL: Grune & Stratton; 145–72.

Jonassen DH, Grabowski BL (1993) Handbook of Individual Differences in Learning and Instruction. Hillsdale, NJ: Lawrence Erlbaum.

Jorm AF (1981) Children with reading and spelling retardation: functioning of whole-word and correspondence-rule mechanisms. Journal of Child Psychology and Psychiatry 22: 171–8.

Jorm AF (1983) The Psychology of Reading and Spelling Disabilities. Routledge & Kegan Paul.

Joyce B, Calhoun E, Hopkins D (1997) Models of Learning-tools for Teaching. Buckingham: Open University Press.

Kamien M (1983) When a Bright Child has Trouble Reading. Booklet: Optometric Extension Program Foundation, California.

Kamil ML, Pearson PD (1979) Theory and practice in teaching reading. University Education Quarterly Winter; 10–16.

Kaufman A (1994) Intelligent Testing with the WISC-III. New York: Wiley.

Kemp M (1987, 1989) Watching Children Reading and Writing: Observational Records for Children with Special Educational Needs. Thomas Nelson, Australia (1987) and Heinemann, USA (1989).

Kephart NC (1960) The Slow Learner in the Classroom. Columbus, USA: CE Merrill.

Kirk SA, McCarthy JJ, Kirk W (1968) The Illinois Test of Psycholinguistic Abilities (revised edition). Urbana, IL: University of Illinois.

Kirk J, Reid G (1999) Adult Dyslexia for Employment and Training (ADEPT). University of Edinburgh.

Kitson N (1994) Please Mrs Alexander: Will you be the robber? Fantasy Play: A case for adult intervention. In: J Moyles (ed). The Excellence of Play. Buckingham: Open University Press; 88–98.

Klein RM, McMullen PA (eds) (1999) Converging Methods for Understanding Reading and Dyslexia. Cambridge, MA: MIT Press.

Korpilahti P, Krause C (1996) Electrophysiological correlates of auditory perception in normal and language-impaired children. University of Turku, Medica-odontologia, D232.

Kovel J (1991) A Complete Guide to Therapy. London: Penguin.

Kress G (1997) Literacy: the changing landscape of communication. In: N McClleland (ed). Building a Literate Nation: The strategic agenda for literacy over the next five years. Stoke-on Trent: Trentham Books.

Landon J (1997) Reading Between Languages: Bilingual Learners and Specific Learning Difficulties. Paper presented at a British Dyslexia Association Seminar on Dyslexia and Bi/Multilingualism, London, October.

Landon J (2001) Multilingualism and dyslexia. In: M Hunter-Carsch, M Herrington (eds). Dyslexia and Effective Learning in Secondary and Tertiary Education. London: Whurr Publishers.

Landon J, Reid G, Deponio P, Mullen K (1999) An Audit of the Processes involved in Identifying and Assessing Bilingual Learners Suspected of being Dyslexic. Paper presented at the BDA's first International Conference of Dyslexia and Multi-lingualism. University of Manchester, June.

Larsen D (1999) Yak-Yak, The Language Processor. Workshop presented at the BDA First International Conference on Multilingualism and Dyslexia, Manchester.

Laumen C, Laumen S, Reid G (1997) Specific Learning Difficulties: A resource book. St Anne's on Sea: Red Rose Publishers.

Lawrence D (1985) Improving self-esteem and reading. Educational Research 27: 194–200.

Layton L, Deeny K (1995) Tackling literacy difficulties: can teacher training meet the challenge? British Journal of Special Education 22: 20–23.

Lazo M, Pumfrey P, Peers I (1997) Metalinguistic awareness, reading and spelling: the roots and branches of literacy. Journal of Research in Reading 20: 85–104.

Lehmkuhle S, Garxia OD, Turner L, Hash T, Baro JA (1993) A defective visual pathway in children with reading disability. New England Journal of Medicine 328: 989–96.

Leong CK (1987) Children with Specific Reading Disabilities. Amsterdam: Swets & Zeitlinger.

Leong CK (1989) Reflections on literacy and knowing. In: M Hunter-Carsch (ed). The Art of Reading. Oxford: Blackwell; 28–38.

Leong CK, Joshi RM (1995) Developmental and Acquired Dyslexia Neuropsychological and Neurolinguistic Perspectives. Amsterdam: Kluwer.

Liberman IY (1983) Should so-called modality preferences determine the nature of instruction for children with reading disabilities? Paper delivered at the International Conference on Dyslexia, Halkidiki, Greece..

Licht R (1989) Reading disability subtypes: cognitive and electrophysiological differences. In: DJ Bakker, H Van der Vlugt (eds). Learning Disabilities. Vol 1. Neuropsychological Correlates and Treatment. Lesse, Netherlands: Swets & Zeitlinger.

Licht R, Spyer G (1995) The Balance Model of Dyslexia: Theoretical and Clinical Progress. Assen: Van Gorcum.

Livingstone MS, Rosen GD, Drislane FW, Galaburda AM (1991) Physiological and anatomical evidence for a magnocellular deficit in developmental dyslexia. Proceedings of the National Academy of Science of the USA, September; 7943–7.

Lovett MW (1999) Defining and remediating the core deficits of developmental dyslexia: lessons from remedial outcome research with reading disabled children. In: RM Klein, PA McMullen (eds). Converging Methods for Understanding Reading and Dyslexia. Cambridge, MA: MIT Press; 111–32.

Mailley S (1997) The Classroom Implications of Visual Perceptive Difficulties: An Exploratory Study including Scotopic Sensitivity Syndrome or Irlen Syndrome. Unpublished MA thesis, Leicester University School of Education.

Mannheim K (1964) In: KH Wolff (ed). Wissenscoziologie. Berlin: Luchterhand; 133, 579.

Mannoni M (1967) The Child, His 'Illness' and the Others. Harmondsworth: Penguin Books.

Markee A (1993) Hands Up for Handwriting. For the Handwriting Interest Group, c/o A Markee, Blackthorn Farm, Snow Lane, Keyham, Leics LE7 9JS, UK.

Maslow AH (1968) Towards a Psychology of Being (second edition). Toronto: D Van Nostrand.

McClelland N (1997) Building a Literate Nation; The Strategic Agenda for Literacy over the Next Five Years. Stoke-on-Trent: Trentham Press.

McGuinness D (1998) Why Children Can't Read and What We Can Do About It. A scientific revolution in reading. Harmondsworth: Penguin.

McLoughlin D (2001) Adult dyslexia: assessment, counselling and training. In: M Hunter-Carsch, M. Herrington (eds). Dyslexia and Effective Learning in Secondary and Tertiary Education. London: Whurr Publishers.

McNab I (1994a) The Benefits of the British Ability Scales 'g-enhanced' Short-form IQ. Windsor: NFER-Nelson.

McNab I (1994b) Specific Learning Difficulties: How severe is severe? British Ability Scales Information booklet. Windsor: NFER-Nelson.

Mellanby J, Anderson R, Campbell B, Westwood E (1996) Cognitive determinants of verbal underachievement at secondary school level. British Journal of Educational Psychology 66: 483–500.

Merry R (1994) Guest Lecture on Differentiation. Presented at a conference on 'Access to Independent Learning'. University of Leicester, 24 October.

Merzenich MM, Jenkins WM, Johnston P, Schreiner C, Miller SL, Tallal P. (1996) Temporal processing deficits of language-learning impaired children ameliorated by training. Science 271: 77–81.

Miles E (1991) Visual dyslexia/auditory dyslexia: is this a valuable distinction? In: M Snowling, M Thomson (eds). Dyslexia: Integrating Theory and Practice. London: Whurr Publishers; 195–203.

Miles E (1996) Teaching Dyslexics in Other Languages Compared with English. Dyslexia Contact November: 33–5.

Miles TR (1983) Dyslexia: The Pattern of Difficulties. Oxford: Blackwell.

Miles TR (1988) Counselling in dyslexia. Counselling Psychology Quarterly 1: 97–107.

Miles TR (1993) Dyslexia: The Pattern of Difficulties (second edition). London: Whurr Publishers.

Miles TR, Varma VP (eds) (1995) Dyslexia and Stress. London: Whurr Publishers.

Miles TR, Miles E (1992) Dyslexia and Mathematics. London and New York: Routledge.

Miles TR, Miles E (1999) Dyslexia: A Hundred Years On (second edition). Buckingham: Open University Press.

Moerland R, Bakker DJ (1991) Hemispheric Stimulation (HEMSTIM). A computer based treatment program for children with P-type or L-type dyslexia. Netherlands: Centrum Informatica voor Gehandicapten.

Montgomery D (1997) Spelling: Remedial Strategies. London: Cassell.

Moreton J, Frith U (1995) Causal modelling: A structural approach to developmental psychopathology. In D. Cicchetti and D.J. Cohen (eds). Manual of Developmental Psychopathology pp 357–390. New York: Wiley.

Morgan WP (1896) A case study of congenital word blindness. British Medical Journal 2: 1378.

Morris J (1984) A Future for Phonics 44. In: M Hunter-Carsch, S Beverton, D Dennis (eds). Primary English in the National Curriculum Oxford: Blackwell; 109–19.

Morris J (1993) Phonics phobia. In: B Hornsby (ed.). Literacy 2000. London: The Hornsby Centre; 29–38.

Moyles J (1995) Beginning Teaching, Beginning Learning in Primary Education. Buckingham: Open University Press.

Mroz M, Hardman F, Smith F (in press) The Discourse of the Literacy Hour. Cambridge Journal of Education 30.

Mutter V, Hulme C, Snowling MJ (1997) Phonological Abilities Test. San Francisco, CA: The Psychological Corporation.

Myers J (1999) Dyslexia: and the Armed Forces - A Training manual Reading, BDA.

Myklebust HR (1971) Progress in Learning Disabilities. New York: Grune & Stratton.

Neisser U (1967) Cognitive Psychology. New York: Appleton Century Crofts.

Nelson TO, Kruglanski AW, Jost JT (1998) Knowing thyself and others. In: VY Yzerbyt, G Lories, B Dardenne (eds). Metacognition: Cognitive and Social Dimensions. London: Sage; 69–89.

Neuman S.B, McCormick S (eds) (1995) Single Subject Experimental Research: afflication for literacy. Newark DE: International Reading Association.

Nicolson RI (1996) Developmental dyslexia: past, present and future. Dyslexia 2(3): 190–207.

Nicolson RI, Fawcett AJ (1990) Automaticity: a new framework for dyslexia research. Cognition 35: 159–82.

Nicolson RI, Fawcett AJ (1995) Dyslexia is more than a phonological disability. Journal of Dyslexia 1: 19–36.

Nicolson RI, Fawcett AJ (1996a) The Dyslexia Early Screening Test. New York: Psychological Corporation.

Nicolson RI, Fawcett AJ (1996b) The Dyslexia Screening Test (6;6 to 16;5 Years). New York: Psychological Corporation.

Nicolson RI, Fawcett AJ (1999) Developmental dyslexia: the role of the cerebellum. Dyslexia: An International Journal of Research and Practice 5: 155–77.

Nicolson RI, Fawcett AJ, Dean P (1995) Time estimation deficits in developmental dyslexia: evidence of cerebellar involvement. Proceedings of the Royal Society of London B 259: 43–7.

Nicolson RI, Fawcett AJ, Moss H, Nicolson MK, Reason R (1999) Early reading intervention can be effective and cost effective. British Journal of Educational Psychology 69: 47–62.

Nicolson RI, Fawcett AJ, Berry EL, Jenkins IH, Dean P, Brooks DJ (1999) Association of abnormal cerebellar activation with motor learning difficulties in dyslexic adults. Lancet 353: 1662–7.

Norwich B (1999) Pupils' reasons for learning and behaving and for not learning and behaving in English and Maths lessons in a Secondary School. British Journal of Educational Psychology Vol 69, no 4, pp. 547–69

O'Connell B (1998) Solution Focused Therapy. London: Sage.

OFSTED (1999) Pupils with Specific Learning Difficulties in Mainstream Schools. A Report of Her Majesty's Chief Inspector of Schools.

Ohlsson S, Lehtinen E (1997) Special edition on Abstraction. International Journal of Educational Research 27: entire issue.

Olson RK, Datta H, Gayan J, DeFries J (1999) A behavioural genetic analysis of reading disabilities and component processes. In: RM Klein, McMullen (eds). Converging Methods for Understanding Reading and Dyslexia. Cambridge, MA: MIT Press; 133–52.

O'Neill H (1999) Managing Anger. London: Whurr.

Orton ST (1937) Reading, Writing and Speech Problems in Children. New York: Norton.

Orton A. (1992) Learning Mathematics. Issues, Theory & Classroom Practice London: Cassell.

Orton Dyslexia Society (ODS) (1994a) Dyslexia: Definition by the Committee of the ODS. Perspectives in Dyslexia, 3015.

Orton Dyslexia Society (ODS)(1994b) Dyslexia: definition by ODS Research Committee. Perspectives in Dyslexia, 3015.

Ott P (1997) How to Detect and Manage Dyslexia. A Reference and Resource Manual. London: Heinemann.

Owen P, Pumfrey P (eds) (1995) Emergent and Developing Reading: Messages for Teachers 1. Children Learning to Read: International Concerns. London: Falmer.

Parents in Education Research Network (PERN): http://www.ioe.ac.uk/pern/

Peer L (1999) Dyslexia/SpLD: a reappraisal as we move into the next century. In: I Smythe (ed). The Dyslexia Handbook. Reading: British Dyslexia Association; 62–6.

Peer L, Reid L (2000) Multilingualism, Literacy and Dyslexia: A Challenge for Educators. London: David Fulton.

Pirozzolo FJ (1979) The Neuropsychology of Developmental Reading Disorders. New York: Praeger Press.

Poussu-Olli HS (1993) Kehityksellinen dysleksia. The Department of Phonetics 38. Finland: University of Helsinki.

Poussu-Olli HS (1996) Aikuisen dyslektikon todellisuutta. Kielikukko 4. Finnish Reading Association.

Presland J (1991) Explaining away dyslexia. Educational Psychology in Practice 6: 215–21.

Pumfrey PD (1977) Measuring Reading Abilities: Concepts, sources and applications. London: Hodder & Stoughton.

Pumfrey PD (1985) Reading: Tests and Assessment Techniques (second edition). Sevenoaks: Hodder & Stoughton in association with the UK Reading Association.

Pumfrey PD (1987) Rasch scaling and reading tests. Journal of Research in Reading 10: 75–86.

Pumfrey PD (1990) Testing and teaching pupils with reading difficulties. In: PD Pumfrey, CD Elliott (eds) (1990) Children's Difficulties in Reading, Spelling & Writing. Basingstoke: Falmer Press; 187–208.

Pumfrey PD (1991) Improving Reading in the Junior School. London: Cassell.

Pumfrey PD (1993) Focus on dyslexia: coloured overlays and tinted spectacles. Special!: 44–6.

Pumfrey PD (1995a) Open dialogue: peer commentary on 'Opening up the quantitative-qualitative divide' by M Hammersley. Education Section Review 19: 13–15.

Pumfrey PD (1995b) Assessing and teaching children with specific developmental dyslexia (SDD): issues and promising practices. In: G Shiel, UN Dhalaigh, B O'Reilly (eds). Reading Development to Age 15. Dublin: Reading Association of Ireland. 3–12.

Pumfrey PD (1995c) The management of specific learning difficulties (dyslexia): challenges and responses. In: I Lunt, B Norwich, V Varma (eds). Psychology and Education for Special Needs: Recent Developments and Future Directions. London: Ashgate; 45–70.

Pumfrey PD (1995d) Specific learning difficulties: implications of research findings for the initial and in-service training of teachers. In: P Mittler, P Daunt (eds). Teacher Education for Special Educational Needs in Europe. London: Cassell; 94–105.

Pumfrey PD (1995e) Reading Standards at Key Stage 1: aspirations and evidence. In: P Owen and PD Pumfrey (eds.) Children Learning to Read: International xxxx, Vol 2. Curriculum and Assessment Issues: Messages for Teachers. London: Falmer Press. 135–54.

Pumfrey PD (1996) Specific Developmental Dyslexia: Basics to back? Leicester: British Psychological Society.

Pumfrey PD (1999) Reading: testing. In: B Spolsky (ed). Concise Encyclopedia of Educational Linguistics. Amsterdam: Elsevier; 459–62.

Pumfrey P, Reason R (1991) Emotional and Social Factors, Specific Difficulties. London: Routledge; 64–74.

Pumfrey PD, Reason R (1992) Specific Learning Difficulties (Dyslexia): Challenges and Responses. London: Routledge.

Pumfrey PD, Reason R (1996) Specific Learning Difficulties (Dyslexia): Challenges and Responses. London: Routledge.

Pumfrey PD, Elliott CD, McNab I, Turner M, Tyler S (1998) Reactions to 'Understanding and managing dyslexia: guidelines for educational psychologists' by RJ (Sean) Cameron. Division of Educational and Child Psychology Newsletter 81: 19-31. DECP Newsletter 84, April: 42–55.

Rack JP (1994) Dyslexia: the phonological deficit hypothesis. In: AJ Fawcett, RI Nicolson (eds). Dyslexia in Children: Multidisciplinary Perspectives. London: Harvester Wheatsheaf; 5–38.

Rack J (1995) Steps towards a more explicit definition of dyslexia. Dyslexia Review 7: 1–13.

Rappaport J, Hunter-Carsch M (1999) Testing rhyme recognition: How does your test measure up? Reading Vol 33(2): 64–71.

Reason R, Boote R (1994) Helping Children with Reading and Spelling: A Special Needs Manual. London: Routledge.

Redl F, Wineman D (1952) Controls from Within: Techniques for the Treatment of the Aggressive Child. The Free Press: Macmillan.

Reeves TC (1999) Home page of Journal of Interactive Learning Research, cited at http://www.aace.org/pubs/jilr/scope.html 12 Feb 2000.

Reid G (Ed.) (1993) Specific Learning Difficulties (Dyslexia). Perspectives on Practice. Edinburgh: Moray House Publications.

Reid G (1994) Dyslexia and Metacognitive Assessment. Paper presented at the Third British Dyslexia Association International Conference on Dyslexia, Manchester University, and in Links II 1: 38–44.

Reid G (1994) Specific Learning Difficulties (Dyslexia): A Handbook for Study and Practice. Edinburgh: Moray House Publications.

Reid G (1996a) (ed). Dimensions of Dyslexia: Volume 1: Assessment, Teaching and the Curriculum. Edinburgh: Moray House Publications.

Reid G (1996b) (ed). Dimensions of Dyslexia Volume 2: Language and Learning, Edinburgh: Moray House Publications.

Reid G (1998) Dyslexia: A Practitioners Handbook (second edition). Chichester: Wiley.

Reid G, Kirk J (2000) Dyslexia in Adults: Education and Employment and Education. Chichester: Wiley.

Reid G, Lyon G, Rumsey JK (1996) Neuroimaging: A Window to the Neurological Foundations of Learning and Behaviour in Children. Baltimore, MD: Paul H Brookes.

Reid M, Webster A, Beveridge M (1995) A conceptual basis for a literacy curriculum. In: P Owen, P Pumfrey (1995) Emergent and Developing Reading: International Concerns, London: Falmer Press; 161–80.

Reitsma P, Verhoeven L (eds) (1998) Problems and Interventions in Literacy Development. London: Kluwer.

Reynolds C (1984) Critical measurement issues in learning disabilities. Journal of Special Education 18: 451–76.

Riddick B (1996) Living with Dyslexia. The Social and Emotional Consequences of Specific Learning Difficulties. London: Routledge.

Riding RJ, Taylor EM (1976) Imagery and prose comprehension in 7 year old children. Educational Psychology in Practice 13(4): 258–265.

Riding R, Rayner S (1998) Cognitive Styles and Learning Strategies: Understanding Style Differences in Learning and Behaviour. London: David Fulton.

Riesman D (1950) The Lonley Crowd. New Haven: Yale University Press.

Rispens J, van Ypern TA, Yule W (1998) Perspectives on the Classification of Specific Developmental Disorders. London: Kluwer.

Robertson J (1999) Dyslexia and Reading: A neuropsychological approach. London: Whurr Publishers.

Robertson J, Pumfrey PD (in press) Differential teaching of pupils with dyslexia: bye-way or highway? British Journal of Special Education 27.

Robinson G, Conway RN (1994) Irlen filters and reading strategies: effect of coloured filters on reading achievement, specific reading strategies and perception of ability. Perceptual and Motor Skills 79: 467–83.

Robinson GL, Roberts TK, McGregor NR, Ellis EB (2000) Investigation of Biochemical Anomalies in People with a Visual Fprm of Dyslexia: Implications for Early Identification and Dietary Intervention. Paper presented at International Special Education Congress 2000. Manchester: UK. Contact the writer at the University of Newcastle NSW, Australia.

Roth I, Frisby JP (1986) Perception and Representation: A Cognitive Approach. Milton Keynes: Open University Press.

Ruddell BR, Ruddell MR (1994) 'Language acquisition and literacy processes. In: BR Ruddell, MR Ruddell, H Singer (eds). Theoretical Models and Processes of Reading (fourth edition). Newark, DA: International Reading Association; 83–103.

Ruddell B, Ruddell MR, Singer H (eds) (1994) Theoretical Models and Processes of Reading (fourth edition). Newark DA: International Reading Association.

Rule J (1999) Dyslexia Contact 18: 2.

Ryden M (1989) Dyslexia, How Would I Cope? London: Jessica Kinsley Publishers.

Sacks O (1995) An Anthropologist on Mars. London: Picador.

Sage R (1995) The Sage Language and Thinking Test (SALT) and the Sage Narrative Tests. Copyright the author, contact via Leicester University School of Education, 21 University Road, Leicester LE1 7RF.

Sage R (2001) Communication. In: M Hunter-Carsch, M Herrington (eds). Dyslexia and Effective Learning in Secondary and Tertiary Education. London: Whurr Publishers.

Salter R, Smyth I (1997) The International Book of Dyslexia. London: World Dyslexia Network Foundation.

Salzberger-Wittenberg I, Henry G, Osborne E (1990) The Emotional Experience of Learning and Teaching. London: Routledge.

Sampson OC (1975a) Fifty years of dyslexia: a review of the literature 1925–75 1; Theory, Research in Education 14: 15–32.

Sampson OC (1975b) Remedial Education. London: Routledge & Kegan Paul.

Sampson OC (1976) Fifty years of dyslexia: a review of the literature, 1925–1975. II: Practice. Research in Education 15: 39–54.

Scheib B, Lillywhite C (1994) Keyboard skills and laptop word processing. In: C Singleton (ed). Computers and Dyslexia. University of Hull: Computer Resource Centre. 88–98.

Scholes RJ (1998) The case against phonemic awareness. Journal of Research in Reading 21: 177–88.

Schonell FJ, Wall WD (1949) Remedial education centre. Educational Review 2: 3–30.

Schonhaut S, Satz P (1983) Prognosis for children with learning disabilities: a review of follow-up studies. In: Rutter M (ed) Developmental Neuropsychiatry, New York: Guildford Press.

Seligman M (1990) Learned Optimism. New York: Pocket Books.

Senge P (1990) The Fifth Dimension. New York: Doubleday.

Seymour P (1994) Variability in dyslexia. In: C Hulme, M Snowling (eds) Reading Development and Dyslexia. London: Whurr Publishers; 65–85.

Seymour PHK, Duncan LG, Bolik FM (1999) Rhymes and phonemes in the common unit task: replications and implications for beginning reading. Journal of Research in Reading 22(2): 113–30.

Shapiro HT (1998) The President's Page. Princeton Alumni Weekly, 21 October.

Sharp P (in press) Emotional Literacy. London: David Fulton.

Sharma MC (1987) Focus On Learning Problems in Mathematics. Framingham: Center for Teaching/Learning Mathematics.

Sharron H (1987) Changing Children's Minds – Feuerstein's Revolution in the Teaching of Intelligence. London and Canada: Souvenir Press.

Singer BR, Singer MR, Ruddell H (1994) Models of Reading. Delaware: International Reading Association.

Singleton C (ed) (1991) Computers and Literacy Skills. University of Hull: Computer Resource Centre.

Singleton CH (ed) (1994) Computers and Dyslexia: Educational applications of new technology. University of Hull: Computer Resource Centre.

Singleton CH (Chair) (1999a) Dyslexia in Higher Education: Policy, provision and Practice. Report of the National Working Party on Dyslexia in Higher Education. Hull: University of Hull.

Singleton CH, Thomas KV, Leedale RC (1996) Cognitive Profiling System (CoPS). Beverley: Lucid Research.

Slade P (1995) Child Play: Its importance for human development. London: Jessica Kingsley.

Slingerland B (1970) The Slingerland Screening Tests of Specific Language Disability. Cambridge, MA: Psychological Testing Corporation.

Slingerland B (1976) Slingerland Screening Tests for Identification of Pupils with Specific Language Disability, USA: Cambridge University Press.

Smith P (1994) Teaching Handwriting. UKRA Mini Book, Royston.

Smythe I (1999) The International Test of Dyslexia. Paper presented at the BDA First International Conference on Multilingualism and Dyslexia, Manchester, June.

Smythe I (ed) (2000) The Dyslexia Handbook 2000. Reading: British Dyslexia Association.

Snowling MJ (1995) Phonological processing and developmental dyslexia. Journal of Research in Reading 18: 132-8.

Snowling MJ (1999) Reading difficulties. In B Spolsky (ed). The Concise Encyclopedia of Educational Linguistics; 451-2.

Snowling MJ, Stothard SE, McClean J (1996) Graded Nonword Reading Test. Bury St Edmunds: Thames Valley Test Company.

Snowling MJ, Nation K (1997) Language, phonology and learning to read. In: C Hulme, MJ Snowling (eds). Dyslexia: Biology, Cognition and Intervention. London: Whurr Publishers; 153-66.

Sotto E (1994) When Teaching Becomes Learning. London: Cassell.

Special Educational Needs Training Consortium (1996) Professional Development to Meet Special Educational Needs. Report to the Department for Education and Employment. SENTC: Institute of Education, University of London.

Springer S, Deutsch G (1997) Left Brain: Right Brain, Perspectives from Cognitive Neuroscience. New York: Freeman.

Stackhouse J, Wells B (1998) Psycholinguistic Assessment of Children with Speech and Literacy Difficulties. London: Whurr Publishers.

Stanovich KE (1980) Toward an interactive–compensatory model of individual differences in the development of reading fluency. Reading Research Quarterly 21: 360–407.

Stanovich KE (1988) The right and wrong places to look for the cognitive locus of reading disability. Annals of Dyslexia 38: 154–77.

Stanovich KE (1991) Discrepancy definitions of reading disability: has intelligence led us astray? Reading Research Quarterly 36: 7–29.

Stanovich KE (1994) Annotation: does dyslexia exist? Journal of Child Psychology and Psychiatry 21: 7–9.

Stanovich KE, Siegel L (1994) Phenotypic profile of children with reading disabilities: a regression-based test of the phonological-core variable – difference model. Journal of Learning Disabilities 21, 590–612.

Stanovich KE, Cunningham AE, Cramer BB (1986) Assessing phonological awareness in kindergarten children: issues of task comparability. Journal of Experimental Child Psychology 38: 175–90.

Stanovich KE, Nathan RG, Val-Rossi M (1986) Developmental changes in the cognitive correlates of reading ability and the development lag hypothesis. Reading Research Quarterly 21: 267–83.

Stanovich KE, Siegel LS, Gottardo A (1997) Progress in the search for dyslexic subtypes. In: C Hulme, M Snowling (eds). Dyslexia: Biology, Cognition and Intervention. London: Whurr Publishers; 108–30.

Stein J, Talcott J (1999) Impaired Neuronal Timing in Developmental Dyslexia: the magno-cellular hypothesis. Dyslexia: An International Journal of Research and Practice 5, no 2: 59–77.

Stein JF, Walsh KE (1997) To see; but not to read. The magnocellular theory of dyslexia. Trends in Neuroscience 20: 147–51.

Strauss A, Werner H, Lehtinen L (1947), Vols 1 and 2: The Psychopathology and Education of the Brain Injured Child. New York: Grune & Stratton.

Street B (1990) Putting Literacies on the Political Agenda. RAPAL Bulletin No 13, University of Lancaster. London: Avanti Publishers.

Street B (1998) Adult Literacy in the United Kingdom: A history of research and practice. University of Lancaster: RAPAL.

Stuart M (1998) Response to Scholes (1998). Let the Emperor retain his underclothes. Journal of Research in Reading 21: 189–94.

Tallal P, Miller S, Fitch RH (1993) Neurobiological basis of speech: a case for the preeminence of temporal processing. Annals of the New York Academy of Sciences: 27–47.

Tallal P, Miller SL, Bedi G, Byma G, Wang X, Nagarajan SS et al. (1996) Language comprehension in language-learning impaired children improved with acoustically modified speech. Science 271: 81–4.

Teacher Training Agency (TTA)(1998) National Standards for Special Educational Needs (SEN) Specialist Teachers. London: Teacher Training Agency.

The Times (1995) Law Report. 30 June.

Tizard J (1972) Children with Specific Reading Difficulties. Report of the Advisory Committee on Handicapped children. London: HMSO.

Topping K (1997) Electronic literacy. In: N McClelland (ed). Building a Literate Nation: The strategic agenda for literacy over the next five years, Stoke-on Trent: Trentham Books.

Torgensen JK, Wagner RK, Raschotte CA (1994) Longitudinal studies of phonological processing and reading. Journal of Learning Disabilities 19: 452–60.

Trieman R (1987) On the relationship between phonological awareness and literacy. Cahiers de Psychologie Cognitive 7: 542–29.

Turner M (1993) Testing times (a two-part review of tests of literacy) Part 1: Special Children 65, April; Part 2. Special Children 66, May.

Turner M (1994) Quantifying exceptionality: issues in the psychological assessment of dyslexia. In: G Hales (ed). Dyslexia Matters. London: Whurr Publishers; 109–26.

Turner M (1995) Assessing reading: layers and levels. Dyslexia Review 7: 15-19.

Turner M (1997) Psychological Assessment of Dyslexia. London: Whurr Publishers.

Tyler S (1990) Sub-types of specific learning difficulty: a review. In: PD Pumfrey, CD Elliott (eds). Children's Difficulties in Reading, Spelling and Writing. London: Falmer Press; 29–39.

Underwood G, Batt V (1996) Reading and Understanding. Oxford: Blackwell.

Vail PL (1992) Learning Styles. Rosemont, NJ: Modern Learning Press.

Valett R (1967) Learning Disabilities. Palo Alto, CA: Fearon Publishers.

Vauras M, Lehtinen E, Kinnunen R, Salonen P (1992) Socioemotional coping and cognitive processes in training learning disabled children. In: B Wong (ed). Intervention Research in Learning Disabilities: An International Perspective. New York: Springer-Verlag.

Vauras M (1996) Linking Research in the Classroom in the Areas of Comprehension, Learning Metacognition and Motivation. Keynote address at the 21st Annual International Conference on Learning Disabilities, Montreal, Canada: Correspondence-Learning Research, University of Turku, FIN-20014, TURKU, Finland.

Vellutino FR (1987) Dyslexia. Scientific American 256: 34–41.

Vellutino FR (1979) Dyslexia: Theory and Research. Cambridge, MA: MIT Press.

Vincent D, De la Mare M (1992) New Macmillan Reading Analysis. London: Hodder & Stoughton.

Vygotsky LS (1962) Thought and Language. Cambridge, MA: MIT Press.

Walker M (1993)Tuition for Adults with Specific Learning Difficulties. Unpublished MA thesis, University of Leicester.

Walker M (2000) cited in Chappell D, Walker M. Effective support for adult learners. In: M Hunter-Carsch, M Herrington (eds). Dyslexia and Effective Support for Learning. London: Whurr Publishers.

Warwick C (1999) A partnership approach. Dyslexia Contact 18: 8–10.

Watkins G, Hunter-Carsch M (1995) Prompt spelling: an approach to paired spelling. Support for Learning 10: 133–7.

Wedell K (1984) Children with Perceptuo-Motor Difficulties. Cambridge: Cambridge University Press.

Weller C, Strawser S (1987) Adaptive behaviour of subtypes of learning-disabled individuals. In: BJ Cratty, RL Goldman (1996) Learning Disabilities, Contemporary Viewpoints. Amsterdam: Harwood Academic Publishers; 101–116.

West TG (1991) In the Mind's Eye, Visual Thinkers, Gifted People with Learning Difficulties, Computer Images and the Ironies of Creativity. Buffalo, NY: Prometheus. (Later edition 1997).

Whitehead AN (1932) The Aims of Education. London: Ernest Benn.

Wilkins A (1993) Reading and visual discomfort. In: DM Willows, R Kruk, E Corcos (eds). Visual Process in Reading and Reading Disabilities. New Jersey: Lawrence Erlbaum Associates; 435–56.

Wilkins A (1997) Discussion with the Writer.

Wilkins A, Nimmo-Smith IM (1987) The clarity and comfort of printed text. Ergonomics 30: 1705–20.

Wilkins A and Lewis L (1999) Coloured overlays, text and texture perception 28: 641–650.

Wilkins A, Evans BJW, Brown JA, Busby AE, Wingfield AE, Jeanes RJ, Bald J (1994) Double-masked placebo-controlled trial of precision spectral filters in children who use coloured overlays. Ophthalmic and Physiological Optics 14: 365–70.

Wilkins A, Milroy R, Nimmo-Smith IM, Wright A, Tyrrell R, Holland K et al. (1992) Preliminary observations concerning treatment of visual discomfort and associated perceptual distortion. Ophthalmic and Physiological Optics 12: 257–63

Wilkins A, Nimmo-Smith IM, Tait A, McManus C, Della Sala S (1984) A neurological basis for discomfort. Brain 107: 989–1017.

Wilkins A, Nimmo-Smith IM, Slater A, Bedocs L (1989) Fluorescent lighting, headaches and eyestrain. Lighting Research and Technology 21: 11–18.

Wilkins AJ, Jeanes RJ, Pumfrey PD, Laskier M (1996) Rate of reading test: its reliability, and its validity in the assessment of the effects of coloured overlays. Ophthalmic and Physiological Optics 16: 491–7.

Willemen FR, Bos WM, Kappers EJ (1992) Scrambler computer program. Rijswijk, Netherlands: CIG.

Willows DM, Kruk RS, Corcos E (eds) (1993) Visual Processes in Reading and Reading Disabilities. Hillsdale, NJ: Lawrence Erlbaum.

Wolfendale S and Bastiani J (2000) The Contribution of Parents to School Effectiveness. London: David Fulton.

Wolfendale S and Topping K (1996) Family Involvement in Literacy. London: Cassell.

Wood D (1998) How Children Think and Learn: The social contexts of Cognitive Development. Oxford: Blackwell.

Wray D (1995) Comprehension monitoring, metacognition and other mysterious processes. In: C Gains, D Wray (eds). Reading: Current Issues. Stafford: NASEN; 43–9.

Young D (1983) The Parallel Spelling Tests. A and B. London: Hodder.

Young P, Tyre C (1983) Dyslexia or Illiteracy? Realising the Right to Read. Milton Keynes: Open University Press.

Ysseldyke J, Algozzine B, Thurlow ML (1992) Critical Issues in Special Education. Boston: Houghton Mifflin.

Yzerbyt VY, Lories G, Dardenne B (1998) Metacognition: Cognitive and Social Dimensions. London: Sage.

Zdzienski D (2000) A learning styles and memory strategies questionnaire for the identification of SpLD (Specific learning diffficulties/dyslexia) in Higher and Further Education. In: M Hunter-Carsch, M Herrington (eds). Dyslexia and Effective Learning in Secondary and Tertiary Education. London: Whurr Publishers.

# Index